Systemic
Fungal Infections
Principles, Pathogenesis and Practice

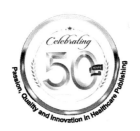

Systemic Fungal Infections
Principles, Pathogenesis and Practice

Editor

Monica Mahajan
MBBS DNB Medicine MNAMS
Medical Director
Max Healthcare, New Delhi
Director (Internal Medicine)
Max Super Specialty Hospital
Saket, New Delhi
I Care Centre
New Delhi, India

JAYPEE BROTHERS MEDICAL PUBLISHERS
The Health Sciences Publisher
New Delhi | London

Jaypee Brothers Medical Publishers (P) Ltd

Headquarters

Jaypee Brothers Medical Publishers (P) Ltd
4838/24, Ansari Road, Daryaganj
New Delhi 110 002, India
Phone: +91-11-43574357
Fax: +91-11-43574314
E-mail: jaypee@jaypeebrothers.com

Overseas Office

JP Medical Ltd
83 Victoria Street, London
SW1H 0HW (UK)
Phone: +44 20 3170 8910
Fax: +44 (0)20 3008 6180
E-mail: info@jpmedpub.com

Website: www.jaypeebrothers.com
Website: www.jaypeedigital.com

Systemic Fungal Infections: Principles, Pathogenesis and Practice

First Edition: 2020

ISBN: 978-93-89188-34-9

Printed at Replika Press Pvt. Ltd.

Contributors

Abhishek Deo FRCP CCT
Principal Consultant
Department of Gastroenterology and Hepatology
Max Super Specialty Hospital
New Delhi, India

Govind Singh Bisht Fellow in Podiatry (USA)
Senior Consultant
Department of Podiatry
Max Hospital
New Delhi, India

Moihhudin Khan MBBS
Fellow, DNB Family Medicine
Max Super Specialty Hospital
New Delhi, India

Nikhil Pal MD Retina Fellow (USA)
Principal Consultant
Department of Ophthalmology
Max Super Specialty Hospital
New Delhi, India

Shaiwal Khandelwal MS FIAGES FICS FMITS
Senior Consultant
Minimally Invasive and Robotic Thoracic Surgery
Max Super Specialty Hospital
New Delhi, India
Fellow in Thoracic Surgery (South Korea)
Robotic Thoracic Surgery (USA)

Sunil Choudhary MBBS
Fellow, DNB Family Medicine
Max Super Specialty Hospital
New Delhi, India

Swati Kapoor MBBS
Fellow, DNB Medicine
Max Super Speciality Hospital
New Delhi, India

Taruna Sharma BA English (Hons)
Deputy Manager
Clinical Directorate Office
Max Super Specialty Hospital
New Delhi, India

Vidit Tripathi MS (ENT)
Senior Consultant ENT
Fortis Hospital
New Delhi, India

Guest Authors

Anandamoyee Dhar
MD (Radiology)
Principal Consultant
Department of Radiology
Max Super Specialty Hospital
New Delhi, India

Ashish Jain
MD
Senior Consultant
Department of Respiratory Medicine
Max Super Specialty Hospital
New Delhi, India

Bansidhar Tarai
MD (Medical Microbiology)
Principal Consultant and Head
Department of Microbiology
Max Super Specialty Hospital
New Delhi, India

Dinesh Khullar
DM (Nephrology) FACP FRCP FISOT
Chairman and Head
Department of Nephrology
Max Super Specialty Hospital
New Delhi, India

Monica Mahajan
MBBS DNB Medicine MNAMS
Medical Director
Max Healthcare, New Delhi
Director (Internal Medicine)
Max Super Specialty Hospital
Saket, New Delhi
I Care Centre
New Delhi, India

Pragnya P Jena
MBBS MD (Medical Microbiology)
Attending Consultant
Department of Microbiology
Max Super Specialty Hospital
New Delhi, India

Pramod Kumar Julka
MD FAMS
Senior Director
Max Institute of Cancer Care
New Delhi, India

Prateek Arora
MS MCh (Plastic Surgery)
Principal Consultant
Max Institute of Reconstructive Aesthetic
Cleft and Craniofacial Surgery (MIRACLES)
Max Super Specialty Hospital
New Delhi, India

Puneet Agarwal
DM (Neurology)
Principal Consultant and Head of Unit
Department of Neurology
Max Super Specialty Hospital
New Delhi, India

Raghav Mantri
MS MCh (Plastic Surgery)
Principal Consultant
Max Institute of Reconstructive Aesthetic
Cleft and Craniofacial Surgery (MIRACLES)
Max Super Specialty Hospital
New Delhi, India

Rajeev Upreti
MRCP (UK) ECFMG (USA) DNB
Registrar
Acute Medicine
George Eliot Hospital, UK

Rohit Jain
MS MCh (Plastic Surgery)
Associate Consultant
Max Institute of Reconstructive Aesthetic
Cleft and Craniofacial Surgery (MIRACLES)
Max Super Specialty Hospital
New Delhi, India

Sahil Bagai
DM (Nephrology)
Associate Consultant
Department of Nephrology
Max Super Specialty Hospital
New Delhi, India

Shaik Maheboob Hussain
MBBS Fellowship Medical Oncology
Senior Resident
Max Oncology Centre
New Delhi, India

Shaunak Dutta
DNB (Gen Surgery) DNB (Plastic Surgery)
Associate Consultant
Max Institute of Reconstructive Aesthetic
Cleft and Craniofacial Surgery (MIRACLES)
Max Super Specialty Hospital
New Delhi, India

Soumya Khanna
MS MCh (Plastic Surgery) DNB (Plastic Surgery)
Associate Consultant
Max Institute of Reconstructive Aesthetic
Cleft and Craniofacial Surgery (MIRACLES)
Max Super Specialty Hospital
New Delhi, India

Sunil Choudhary
MS FRCSEd
Senior Director and Chief
Max Institute of Reconstructive Aesthetic
Cleft and Craniofacial Surgery (MIRACLES)
Max Super Specialty Hospital
New Delhi, India
Fellow of European Board of Plastic Reconstructive
and Aesthetic Surgery (EBOPRAS)

Tanmay Trivedi
DNB (Internal Medicine) Senior DNB
Resident
Department of Neurology
Max Super Specialty Hospital
New Delhi, India

Tarun Mohindra
MD Fellow (Oncology)
Attending Consultant
Max Institute of Cancer Care
Max Super Specialty Hospital
New Delhi, India

Preface

There have been major advances in the realm of medical mycology in the past decade. New fungal species have been identified and there have been new additions to the list of human fungal pathogens. The nomenclature of fungi has changed based on their genetic analysis. Fungal infections are not limited to the skin. Systemic fungal infections are responsible for global mortality with statistics matching lives lost due to malaria and tuberculosis. The pool of immunocompromised hosts has increased to include an increasing number of bone marrow and solid organ transplant recipients, HIV, steroids and monoclonal antibodies use in 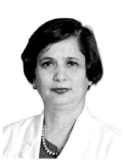 rheumatological disorders. Opportunistic and endemic fungi cause invasive fungal infections in immunocompromised as well as immunocompetent individuals. Improved survival and longevity entail higher incidence of fungal infections. Systemic mycosis has become an important public health problem. They are difficult to diagnose and have limited therapeutic options. Treatment is expensive and has major toxicities. More than 1.5 million deaths are attributed to fungal infections annually. The actual number may be much higher due to under-diagnosis and under-reporting.

Gone are the days when diagnosis of fungal infections was limited to the use of conventional techniques of fungal staining and culture. Serodiagnosis and molecular methods have improved diagnosis of IFI. Imaging techniques including CT and MRI have aided in defining the extent of the disease and in planning a rational treatment approach.

Polyenes were the first class of antifungals that emerged in the late 1950s with amphotericin B being introduced in 1958. Today, three classes of antifungals are the cornerstone of therapy—the polyenes, azoles and echinocandins. Amphotericin B remains the gold-standard for management of a number of systemic fungi. Azoles include the most diverse group of drugs and include newer triazoles including voriconazole, posaconazole and isavuconazole displaying a wide spectrum of activity. The echinocandins are the newest antifungals and look the most promising due to their low toxicity. The challenge with using all these drugs includes need for hospitalization, prolonged use, toxicity, drug interactions and the cost of therapy. Newer azoles and echinocandins have been added to the armamentarium but very few agents are in the research pipeline. The pace of research is not matching the recent surge in the cases of fungal infections. Combination therapy and improvements in existing formulations are being explored.

Antifungal resistance and its clinical impact on outcomes is a major concern. Some of the fungal pathogens have become multidrug resistant to more than one class of antifungals. Standard guidelines are being updated for antifungal susceptibility testing. The Clinical and Laboratory Standards Institute has published reference methods for susceptibility testing.

However, *in vitro* susceptibility patterns may not replicate in terms of treatment success in a critically ill patient. A number of host factors result in clinical resistance in the absence of microbiological resistance. Molecular mechanisms and alteration in gene expression result in resistance to antifungals. These have been better understood for azoles compared to polyenes and echinocandins. Research is critical to further elaborate on these resistance mechanisms and patterns so that the antifungals do not meet the same fate that the antibiotics are meeting with widespread antimicrobial resistance among bacteria.

Nanobiotechnology is a beacon of hope in improving efficacy of existing antifungals, targeted drug delivery, enhanced biodistribution and reduced toxicity. Drug delivery systems using nanoparticles have been developed and nanoantifungals are the way forward. Polymeric nanoparticles, solid lipid nanoparticles, liposomes and magnetic nanoparticles are being investigated for pharmacological purposes.

There are advances being made in developing fungal vaccines and universal immunization against fungi. Various candidate vaccines are in different phases of clinical trials. The majority of patients requiring protection against fungi are immunocompromised. The vaccines may exacerbate rather than protect against opportunistic infections in these hosts. As of now, there is no approved antifungal vaccine licensed for clinical use but vaccines, their adjuvants and immunotherapy are going to be the new frontier for combating fungal infections.

There is very little emphasis on teaching of mycology as part of the undergraduate medical curriculum. The diagnosis of systemic mycosis has become so frequent that we need to keep abreast with the diagnosis and treatment options. This book is an endeavor to demystify medical mycology and to provide simple and practical information on managing these infections. It is aimed at providing information to medical students, microbiologists, clinicians and intensive care specialists.

I would like to thank my colleagues Bansidhar Tarai, Pragnya P Jena, and Rajeev Upreti for helping me in this academic project. A special thanks to Dr Sunil Choudhary for designing the book cover. Honored to receive contributions from the guest authors who are experts in their fields with vast experience. This book would not be possible without my pillars of strength—my parents, my life-partner Sanjiv and children Sidhaant and Sadhika. Thanks to M/s Jaypee Brothers Medical Publishers (P) Ltd, New Delhi, India, for showing confidence in me. Hope this book is a useful medical contribution in serving our patients better.

Monica Mahajan

Acknowledgments

I am thankful to Shri Jitendar P Vij (Group Chairman), Mr Ankit Vij (Managing Director), Mr MS Mani (Group President), Ms Chetna Malhotra Vohra (Associate Director—Content Strategy) and Ms Pooja Bhandari (Production Head) of M/s Jaypee Brothers Medical Publishers (P) Ltd, New Delhi, India, for giving a go-ahead at the very beginning and helping me in every way possible to bring out this book.

I wish to express my gratitude to Ms Prerna Bajaj (Development Editor) of M/s Jaypee Brothers Medical Publishers for her earnest efforts and valid suggestions towards publishing this book.

Contents

Section 3: Antifungal Drugs

Section 4: Specific Fungal Infections

Section 5: Invasive Fungal Infections

Section 6: New Frontiers in Mycology

Abbreviations

AAS	Allergic *Aspergillus* sinusitis	CYP450	Cytochrome-P450
ABCD	Amphotericin B colloidal dispersion	DNA	Deoxyribonucleic acid
ABD	Amphotericin B deoxycholate	ECIL	European Conference on Infections in Leukemia
ABLC	Amphotericin B lipid complex	ELISA	Enzyme-linked immunosorbent assay
ABPA	Allergic bronchopulmonary aspergillosis	ESRD	End-stage renal disease
AFST	Antifungal susceptibility testing	EUCAST	European Committee on Antibiotic Susceptibility Testing
ANC	Absolute neutrophil count		
APACHE II	Acute Physiologic Assessment and Chronic Health Evaluation II scoring system	5-FC	5-Fluorocytosine
		FDA	Food and Drug Administration
		FDG	Fluorodeoxyglucose
APECED	Autoimmune polyendocrinopathy-candidosis-ectodermal dystrophy	FISH	Fluoroscence *in situ* hybridization
		GCSF	Granulocyte colony-stimulating factor
ARDS	Acute respiratory distress syndrome	GM	Granulocyte macrophage
BAL	Broncho-alveolar lavage	CSF	Colony-stimulating factor
CCPA	Chronic Cavitary Pulmonary Aspergillosis	GMS	Gomori methenamine silver
		GPI	Glycosylphosphatidyl inositol
CDC	Centre for Disease Control	GVHD	Graft-versus-host disease
CE	*Candida* endocarditis	HAART	Highly active antiretroviral therapy
CEUS	Contrast-enhanced ultrasound	H&E	Hematoxylin and eosin
CFT	Complement fixation test	HIV	Human immunodeficiency virus
CGD	Chronic granulomatous disease	HSCT	Hematopoietic stem cell transplant
CIE	Counter immunoelectrophoresis	HSP90	Heat shock protein 90
CLSI	Clinical and Laboratory Standards Institute	IA	Invasive aspergillosis
		ICA	Internal carotid artery
CMC	Chronic mucocutaneous candidiasis	ICAM	Intercellular adhesion molecule
		ID	Immunodiffusion
CMV	Cytomegalovirus	IDSA	Infectious Diseases Society of America
CNPA	Chronic necrotizing pulmonary aspergillosis		
		IFD	Invasive fungal disease
COMT	Catechol-o-methyl transferase	IFI	Invasive fungal infection
COPD	Chronic obstructive pulmonary disease	IFN-γ	Interferon-γ
		IRIS	Immune reconstitution inflammatory syndrome
CrCl	Creatinine clearance		
CSF	Cerebrospinal fluid	IVIG	Intravenous immunoglobulin
CT	Computed tomography	LA	Latex agglutination
CVC	Central venous catheter	LAmB	Liposomal amphotericin B

LAMP	Loop-mediated isothermal amplification	PJP	*Pneumocystis jirovecii* pneumonia
LDH	Lactate dehydrogenase	PNA Probes	Peptide nucleic acid probes
LFA	Lateral flow assay	RAPD	Random amplified polymorphic DNA
MAC	*Mycobacterium avium* complex	RDBH	Reverse dot-blot hybridization
MALDI-TOF	Matrix-assisted laser desorption ionization/time-of-flight	RIA	Radioimmunosorbent assay
MEC	Minimal effective concentration	ROS	Reactive oxygen species
MIC	Minimal inhibitory concentration	SDA	Sabouraud dextrose agar
MRI	Magnetic resonance imaging	SJS	Stevens-Johnson syndrome
MT-PCR	Multiplex tandem polymerase chain reaction	SOT	Solid organ transplant
		TDM	Therapeutic drug monitoring
NSIP	Nonspecific interstitial pneumonia	TEN	Toxic epidermal necrolysis
OD index	Optical density index	TMP-SMX	Trimethoprim-Sulfamethoxazole
PAS	Periodic acid-Schiff	T1WI	T1-weighted image
PCR	Polymerase chain reaction	T2WI	T2-weighted image
PET	Positron emission tomography	VCAM1	Vascular cell adhesion molecule-1
PFT	Pulmonary function test	VVC	Vulvovaginal candidiasis

Section 1

INTRODUCTION

1

Introduction to Mycology

Monica Mahajan

▧ INTRODUCTION

Fungi are eukaryotic, unicellular or multicellular, thick-walled heterotrophs which are mostly saprophytic in nature. They are responsible for degradation of organic compounds. Out of about 2,50,000 fungal species identified till date, only about 150–200 are known to be human pathogens.

▧ STRUCTURE OF FUNGI

Fungi have a complex cellular organization and the fungal cell contains a membrane-bound nucleus where the DNA is wrapped around histone proteins. Yeast cells are uninucleate, while filamentous fungi may be uninucleate or multinucleate. The cell organelles include endoplasmic reticulum and Golgi body. In contrast to plant cells, fungi lack chloroplasts or chlorophyll. The fungi may exhibit a range of colors—red, green, or black—due to pigments, such as carotenoids, melanins, flavins, and indigo associated with the cell wall.

The fungal cell wall has a complex structure. It contains chitin, $(1,3)/(1,6)$-β-glucans, mannans, and mannoproteins. Glucan is a polymer of glucose, whereas mannan is a polymer of mannose. These maintain the cell wall integrity. Chitin is a unique cell wall component of fungi. It is a polysaccharide homopolymer of $\beta(1,4)$ *N*-acetyl-glucosamine, which occurs as microfibrillar units. The amount of chitin in the cell wall of various fungi is variable. In some fungi such as the zygomycetes, chitin molecule is converted partially to chitosan. It is absent in humans. It provides structural strength to the cell wall and prevents the cell from desiccation. It protects the fungus during stressful environmental conditions. It may play a role in immune activation and attenuation. Chitin is also found in the exoskeleton of insects, such as mosquitoes, sandflies, and ticks, performing a similar function in them. Fungal capsules are composed of extracellular polysaccharides.

The plasma membrane of fungal cells is predominantly made of sterols, glycerophospholipids, and sphingolipids. Major families of proteins include ATPase family along with transport and signal transduction proteins. Ergosterol is a special fungal sterol that is the main component of the cell membrane. It plays a role similar to cholesterol in animals and phytosterols in plants. Since it is absent in animals, it serves as a target for antifungal drugs.

■ GROWTH

The unicellular or multicellular undifferentiated vegetative or assimilative body of a fungus is a *thallus*. Thallus is unicellular in yeasts, multicellular in filamentous fungi, or both in dimorphic fungi, since they exist in both yeast and filamentous forms.

Fungi display two morphological stages:
1. Vegetative
2. Reproductive

Hyphae

The vegetative stage of fungi consists of fine, long filaments called hyphae.

Mycelium

A collection of branching filamentous hyphae is called mycelium. Mycelia can grow on decaying material, soil, or in living tissues.

Septate Hyphae

Hyphae are divided into discrete cells by septa. These septa contain tiny holes or perforations that permit flow of nutrients from cell to cell in a hypha.

Coenocytic Hyphae

Arrangement of aseptate fungi having large cells with multiple nuclei.

■ REPRODUCTION

Perfect Fungi

Mode of reproduction is both sexual and asexual.

Imperfect Fungi

Undergo asexual reproduction by mitotic cell division.

Asexual Reproduction

Fungi reproduce asexually by the following methods:
1. Fragmentation
2. Budding
3. Spore formation

Fragmentation

Fragmentation of mycelia and hyphae results in growth of new colonies from each component.

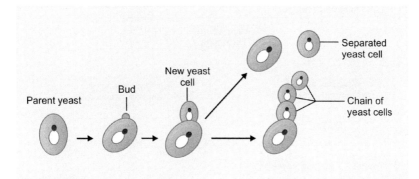

Fig. 1.1: Budding in yeast.

Budding

Somatic cells in yeast form buds. The cell develops a bulge. The nucleus undergoes mitotic division. Subsequent to cytokinesis, the bud separates from the mother cell (Fig. 1.1).

Spore Formation

This is the most frequent method by which fungi undergo asexual reproduction. A single parent cell undergoes mitosis to form spores. Spores are reproductive particles with same genetic composition as their parent, which help colonize new environment. Spores can be present inside a special reproductive sac called sporangium or can be directly released from the parent thallus. Sporangiospores are produced in a sporangium. Single-celled or multicellular conidiospores arise from the tip or side of the hyphae and germinate to produce new mycelia.

Sexual Reproduction

Sexual reproduction produces genetic variation in fungal population. It occurs when the fungi are subjected to unfavorable natural conditions.

There are two different mating types:
1. *Homothallic*: When both mating types coexist in the same mycelium or self-fertile
2. *Heterothallic*: Requires two compatible mycelia to reproduce sexually

Sexual reproduction includes the three stages:
1. *Plasmogamy*: Fusion of two haploid cells
2. *Karyogamy*: Two nuclei fuse together to form diploid zygote nucleus
3. *Meiosis*: Gametes of different mating types are produced and spores are disseminated into the environment

▦ NUTRITION

Fungi are heterotrophs. They cannot use carbon dioxide from the atmosphere and utilize carbon-containing organic compounds as a source of carbon. They cannot fix atmospheric nitrogen and obtain it from their diet.

Flowchart 1.1: Classification of fungi.

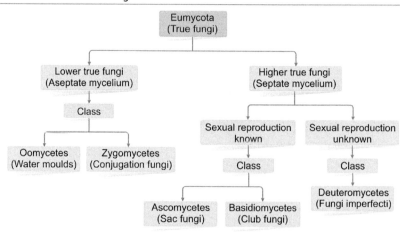

In fungi, digestion precedes the ingestion of food. Isoenzymes are transported out of the hyphae to digest food in the outside environment. The smaller molecules produced are absorbed from the large mycelial surface. Food is stored as glycogen unlike plants which store food as starch. Fungi are mostly saprophytic in nature.

■ CLASSIFICATION OF FUNGI (FLOWCHART 1.1)

Fungi are classified as follows:
1. *Zygomycota*: Conjugated fungi
2. *Ascomycota*: Sac fungi
3. *Basidiomycota*: Club fungi
4. *Deuteromycota*: Imperfect fungi

Zygomycota: Conjugated Fungi

Zygomycetes belong to the phylum Zygomycota. These are saprophytic fungi e.g. *Rhizopus* spp. The usual mode of reproduction is asexual by formation of sporangiospores in sporangia. During unfavorable environmental conditions, these fungi reproduce sexually by conjugation of two opposing mating strains. A diploid zygospore is formed which is protected from desiccation by a thick coat. When environmental conditions improve, the zygospore undergoes meiosis to form haploid spores. These are released to form a new organism.

Ascomycota: Sac Fungi

Fungi of this phylum are characterized by the presence of an ascus. Ascus is derived from the Greek word "askos" meaning sac-like. This microscopic sexual structure contains nonmotile haploid ascospores. Most fungi belong to this phylum e.g. *Aspergillus* spp. Baker's yeast and wine-fermenting yeasts belong to this phylum. They are filamentous and have septate hyphae.

Ascomycetes reproduce asexually to form conidiophores that release conidiospores. During sexual reproduction, mating strains of two different types are involved. The male strain produces a haploid antheridium, which contains the male gamete; and, the female strain develops the female organ ascogonium. Mating of antheridium and ascogonium results in fertilization to form haploid ascospores after meiosis. The ascocarp is the fruiting body that releases the spores.

Basidiomycota: Club Fungi

The basidiomycota contain more than 30,000 fungal species, including mushrooms and single-celled yeasts. Both edible and wild mushrooms belong to this phylum. Some mushrooms contain a toxin phalloidin. Pathogenic fungi "rusts" (Uredinales) and "smuts" (Ustilaginales) are symbiotic basidiomycota, which cause disease in wheat and crops. These reproduce sexually. The most salient characteristic is a club-shaped fruiting body called basidium from which sexual spores are produced. Karyogamy and meiosis occur in the basidium to produce haploid basidiospores. Pathogenic fungi including *Cryptococcus neoformans* are basidiomycetes.

Deuteromycota: Imperfect Fungi

These fungi do not possess the morphological sexual structures and do not display a sexual phase. It is not a true phylum as it is a polyphyletic group. The closest group is ascomycetes. *Aspergillus* was earlier classified as deuteromycetes and now reclassified as ascomycetes. A number of fungal species in this group have a close relationship to fungi in other phyla and do not fit well into the taxonomic classification. Most deuteromycota have visible mycelia. Fungi reproduce asexually by sporogenesis. Recombination of genetic material between different nuclei occurs subsequent to recombination of some hyphae e.g. *Penicillium* spp. These fungi play an important role in antibiotic (penicillin) production, edible fungi in cheese, or in human fungal infections e.g. athlete's foot.

▨ CLASSIFICATION OF MYCOSES ON THE BASIS OF SITE OF INFECTION

On the basis of site of infection, mycoses or fungal infections are classified as:
- Superficial
- Cutaneous
- Subcutaneous
- Systemic/deep

Superficial Mycoses

Dermatophytoses

Caused by agents of the genera *Trichophyton, Epidermophyton,* and *Microsporum* species (Table 1.1).

Table 1.1: Superficial mycoses		
Superficial mycoses	*Agent*	*Clinical features*
Pityriasis versicolor	*Malassezia furfur*	Hyperpigmented or hypopigmented patches on skin of neck, chest, and back
White piedra	*Trichosporon beigelii*	Friable, soft, beige nodule of distal end of hair shaft
Black piedra	*Piedraia hortae*	Black, firm nodule involving hair shaft
Tinea nigra	*Exophiala werneckii*	Brown/black silver nitrate-like stain on palms/soles

Cutaneous Mycoses

Dermatomycoses

Cutaneous infections due to other fungi, the most common being *Candida* spp.

Subcutaneous Mycoses

Subcutaneous mycoses are caused by direct inoculation of subcutaneous tissue with spores at the site of trauma. These can be of three types:
1. Chromoblastomycosis
2. Mycetoma
3. Sporotrichosis

Chromoblastomycosis

It presents as verrucoid lesions involving the lower limbs. Histopathological examination shows muriform cells with perpendicular septations called "copper pennies" appearance. The underlying muscle and bone are spared. Fungi causing chromoblastomycosis include *Fonsecaea pedrosoi, Fonsecaea compacta, Cladosporium carrionii*, and *Phialophora verrucosa*.

Mycetoma

It is a suppurative, granulomatous, and subcutaneous fungal infection with formation of draining sinus tracts. Pigmented granules visible to the naked eye extrude out of the tract. These granules are formed by the microcolonies of the fungus responsible for the infection. There is destruction of underlying muscle, tendon, and bone. Mycetoma can be eumycotic mycetoma or actinomycotic mycetoma. The most frequent pathogen of eumycotic mycetoma is *Pseudallescheria boydii*; while that for actinomycotic mycetoma, is *Nocardia brasiliensis*.

Sporotrichosis

This is a subcutaneous infection caused by *Sporothrix schenckii* that spreads along the cutaneous lymphatics of the involved limb.

Systemic/Deep Mycoses

The pathogens causing deep mycoses can be classified as:
1. Primary pathogens (Table 1.2)
2. Opportunistic fungal pathogens (Table 1.3)

Table 1.2: Primary pathogenic fungi

Systemic mycosis	Pathogenic fungus
Histoplasmosis	Histoplasma capsulatum
Blastomycosis	Blastomyces dermatitidis
Paracoccidioidomycosis	Paracoccidioides brasiliensis
Coccidioidomycosis	Coccidioides immitis

Table 1.3: Opportunistic fungal pathogens

Systemic mycosis	Opportunistic fungus
Cryptococcosis	Cryptococcus neoformans
Aspergillosis	Aspergillus species
Zygomycosis	Mucor, Rhizopus
Systemic candidiasis	Candida species

Primary Pathogenic Fungi/Primary Mycoses

These infections occur in patients with normal immunity living in the endemic areas. The patient may be asymptomatic or may experience mild symptoms. Most fungi gain access to the host by inhalation of spores.

Opportunistic Fungal Pathogens

These opportunistic pathogens cause infection in immunocompromised patients. The fungus may gain access through the respiratory passages, gastrointestinal tract, or intravascular devices.

FUNGAL DIMORPHISM

A change in environment causes certain fungi to convert from one phenotype to another yeast form or mold. The fungi which get affected by the prevailing temperature are called thermal dimorphic. Other factors influencing fungal dimorphism include amino acids, carbohydrates, trace elements, or genetic characteristics. Fungi which demonstrate dimorphism include *Coccidioides immitis, Histoplasma capsulatum, Blastomyces dermatitidis, Paracoccidioides brasiliensis, S. schenckii*, and opportunistic fungi including *Candida albicans* and *P. marneffei*.

The primary pathogens and *S. schenckii* transform from a hyphal form to a yeast-like form in tissue. *C. immitis* transforms into a spherule. *C. albicans* transforms from a budding yeast-like structure called blastoconidia to filamentous structures known as germ tubes. *P. marneffei* undergoes dimorphic conversion into sausage-shaped cells. *H. capsulatum* grows in its yeast form at 37°C, but switches to mold form at 20–25°C.

▓ SUGGESTED READING

1. Blackwell M, Vilgalys R, James TY, et al. Eumycota: mushrooms, sac fungi, yeast, molds, rusts, smuts, etc. 2012. http://tolweb.org/Fungi/2377/2012.01.30. [Version January 30, 2012].
2. Brandt M, Warnock D. Taxonomy and classification of fungi. In: Jorgensen J, Pfaller M, Carroll K, Funke G, Landry M, Richter S, Warnock D (Eds). Manual of Clinical Microbiology, 11th edition. Washington, DC: ASM Press; 2015. pp. 1935-43.
3. Carris LM, Little CR, Stiles CM. Introduction to fungi. The Plant Health Instructor. American Phytopathological Society; 2012. doi: 10.1094/PHI-I-2012-0426-01.
4. Talaro KP, Chess B. The fungi of medical importance. In: Foundations in Microbiology, 9th edition. New York, NY: McGraw-Hill Education; 2015. pp. 663-92.

Section 2

DIAGNOSIS OF FUNGAL INFECTIONS

2

Diagnosis of Fungal Infection

Monica Mahajan

INTRODUCTION

The diagnosis of fungal infection is majorly dependent on choosing the appropriate specimen, proper collection, and investigations ordered. Traditional techniques including direct microscopy, histopathology, and culture are dependent on trained personnel. With recent advances in mycology, newer methods of fungal identification including molecular methods and antigen detection are being developed as surrogates for culture in the diagnosis of fungal diseases.

Diagnosing invasive fungal infections correctly is of paramount importance due to the following reasons:

- New fungal species are being identified and fungal taxonomy is changing.
- The armamentarium of antifungal agents is expanding.
- There is emerging resistance to antifungal drugs.
- With increase in number of immunocompromised hosts and increasing lifespan, advances in chemotherapy and organ transplant, there is a significant rise in cases of invasive fungi.
- A patient may be simultaneously infected with bacteria and fungi or even multiple fungi.

Thus, the best option to make a rapid and definite diagnosis of invasive fungi is to combine conventional methods with modern diagnostic tools.

SPECIMENS FOR DIAGNOSIS

- Skin scrapings, nail clippings and plucked hair
- Scrapings from mucosal membranes including oral mucosa and vagina
- Aspirated pus
- Tissue biopsy
- Blood
- Cerebrospinal fluid (CSF)
- Pleural fluid
- Sputum
- Bronchoalveolar lavage (BAL)
- Urine
- Bone marrow
- Ocular specimen

Collection of Specimens

Skin

Clean with 70% alcohol to remove oil, dirt, ointments, and surface saprophytes. Scrape outward from the margin of the lesion using a blunt scalpel. Cello tape adhesive strip may be pressed against the lesion and peeled off, and then place the adhesive side down on a clean glass slide.

Nails

Discolored, dystrophic, or brittle parts of nail are usually clipped after cleaning as above, and the specimen should include full thickness of the nail. The specimens need to be minced before inoculating on media.

Oral Cavity

Specimens from oral cavity include smears from mucosal swabs, saliva, imprint culture, concentrated oral rinse and mucosal biopsy. Swabs should be moistened with sterile water or saline prior to taking the sample.

Hair

Using a Wood's lamp, hair is obtained from the edge of infected area by plucking, brushing, or with a sticking tape. Pluck hair from the scalp with forceps. Hair plucked without roots are not suitable for diagnosis.

Body Fluids

Collect specimens through sterile procedure in containers with small amount of heparin to prevent blood clotting; drained fluid from continuous peritoneal dialysis patients should be collected without heparin.

Blood

20–30 mL blood divided into two culture bottles (Fig. 2.1).

Cerebrospinal Fluid

About 3–5 mL specimen centrifuged and the supernatant fluid used for serological tests, and sediment used for microscopic examination and culture.

Ocular Specimens

Scraping from corneal ulcer using a sterile platinum spatula in suspected fungal endophthalmitis. Vitreous humor should be centrifuged and the sediment should be examined. Preferably avoid collecting swabs from corneal lesions.

Ear

Scrapings or swabs from ear canal.

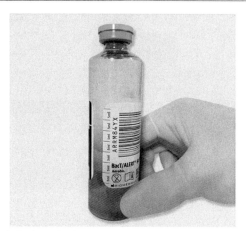

Fig. 2.1: Blood culture bottle for fungal culture.

Urine

Fresh mid-stream specimen, ensuring that vaginal or perineal secretions do not contaminate. In the case of prostatitis, prostatic massage must be done prior to the collection of urine sample.

Sputum

Fresh, early morning sputum or induced sputum by nebulizing with normal saline; ideally three sputum samples are better than a 24-hour collection. N-acetyl-L-cysteine as a mucolytic agent improves chances of recovering the fungus.

Bronchoalveolar Lavage

Ideal for collecting lower respiratory tract secretions in immunocompromised patients.

Pus

Aspirated with a sterile needle and syringe; if grains are visible in pus (mycetoma), these should be collected. If swab is used, take deeper material from the lesion.

Bone Marrow

For deep fungal infections, collect aspirate in sterile container with heparin.

Tissue

Collected in sterile saline without heparin.

Medical Devices

These include stents, replacement joints, surgical implants, and contact lenses and these should be collected in sterile container (Fig. 2.2).

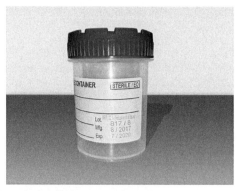

Fig. 2.2: Sterile container for sample collection.

Swabs are convenient but have the disadvantage that only a limited amount of specimen can be obtained. Moreover, swabs get easily contaminated. In case, it is not possible to collect specimens by other means, swabs can be used; but this should be an infrequent practice and not the norm.

Transportation of Laboratory Specimens

Specimens must be preferably transported and processed within 2 hours of collection. In case of delay in processing, they should be stored under refrigeration at 4°C for no longer than 24 hours. This reduces growth of contaminants and maintains viability of the pathogens.

Delays may result in the death of fastidious organisms. Refrigeration preserves the relative proportion of pathogenic fungi which is important in the case of semi-quantitative/quantitative cultures of urine and sputum. Blood specimens should not be refrigerated and should be kept in an incubator at 35°C. CSF should be transported at room temperature. Some fungi including *Cryptococcus neoformans* and *Blastomyces dermatitidis* do not survive well in frozen specimens.

Hair and nails are transported in a dry envelope. Other specimens are usually stored and transported in dry ice. Cultures must be developed in tubed media and not on culture plates. Packaging must meet biohazard regulations. The inside labeling should include the patient details, specimen source, and suspected organism. The outside labeling on the package should mention potential pathogen warning (Fig. 2.3).

Processing of Specimens

Skin/Hair/Nails

Direct examination following KOH preparation.

Blood/Bone Marrow

Inoculate to BHI broth/slant (Fig. 2.1).

Tissue Specimens

Examine the specimen for pus, caseous material, or granules. Mince the tissue material aseptically and inoculate on appropriate media.

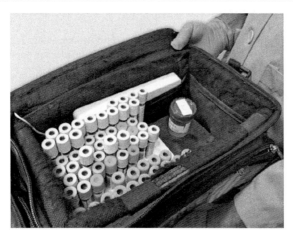

Fig. 2.3: Sample transport container.

Wound Abscess/Pus

Culture anaerobically if actinomycosis is suspected.

Cerebrospinal Fluid

Centrifuge, examine the sediment under microscope and inoculate on culture media.

Sputum/Pleural Fluid/BAL/Ascitic Fluid

Specimen should not be stored for longer periods to prevent overgrowth of pathogens.

Genitourinary Specimens

Centrifuge first morning sample and inoculate on media.

METHODS OF FUNGAL ISOLATION

Direct microscopic examination • *Wet mount*: –KOH, Calcofluor White, India ink • Fluorescent antibody testing • Histopathology
Fungal culture
Nonculture methods *Serology*: Antibody detection, antigen detection, immunohistochemistry
Tests for cell-mediated immunity • Skin tests • *In vitro* tests
Molecular methods • Polymerase chain reaction • Microassays

SUGGESTED READING

1. Kozel TR, Wickes B. Fungal diagnostics. Cold Spring Harb Perspect Med. 2014;4(4):a019299.
2. Mennink-Kersten MA, Verweij PE. Non-culture-based diagnostics for opportunistic fungi. Infect Dis Clin North Am. 2006;20(3):711-27, viii.
3. Ramanan P, Wengenack NL, Theel ES. Laboratory diagnostics for fungal infections: a review of current and future diagnostic assays. Clin Chest Med. 2017;38(3):535-54.

3

Conventional Methods for Direct Examination of Fungi

Monica Mahajan

INTRODUCTION

Direct examination of biological material for fungi is a valuable diagnostic procedure to provide a tentative and sometimes a definite diagnosis even before the culture shows the growth of a fungus. It demonstrates various fungal elements including mycelia, hyphae, spores, budding yeast, and mycotic granules. The advantage of examining a wet mount is that one can examine the yeast in its natural environment and it causes least damage to its fragile structure (Table 3.1).

The specimen to be examined is placed on a slide and a drop of 10–20% potassium hydroxide is added to dissolve the keratin and cellular material without affecting the fungi. It is then covered with a coverslip, left for 20 minutes, incubated at 37°C and then examined under the microscope. Preparations for direct examination include KOH, calcofluor white, India ink, periodic acid–Schiff (PAS), and Giemsa.

On examination, *Candida* presents as yeasts and hyphae in the same microscopic field. *Aspergillus* has thin, septated hyphae that branch at acute angles. Mucorales are nonseptated, broad, ribbon-like hyphae that branch at right angles.

The disadvantage of using KOH is that it reacts with pus, sputum, or skin, and produces artifacts that superficially resemble hyphae or budding fungi. Crystals can form on standing and it becomes difficult to interpret the slide.

Table 3.1: Methods for direct examination of fungi and their utility.

Method	Utility
Gram stain	Most fungi gram positive, *Actinomyces*, and *Nocardia* gram variable (Fig. 3.1)
KOH mount	For keratinous material, adding blue ink improves contrast (Fig. 3.2)
India ink	Useful for indicating presence/absence of extracellular polysaccharide capsule of fungal cells, negative stain; for detection of encapsulated organisms, for example, *C. neoformans* in cerebrospinal fluid (Fig. 3.3)
Lactophenol cotton blue (LPCB)	Most widely used; phenol kills any live organisms, lactic acid preserves fungal structure, cotton blue stains chitin in cell wall (Fig. 3.4)

Contd...

Contd...

Method	Utility
Giemsa	Methylene blue and eosin stain for trophozoites of *P. jiroveci*, yeast, and *Histoplasma* species
Calcofluor white, Blankophor P, Uvitex 2B	Fluorescent dyes, chalk white, or brilliant apple-green fluorescence; needs fluorescence microscope (Fig. 3.5)
Gomori's methenamine silver (GMS)	Stains fungal cell wall; silver nitrate outlines fungi in brown black, silver precipitates on the fungal cell wall wherever aldehydes are located
Periodic acid–Schiff (PAS)	Stains fungal cell wall polysaccharide, fungi stain pink red with blue nuclei
Mucicarmine (Mayer)	For mucin, stains capsule of *C. neoformans* deep rose
Fontana-Masson stain	For melanin
Papanicolaou stain	For initial differentiation of dimorphic fungi, good for sputum smears
Acid-fast stain (modified Kinyoun method)	To differentiate acid-fast *Nocardia* from other aerobic *Actinomyces*. Some of the filaments stain red with carbol-fuchsin stain (Fig. 3.6)

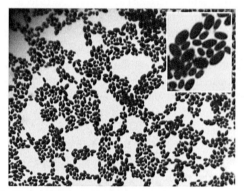

Fig. 3.1: Budding yeast cells, Blastoconidia on Gram stain.

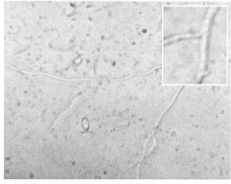

Fig. 3.2: Hyaline, branched fungal hyphae on KOH mount.

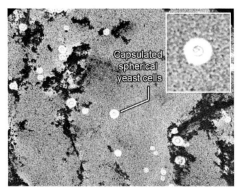

Fig. 3.3: *Cryptococcus* species on India ink mount.

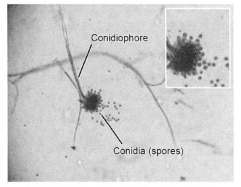

Fig. 3.4: Mycelium on LPCB mount (LPCB: Lactophenol cotton blue stain).

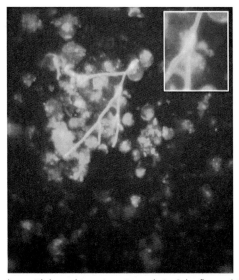

Fig. 3.5: Septate fungal hyphae with branching at acute angle in Calcofluor white stain.

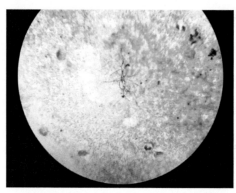

Fig. 3.6: *Nocardia* species in modified ZN stain (ZN: Ziehl–Neelsen stain/Kinyoun stain).

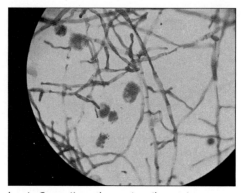

Fig. 3.7: Septate fungal hyphae in Gomori's methenamine silver stain.

Gomori's methenamine silver (GMS) stain (Grocott's modification) is based on the liberation of aldehyde groups and their subsequent identification by the reduced silver method (Fig. 3.7). The fungi and bacteria are stained brown to black due to precipitation of silver, cytoplasm stains old rose, and the tissue pale green. The GMS stain is better than other fungal stains on account of the following two reasons:

1. It stains both live and dead fungi in contrast to PAS which stains only living things.
2. It also stains the higher bacteria (nocardia and actinomyces) that are not stained by other fungal stains.

India ink should be free from granular carbon particles to ensure a good preparation. *Cryptococcus* appears as a yeast in tissues and shows a capsule with contrast provided with an India ink preparation. *Blastomyces* is a yeast that has a broad budding pattern resembling a figure of eight. The pathognomic appearance of *Coccidioides immitis* is a spherule with endospores. WBC may be mistaken with fungi with India ink. They can be distinguished from *C. neoformans* by the halo effect—a dark background that highlights hyaline yeast cells and capsular material.

The disadvantage of using special stains to detect fungi is that they mask the natural color of the fungus, thereby making it difficult to distinguish between naturally pigmented and hyaline fungi.

PRESUMPTIVE IDENTIFICATION OF FUNGI BY DIRECT MICROSCOPIC EXAMINATION (TABLE 3.2)

Table 3.2: Fungal identification by microscopic examination.

Fungi	Microscopic features
Aspergillus species	Small and regular size hyphae, distinct cross-septa, dichotomously branching at 45° (Figs. 3.8A and B)
Zygomycetes	Irregular, larger hyphae, ribbon-like, septa absent (Figs. 3.9A and B)
Dermatophytes	Hyphae small, regular, rectangular arthrospores occasionally, some branching, only in skin, hair, and nail scrapings
Microsporum species	Hyphae and pseudohyphae (sausage appearance), budding yeast forms (blastospores)
Candida species	Yeast cell spherical, irregular size, nonencapsulated
Cryptococcus neoformans	Encapsulated yeast
Histoplasma capsulatum	Uniform sized, small budding yeast with a single bud attached by a narrow base, extracellular or within macrophages
Blastomyces dermatitidis	Large yeast cells with thick, double-contoured wall, with a single bud attached by a broad base—figure-of-eight appearance

HISTOPATHOLOGY

Histopathologic examination of biopsy specimens gives vital information regarding the invasive fungi and the possible response generated including phagocytosis and granulomatous

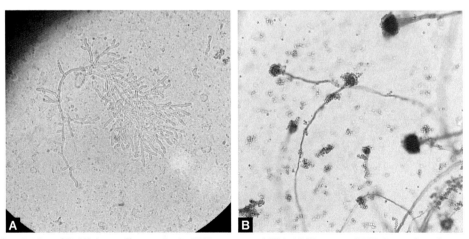

Figs. 3.8A and B: (A) *Aspergillus* species in KOH mount, and (B) in LPCB mount (LPCB: Lactophenol cotton blue stain).

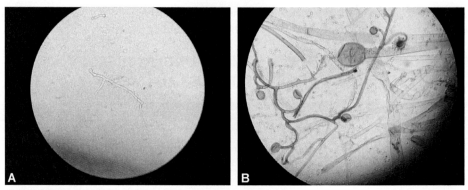

Figs. 3.9A and B: (A) Zygomycetes (aseptate fungal hyphae with branching at right angle) in KOH mount, and (B) in LPCB mount (LPCB: Lactophenol cotton blue stain).

reaction. A basic hematoxylin and eosin (H&E) stain can be used to stain the sections. Silver impregnation stains are better as these stain the fungi strongly without staining the cells.

It is pertinent to ask for special fungal stains if there is a high index of suspicion before the tissue is subjected to routine histopathology exam.

■ SUGGESTED READING

1. El-Aal A, El-Mashad N, Mohamed A. Revision on the recent diagnostic strategies of fungal infections. Open J Med Microbiol. 2017;7:29-40.
2. Haldane DJ, Robart E. A comparison of calcofluor white, potassium hydroxide, and culture for the laboratory diagnosis of superficial fungal infection. Diagn Microbiol Infect Dis. 1990;13:337-9.
3. Posteraro B, Torelli R, De Carolis E, et al. Update on the laboratory diagnosis of invasive fungal infections. Mediterr J Hematol Infect Dis. 2011;3(1):e2011002.

4

Fungal Culture

Monica Mahajan, Bansidhar Tarai, Pragnya P Jena

INTRODUCTION

Fungi take more time than bacteria to grow on culture. Since fungal cultures may require incubation periods ranging from days to weeks, the rapidly growing bacteria in the specimen may interfere with the isolation of fungi. Hence, fungal culture media are designed to favor the growth of fungi over bacteria.

The media are either in petri dishes or tubes. The advantages of tubed media over petri dishes are as follows:

- Easier storage and transport
- Less chances of dehydration
- Less chances of release of spores into the environment.

The disadvantage of screw-top tubes is the difficulty in preparing stained mounts for microscopic examination. However, petri dishes provide a larger surface for growth resulting in better separation of colonies. This makes it easier to subculture and to tease mounts or make transparent tape preparations. Petri dishes are more prone to dehydration.

FUNGAL GROWTH REQUIREMENTS

Temperature

Many fungi have an optimum growth at temperatures below 37°C. Therefore, culture tubes (Fig. 4.1) are incubated at two temperatures:
1. One tube at 25°C (room temperature)
2. One tube at 37°C (incubator)

This is essential to study fungal dimorphism. Any fungus that is capable of growth at 37°C is always considered pathogenic. *Nocardia* spp. and some dimorphic fungi grow best at 37°C.

The ability to withstand freezing and thawing or tolerating refrigeration varies among different fungi. *Histoplasma capsulatum* and *Mucorales* are especially susceptible, and can be killed/inhibited on storage of samples at low temperatures.

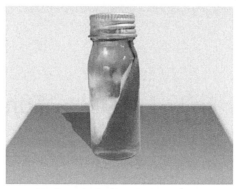

Fig. 4.1: Sabouraud dextrose agar (SDA) media for fungal culture.

Atmosphere

True fungi are aerobes, whereas few bacteria-like fungi are anaerobes.

Time

Fungi may require days to weeks of incubation before the initial growth occurs. Cultures should be examined for fungi for at least 4 weeks. Saprophytes grow fastest, and the growth may be visible over a span of days. *Paracoccidioides* brasiliensis grows over 4–5 weeks, and *Histoplasma capsulatum* may require up to 10 weeks for growth.

■ FUNGAL CULTURE MEDIA (TABLE 4.1)

Table 4.1: Culture media and their characteristics.

Culture media	Characteristics
Sabouraud's dextrose agar	Classic media for all fungi, contains glucose and peptones, pH 5.6, insufficiently rich to recover fastidious pathogenic species/dimorphic fungi
Sabouraud's dextrose agar with chloramphenicol	Inhibits bacterial growth; alternatively, streptomycin or penicillin may be used
Mycosel agar	Commercially prepared agar containing chloramphenicol and cycloheximide that inhibits saprophytic fungi and some yeasts including *C. neoformans*
Brain heart infusion (BHI) slant	More enriched than Sabouraud's dextrose, for recovery of *H. capsulatum*
Potato dextrose agar (PDA), corn meal agar	Used in microcultures to induce sporulation; may be too rich for some fungi and cause excessive mycelial growth rather than sporulation
Caffeic acid agar	Photosensitive, protect from light. *C. neoformans* produces black colonies due to melanin

Contd...

Contd...

Culture media	Characteristics
Bird seed agar	To isolate *C. neoformans* from contaminated cultures
Kelley agar/KT medium	To convert dimorphic fungus *Blastomyces dermatitidis* from mycelial to yeast form
Levine's modified converse liquid medium	To promote spherule production by *Coccidioides immitis*

Antimicrobials including chloramphenicol, streptomycin, gentamycin, and penicillin inhibit bacterial growth, whereas cycloheximide inhibits saprophytic growth. Culture media may be enriched with 5–10% sheep blood to support the growth of certain fungi.

CHARACTERISTICS FOR CLASSIFICATION OF FUNGI BASED ON CONVENTIONAL METHODS

- Colony morphology
- Chlamydospore formation
- Germ tube formation
- Adhesive tape preparation
- Microculture
- *Biochemical features*: Carbohydrate fermentation, carbohydrate assimilation, and urease test.

IDENTIFICATION OF FUNGI

The visible colonies are inspected for their morphology.

Yeasts can be identified on the basis of their growth pattern, color, colony morphology on chromogenic media, and biochemistry testing (Figs. 4.2 and 4.3). Filamentous fungi are

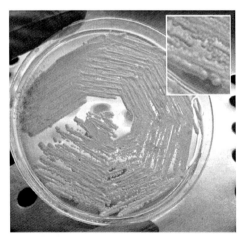

Fig. 4.2: Creamy, smooth, and pasty colony of yeast.

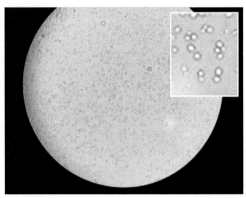

Fig. 4.3: Budding yeast cells on KOH mount.

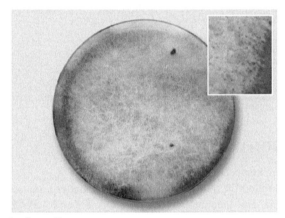

Fig. 4.4: Cottony growth of mycelium.

more difficult to identify. Without spores, the only real distinction is whether the hyphae are septate or not. Media that assist in sporulation include potato dextrose agar. Once the colony has sporulated, staining with lactophenol cotton blue helps identify the genus.

Colony Morphology

Macroscopic and microscopic feature.

Surface Topography

Free-growing fungi cover the entire surface of agar, whereas other fungi grow in a restricted manner (Fig. 4.4).

Surface Texture

It may be cottony or woolly (floccose), chalky, granular, powdery, velvety, silky, glabrous, or waxy. Yeast colonies are generally smooth, creamy, viscous, or pasty in appearance. Dimorphic fungi grow in 7–14 days and have a cobweb aerial mycelium.

Pigmentation

Fungi vary from colorless to brightly colored. Color may be visible from the fungus itself, its sporulating apparatus on the agar, or on the bottom of the colony called "reverse pigmentation."

▨ MICROSCOPIC EXAMINATION

Wet Mount-teased Preparation

Adhesive/Scotch Tape Preparation Method

The adhesive side of a small length of transparent tape is touched to the surface of the colony. The tape is adhered to the surface of a microscope slide, stained with lactophenol cotton blue, and observed (Fig. 4.5). The spores remain intact by this technique and their arrangement can be useful in species identification.

▨ BIOCHEMICAL STUDIES

To identify yeast and yeast-like organisms.

Carbohydrate Fermentation

Yeast metabolizes sugars both aerobically and anaerobically. The growth of yeast and utilization of carbohydrate under anaerobic conditions is studied by inoculating the specimen under a broth. The production of acid and gas by the process of fermentation is observed.

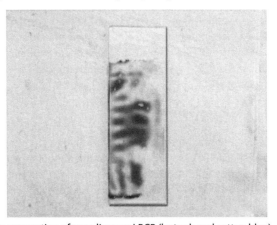

Fig. 4.5: Adhesive tape preparation of mycelium on LPCB (lactophenol cotton blue).

Carbohydrate Assimilation

It is used for definite species identification of *Candida* and a few other fungi. It determines the ability of a fungus to utilize a carbohydrate (glucose, maltose, lactose, sucrose, etc.) as the only source of carbon. In case of positive test, bromocresol indicator turns from purple to yellow. Tubes unchanged after 10 days are negative.

Nitrogen Assimilation

Bromothymol blue turns yellow on utilization of nitrogen by fungi.

Rapid Urease Test

This test is used to detect the presence of urease enzyme by different *Candida* species. Christensen's urea agar slants are studied for a color change. Urea is hydrolyzed by the yeast to form ammonia, which increases the pH and turns media from yellow to dark pink.

▓ SPECIAL TESTS

- *Germ-tube formation/Reynold–Braude phenomenon*: It is a rapid, efficient, and economic presumptive test for *C. albicans*. True germ tube is defined as hyphal projections from the germinating yeast cell, lacking any constriction at the point of origin from the parent cell. Several colonies of yeast are incubated into a substrate at 37°C. *C. albicans* forms germ tubes within 3–4 hours, while other species do not form germ tubes in that time period.
- *Demonstration of chlamydospores formation for Candida*: Suspected *Candida* species are inoculated on plates or slides with chlamydospore agar (cornmeal with Tween-80), incubated for 3 days, and observed every 24 hours for formation of chlamydospores. *C. albicans* produces abundant chlamydospores.

▓ MALDI-TOF

Many fungi can now be speciated with matrix-assisted laser desorption/ionization time-of-flight (MALD-TOF) mass spectrophotometry. Colonies from a positive culture are mixed with a specialized reagent and directly analyzed in the mass spectrometer. The time to result is approximately 1 minute. MALDI-TOF reduces turn around time and need for subculture (For further details, refer to Chapter 6).

▓ AUTOMATED FUNGAL CULTURES

A number of automated commercial systems are now available. They are continuously monitored systems and have special culture media to enhance fungal growth. They have largely replaced the lysis centrifugation method that was more cumbersome and involved lysis of RBC and centrifugation of blood to isolate *Candida*. The time of positivity of culture will depend on the automatic blood culture system and the causative species. BACTEC 9240 is one of the most validated systems, and the addition of Mycosis–IC/F, a selective medium for fungi, enhances the sensitivity of fungal detection.

■ INTERPRETATION OF POSITIVE FUNGAL CULTURES

The growth of fungus on a culture does not necessarily mean it is pathogenic. The results have to be interpreted with caution and compared with the microscopic examination of the specimen. Isolation of an opportunistic fungal pathogen from sterile sites, i.e. blood and CSF is always considered significant. However, the isolation of fungus from an unsterile site such as urine, sputum, or pus must be interpreted in light of the clinical scenario.

Limitations of Fungal Culture

Failure to isolate fungi on an appropriate culture media may be due to the following factors:
- Inadequate specimen
- Inappropriate specimen
- Delayed transport of specimen
- Incorrect isolation procedure
- Inadequate periods of incubation.

The isolation of molds and yeasts can take several weeks, and the results may be available too late. Therefore, there is a need for more automated systems with chromogenic agars for early detection and identification of fungi. Serological tests may be valuable in early diagnosis.

■ SUGGESTED READING

1. Borman AM, Johnson EM. Interpretation of fungal culture results. Curr Fungal Infect Rep. 2014; 8(4):312-21.
2. Bosshard PP. Incubation of fungal cultures—how long is long enough? Mycoses. 2011;54(5):e539-45.
3. Fernandez R, Lopansri BK, Dascomb K, et al. Clinical effectiveness of fungal blood cultures: a 10-year retrospective analysis [abstract]. Open Forum Infect Dis. 2014;1(suppl):S377-8.
4. Kirby JE, Delaney M, Qian Q, et al. Optimal use of Myco/F Lytic and standard BACTEC blood culture bottles for detection of yeast and mycobacteria. Arch Pathol Lab Med. 2009;133:93-6.
5. Murray PR, Masur H. Current approaches to the diagnosis of bacterial and fungal bloodstream infections in the intensive care unit. Crit Care Med. 2012;40:3277-82.
6. Vyzantiadis TA, Johnson EM, Kibbler CC. From the patient to the clinical mycology laboratory: how can we optimise microscopy and culture methods for mould identification? J Clin Pathol. 2012;65:475-83.

5

Serodiagnosis in Mycology

Monica Mahajan, Bansidhar Tarai, Pragnya P Jena

INTRODUCTION

Fungal culture remains the gold standard for diagnosing invasive fungal infection but the limitations are low sensitivity and the cultures becoming positive only late in the course of the infection. It may be difficult to obtain specimens for microbiological tests and histopathology to identify the etiological agent.

The nonculture-based techniques for fungal diagnosis include the following:
- Detection of specific host immune responses by antigen and antibody tests using immunological agents
- Detection and quantification of specific fungal metabolite products
- Amplification and detection of specific fungal nucleic acid sequences by PCR.

The advantages of serologic tests include the rapidity of obtaining results and significant reduction in morbidity and mortality by early initiation of antifungals. They also serve as prognostic indicators during the management of patients.

Targets for serological tests are as follows:
- Detection of fungal antigen
- Detection of fungal antibody
- Detection of fungal metabolites.

Serological tests in use:
- Latex agglutination (LA) (Fig. 5.1)
- Immunodiffusion (ID)
- Complement fixation test
- Enzyme-linked immunosorbent assay (ELISA) (Figs. 5.2A and B)
- Lateral flow assay (LFA) (Fig. 5.3)
- Counter immuno-electrophoresis (CIE)
- Radioimmunosorbent assay (RIA).

All reports have to be interpreted in light of the clinical and radiological findings and fungal culture reports.

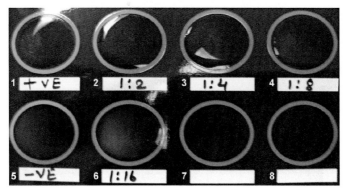

Fig. 5.1: Detection of Cryptococcal antigen with titre by Latex agglutination method.

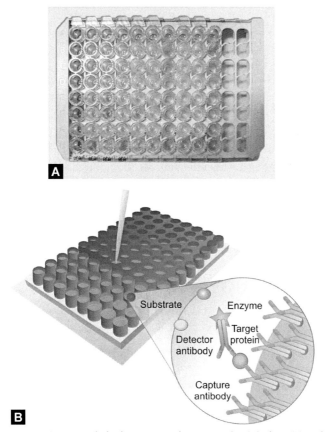

Figs. 5.2A and B: ELISAs. (A) Enzyme-linked immunosorbent assay (ELISA) plate; (B) Architecture of ELISA in closed view.

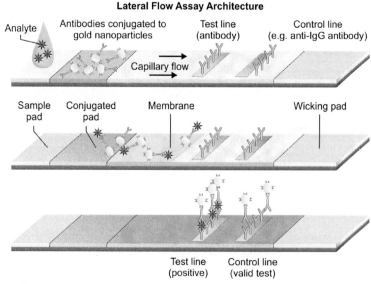

Lateral Flow Assay Architecture

Fig. 5.3: Lateral flow assay.

■ ANTIBODY TESTING FOR FUNGAL INFECTIONS

Tests for fungal antibodies are useful in diagnosis of endemic fungal infections, such as:

- Diagnosis of acute (seroconversion) and chronic histoplasmosis
- Diagnosis and monitoring the treatment of coccidioidomycosis
- Antibody tests are used for diagnosis of allergic bronchopulmonary aspergillosis (ABPA) and chronic pulmonary aspergillosis, chronic and granulomatous *Aspergillus* rhinosinusitis
- Diagnosis of paracoccidioidomycosis
- Tests for detection of anti-*Pneumocystis* antibody and anti-*Cryptococcus* antibody are useful for research studies
- Anti-mannan antibodies for *Candida* are combined with mannan antigen testing to improve sensitivity
- Diagnosis of rare fungal infections such as anti-*sporothrix* antibodies in CSF, anti-*Scedosporium* antibodies in mycetoma.

It is important to test paired sera specimens, both acute and convalescent, to determine whether the antibody titers are increasing or decreasing.

However, antibody testing has the following limitations:

- Compared to immunocompetent patients, immunocompromised individuals may not be able to generate sufficient humoral response and develop detectable antibody levels
- The infection may be too fulminant to provide sufficient time for developing significant antibody titers
- Antibodies may be present in colonized but uninfected individuals

Antigens for Antibody Testing

Unpurified or semi-purified antigens previously used for antibody testing were flawed due to cross-reactions owing to the presence of determinants shared among pathogenic fungi. Standardized antigens derived by recombinant techniques have largely replaced these as the results provided with the purified antigens are more reliable and reproducible.

Immunodiffusion (ID) is simple and inexpensive method for detecting precipitating antibodies. Counter-immunoelectrophoresis (CIE) is utilized for detection of precipitins. Complement fixation (CF) is a quantitative technique but more cumbersome to perform. Almost all tests detect IgG or IgE antibodies with the exception of IgM for coccidioidomycosis.

■ ANTIGEN TESTING FOR FUNGAL INFECTIONS

Antigen testing may prove useful in the following scenarios:
- Mannan test for candidiasis
- Galactomannan test for invasive aspergillosis
- *Cryptococcus neoformans* capsular antigen.

Antigen testing is limited by the following:

Antigenemia may be ill-sustained in candidiasis and invasive aspergillosis as antigens are rapidly cleared from the circulation by receptor-mediated endocytosis in the liver. Hence, serial samples need to be tested.

Antibodies for Antigen Testing

Polyclonal antibodies result in significant cross-reaction. Monoclonal antibodies have less batch-to-batch variability and can be generated in unlimited quantities.

LA and ELISA remain the primary techniques for antigen detection. Radioimmunoassay (RIA) is sensitive but disposal of radioactive isotopes is a limitation.

■ PAN-FUNGAL DETECTION OF β-D-GLUCAN

1,3-β-D-glucan, a cell wall component of many fungi, is detected by the β-D-glucan assay. Fungitell assay has been cleared by the Food and Drug Administration (FDA) as an aid to diagnose invasive fungal infections with the exception of *Mucorales* and *C. neoformans*. β-D-glucan triggers coagulation cascade of amebocyte cells in North American horse-shoe crab (*Limulus polyphemus*) through Factor G. The output of the serum assay is based on spectrophotometer readings, in which optical density (OD) is converted to β-D-glucan concentrations. The results are interpreted as negative (range <60 pg/mL), indeterminate (60–79 pg/mL), or positive (>80 pg/mL). These cutoffs are clinically relevant for invasive candidiasis but need to be defined better for invasive aspergillosis. The β-D-glucan assay is positive in patients with a variety of invasive fungal infections, including *Candida* spp., *P. jirovecii*, *Aspergillus* spp., *Fusarium, Trichosporon,* and *Saccharomyces*. The test is typically negative in patients with mucormycosis or cryptococcosis.

The β-D-glucan assay may be used as a screening tool for presumptive diagnosis of invasive fungal infections early in the course of infection, prior to the onset of overt clinical symptoms and signs. The test has a strong negative predictive value (NPV). This makes it useful for excluding a diagnosis of invasive fungal infection. False-positive results have been reported with the following:

- Albumin
- IVIG
- Cellulose filters for intravenous administration
- Intravenous amoxicillin–clavulanic acid
- Hemodialysis with cellulose membranes
- Infection with bacteria such as *Pseudomonas aeruginosa* that contain cellular β-glucans.

SPECIFIC SERODIAGNOSTIC TESTS

Aspergillosis

Diagnosis of invasive aspergillosis is a major challenge since the clinical, microbiological, and radiological findings may not correlate. It is difficult to differentiate *Aspergillus* colonization from true infection. Diagnosis of aspergillosis by non-culture techniques may improve prognosis by early initiation of treatment.

Antibody Detection Tests for Aspergillosis

Multiple tests are available for testing IgG antibody to detect *A. fumigatus* in serum. Fewer incompletely validated tests are available for other species of *Aspergillus*. About 30–50% of patients with ABPA have low titers of detectable antibodies to *A. fumigatus*. In case of high titers, chronic pulmonary aspergillosis should be suspected. The best IgG assays for chronic pulmonary aspergillosis and aspergilloma due to *A. fumigatus* have a 90–95% sensitivity. *A. flavus* IgG antibody is a useful confirmatory evidence in fungal sinusitis, especially if histology is positive and culture is negative. Patients with *Aspergillus* bronchitis have positive IgG antibodies and negative IgE antibodies. Patients with cystic fibrosis may have higher baseline IgG antibody titers.

IgE antibody testing against *A. fumigatus* is useful to detect *Aspergillus* sensitization. The skin-prick test is more sensitive than blood testing. Usually, both are positive but either may be conducted to diagnose ABPA.

Antigen Detection Tests for Aspergillosis

Galactomannan: The galactomannan assay was developed in the Netherlands by Stynen et al. in 1992. Galactomannan is a heteropolysaccharide composed of a mannan core and a lactoferrin side chain. It is a major structural glycoprotein primarily found in the cell wall of mold-like fungi especially in *Aspergillus* spp. and *Penicillium* spp. It is shed in the blood stream and tissues during hyphal growth. Although several potential *Aspergillus* antigens have been studied, galactomannan correlates best with the extent of infection.

A rat monoclonal antibody EB-A2 is used to detect circulating *Aspergillus* galactomannan either by LA or by sandwich ELISA technique. The limitation of LA test (Pastorex *Aspergillus*, France) is its low sensitivity. It detects galactomannan levels only if more than 15–20 ng/mL. Moreover, it detects galactomannan only during the late stage of the disease. It cannot be used to detect galactomannan in urine due to high false-positive results. A newer and superior technique for galactomannan detection is the sandwich ELISA (Platelia *Aspergillus*). This test is more sensitive than LA and detects galactomannan levels as low as 0.5–1.0 ng/mL. The higher sensitivity of this test is attributed to the fact that EB-A2 functions both as a captor and as a detector. The test has been approved by the US–FDA. The test becomes positive even before overt signs and symptoms of the disease develop.

The Platelia *Aspergillus* ELISA results are reported as a ratio between the OD of the patient's sample and that of a control with a low but detectable amount of galactomannan. This ratio is called the OD index. A serum sample is considered positive at a cutoff index of 0.5 based on testing of two aliquots of the same sample, and another sample collected at a subsequent time point. The optimal cutoff value of 0.5 is used to consider a test positive, and the same has been accepted by the FDA. The test has a higher NPV (92–98%) than a positive predictive value (PPV 25–62%) and is better at ruling out the diagnosis of aspergillosis rather than confirming the diagnosis of the same. The amount of galactomannan released varies according to the species of *Aspergillus*. The amount of galactomannan released by *A. fumigatus* is lesser than that of other species. Serial galactomannan monitoring may be useful in assessing the therapeutic response to antifungal agents and predicting clinical outcomes in high-risk patients.

The results obtained by the Platelia *Aspergillus* ELISA get influenced by a number of factors including:

- Prior use of azoles reduces test sensitivity
- The stage of disease at the time of testing
- Prevalence of aspergillosis in the population being studied
- Age of population being studied as more false-positive results have been reported in pediatric hematopoietic stem cell transplantation (HSCT) and lung transplant recipients. False-positive results are more often noted during the first 100 days following HSCT
- Cutoff values and significance of serial test values.

The monoclonal antibody EB-A2 cross-reacts with a number of other organisms including *Penicillium* spp., *Paecilomyces* spp., and *Alternaria* spp. Other causes of false-positive results include infant milk formulas, gastrointestinal colonization with *Bifidobacterium bifidum*, and enteral feeding with a formula containing soybean protein. The test has cross-reactivity with antimicrobials including piperacillin and amoxicillin. False-positive results with piperacillin–tazobactam and other β-lactam antibiotics may persist for up to 5 days after discontinuation of these drugs. These antibiotics are derived from *Penicillium* spp. that contain galactomannan in the cell wall. False-positive results are more likely in patients with gastrointestinal mucositis due to chemotherapy or graft versus host disease (GVHD).

The use of *Aspergillus* ELISA for other body fluids including CSF and BAL fluids needs more prospective studies. The test performed on BAL fluid provides additional sensitivity compared with culture.

Candidiasis

Diagnosis of invasive candidiasis is challenging due to its nonspecific presentation, frequent colonization, long incubation period, and low sensitivity of blood cultures.

Antibody Detection for Candidiasis

Candida antibodies can be detected by techniques including ID, CIE, RIA, and ELISA. However, the usefulness of these tests remains uncertain as patients with mucosal colonization may have these antibodies. Immunocompromised patients may have false-negative results. All normal individuals possess antibodies to mannan, the major cell wall mannoprotein of *Candida* species. ELISA to detect circulating anti-*Candida albicans* mannan antibodies is now being marketed in a number of countries (Platelia *Candida* antibody). Antibodies to the 48 kDa enolase antigen of *C. albicans* have been detected in patients with invasive candidiasis. Mycelia-form-specific antigens of *C. albicans* and antigens on the surface of germ tubes of *C. albicans* have been evaluated for detecting *Candida* antibodies in patients with invasive candidiasis.

These tests are insensitive and nonspecific. However, combining the results for ELISA for detection of antimannan antibodies with those of an ELISA for detection of circulating *C. albicans* mannan antigen increases both sensitivity and specificity.

Antigen Detection for Candidiasis

Various antigen tests have been evaluated for diagnosis of invasive candidiasis including cell wall mannan and mannoproteins, heat shock protein (HSP) 90, enolase, and proteinase.

Mannan: Mannan is the most extensively researched and evaluated rapid diagnostic test for invasive candidiasis. Mannan or mannoprotein is a surface antigen of *C. albicans* released from the *Candida* cell wall during infection. Mannan circulates in the form of immune complexes that must first be dissociated for optimal detection of the antigen. This can be achieved by boiling in the presence of EDTA. Since mannan has a rapid clearance from the blood circulation by endocytosis in the spleen and liver, multiple serum samples are essential to optimize sensitivity of the test.

The LA is easier to perform than ELISA and has a variable sensitivity ranging from 38% to 81%. More recently, a sandwich ELISA (Platelia *Candida* Antigen) has been developed. It uses EB-CA1 as a monoclonal antibody and appears to be more sensitive than the LA test. By combining the results of *Candida* antigen ELISA with the antimannan antibody ELISA, the sensitivity increases to 80% and specificity to 93%. The median time interval between serologic testing and blood culture is 6 days for antigen detection. Non-neutropenic surgical patients tend to present first with positive antibody tests, while hematologic patients tend to present with antigenemia. Since the α-linked oligomannose residues are cleared rapidly from the circulation, the test to detect circulating mannan needs to be repeated frequently.

Other tests for rapid diagnosis of invasive candidiasis include the following:
- Detection of (1-3)-β-D-glucan
- Detection of D-arabinitol.

PCR-based DNA detection techniques have variable sensitivity and specificity. Blood cultures are unreliable in diagnosis of invasive candidiasis. Serial samples for non-culture-based tests along with blood culture results is the best option for diagnosis of invasive candidiasis.

Cryptococcosis

Antibody Detection for Cryptococcosis

Antibodies to *C. neoformans* are rapidly neutralized by large amounts of capsular antigen released during infection, and tests for antibody detection are of limited value during early infection. Detection of cryptococcal antibodies after a successful treatment indicates a good prognosis.

Antigen Detection for Cryptococcosis

The development of an LA test for detection of *C. neoformans* capsular polysaccharide antigen in serum and CSF has become a vital tool in diagnosis of cryptococcal meningitis and disseminated cryptococcosis. It is most often utilized for screening serum and CSF specimens but other body fluids including bronchoalveolar lavage fluid can also be tested. The LA test has a sensitivity and specificity of around 95%.

Causes of false-positive results for cryptococcal antigen include the following:
- Nonspecific interference with rheumatoid factor eliminated by prior treatment of the sample with proteolytic enzyme pronase
- HIV-infected patient due to unidentified factors eliminated with 2-β-mercaptoethanol, but not with pronase
- Infection with *Trichosporon asahii* due to cross-reacting antigens with *C. neoformans*
- Several bacterial infections.

Causes of false-negative results for cryptococcal antigen include the following:
- In patients with AIDS even with culture-confirmed cryptococcal meningitis
- Low organism load
- If organisms are not well encapsulated
- In serum and CSF specimens owing to a prozone effect, but this can be deleted by dilution of the sample.

A number of LA tests for *C. neoformans* antigen detection are available which utilize polyclonal antibodies to detect capsular antigen but a more recent commercial LA test uses a murine monoclonal antibody specific for *C. neoformans* polysaccharide. The commercial LA tests have a detection limit of 5–20 ng of polysaccharide per mL of sample. The LA titer results may vary based on the commercial kit being used. Therefore, it is important to analyze sequential samples from a patient using the same commercial kit each time.

EIA is able to detect much lower concentrations of the cryptococcal antigen than LA but it has not replaced the older, simpler LA methods. The EIA is also advantageous as it is unaffected by prozone reactions, does not react with rheumatoid factor, or requires pronase treatment.

An increasing or unchanged CSF antigen titer in a patient of cryptococcal meningitis may indicate clinical and/or microbiological treatment failure. Rising CSF antigen levels during maintenance treatment may predict relapse.

Blastomycosis

Antibody Detection for Blastomycosis

Antibody detection tests for *Blastomyces dermatitidis* use ID although other procedures including ELISA, CF, and RIA have also been evaluated. The ID tests for antibodies utilize a purified antigen of *B. dermatitidis* termed the A antigen. Another immunodominant surface protein antigen of *B. dermatitidis* is named WI-1. It is a unique antigen found only in *B. dermatitidis* and absent in *H. capsulatum* and *C. albicans*. A RIA employing WI-1 has been developed.

Antigen Detection for Blastomycosis

A sandwich ELISA using rabbit polyclonal antibodies to detect *B. dermatitidis* antigen in urine is being evaluated.

Coccidioidomycosis

Antibody Detection for Coccidioidomycosis

Antibody detection for *Coccidioides immitis* utilizes the CF technique, ID, LA or an ELISA-based test.

The CF test uses a heat labile antigen derived from Coccidioidin—a filtrate of autolyzed *C. immitis* mycelial cultures. The test becomes positive between 4 and 12 weeks after infection and detects IgG antibodies. Titers of >1:16 indicate spread of the disease beyond the respiratory tract. Titers above 1:32 are suggestive of disseminated disease. Early or residual disease will result in low titers. Patients with HIV or other immunocompromised states may have false-negative results. Titers should fall during course of treatment. The test can be performed on serum, CSF, pleural fluid, or synovial fluid.

The ID test is a useful screening method. It uses heated coccidioidin antigens to detect IgM antibodies to *C. immitis* and unheated coccidioidin to detect IgG antibodies. LA tests (LA-Cocci-antibody System) is simple and faster and detects IgM antibodies. Due to high false-positive rates, a positive result should be confirmed using the ID method. It is not recommended for CSF screening. An ELISA test is now available for detection of both IgM and IgG antibodies to *C. immitis* in serum and CSF with high sensitivity and specificity rates. A recombinant chitinase antigen which is more sensitive than coccidioidin has reduced cross-reactivity with sera from blastomycosis and histoplasmosis patients.

Antigen Detection for Coccidioidomycosis

Antigen detection tests are not available as a routine. An inhibition ELISA detecting antigens derived from spherulin—a filtrate of autolyzed *C. immitis* spherule-phase cultures—appears promising.

Histoplasmosis

Antibody Detection for Histoplasmosis

It takes 2–6 weeks to generate sufficient antibody response in cases of acute pulmonary histo-plasmosis. Serologic tests are more useful in the following scenarios:

- *Histoplasma* meningitis—antibodies to *H. capsulatum* in CSF may be the only positive diagnostic test
- In patients with chronic pulmonary histoplasmosis
- Disseminated histoplasmosis.

Tests may be positive in 100% immunocompetent patients and 80% of immunocom-promised patients. The major antigen used for detection of *histoplasma* antibodies is histoplasmin. It is a soluble filtrate of *H. capsulatum* mycelial cultures. Histoplasmin antigen has two components:

1. H antigen—antibodies against H antigen are formed during acute histoplasmosis.
2. M antigen—antibodies against M antigen are produced during all phases of the disease.

The ID test is qualitative test, while CF test is a quantitative test for detecting antibodies. The ID test is more specific than CF. CF titers of 1:32 or greater and rising titers when serial samples are tested are diagnostic of histoplasmosis. Antibodies may persist from few months to several years following exposure. Recombinant H and M antigens have been developed to improve the detection of histoplasmosis. Since antibody production in AIDS may be insufficient, it may be more appropriate to use antigen detection tests in these patients.

Antigen Detection for Histoplasmosis

Antigen detection is a vital diagnostic tool for histoplasmosis in immunocompromised patients and in cases of disseminated histoplasmosis. Specimens for detection of the *Histoplasma* polysaccharide antigen include serum, CSF, urine, and BAL. Effective treatment should reduce the antigen concentrations, whereas failure of levels to fall indicate treatment failure. Relapse will result in an increase in the level of antigen subsequent to a previous decline.

Antigen tests are useful for early diagnosis since antibodies to *H. capsulatum* take at least a month to appear. Antigenuria can be detected in early phase of the disease. RIA, sandwich ELISA, and inhibition ELISA have been used for *Histoplasma* antigen detection. The use of monoclonal antibodies has increased the sensitivity of the test. There is cross-reactivity with blastomycosis, paracoccidioidomycosis, and *Penicillium marneffei*.

PCR-based molecular detection methods may be useful for the detection of *H. capsulatum* in tissues but is inferior to detection of antigen in urine.

Paracoccidioidomycosis

Antibody Detection for Paracoccidioidomycosis

IgG antibodies to *P. brasiliensis* are elevated in patients with paracoccidioidomycosis and decline on initiating treatment. The antibody levels may be low in patients with AIDS. The serologic tests use ID, CF, or ELISA. The antigens used are derived from the yeast cell wall, cytoplasm, or culture filtrates. ID is more specific than CF in diagnosis. Cross-reaction can occur with serum from patients with histoplasmosis.

Antigen Detection for Paracoccidioidomycosis

Antigen testing can be useful to detect paracoccidioidomycosis in serum, urine, CSF, and BAL. An inhibition ELISA uses monoclonal antibodies directed against the 87 kDa HSP antigen of *P. brasiliensis*. It cross-reacts with serum of patients with histoplasmosis and aspergillosis. Serial antigen testing is useful in monitoring therapeutic response.

Penicilliosis

Antibody Detection for Penicilliosis

P. marneffei antigens of different molecular masses are used as reagents for antibody detection in cases of disseminated penicilliosis.

Antigen Detection for Penicilliosis

Dot blot ELISA and LA tests are utilized for detecting *P. marneffei* antigenuria. These use a polyclonal anti-*P. marneffei* antibody. Different clones of monoclonal antibodies are being studied.

Sporotrichosis

An LA test for sporotrichosis is commercially available (LA-Sporo-antibody system) to detect antibodies in serum and CSF.

Serologic tests for zygomycosis need further evaluation.

■ SUGGESTED READING

1. Arendrup MC, Boekhout T, Akova M, et al. ESCMID and ECMM joint clinical guidelines for the diagnosis and management of rare invasive yeast infections. Clin Microbiol Infect. 2014;20(Suppl. S3):76-8.
2. Arvanitis M, Anagnostou T, Fuchs BB, et al. Molecular and non-molecular diagnostic methods for invasive fungal infections. Clin Microbiol Rev. 2014;27:490-526.
3. El-Aal A, El-Mashad N, Mohamed A. Revision on the recent diagnostic strategies of fungal infections. Open J Med Microbiol. 2017;7:29-40.
4. Marcos JY, Pincus DH. Fungal diagnostics: review of commercially available methods. Methods Mol Biol. 2013;968:24-45.
5. Richardson MD, Page ID. *Aspergillus* serology: have we arrived yet? Med Mycol. 2017;55(1):48-55.

6

Molecular Techniques for Diagnosis of Systemic Fungal Infections

Monica Mahajan, Bansidhar Tarai, Pragnya P Jena

INTRODUCTION

Recent advances in molecular technology are revolutionizing the identification of newer fungi producing diseases in humans and animals. The reason for this rapidly advancing application in clinical mycology is the accumulation of newer protein and DNA sequence data on a daily basis and extensive research being done in this field.

NUCLEIC ACID DETECTION

Fungal cultures are time-consuming and have low sensitivity. Molecular methods for fungal identification give best results when fungi grow on culture media. However, they can still be utilized in the fixed tissue specimens, if they contain template nucleic acid in the absence of viable cells. Nucleic acid detection involves amplification of the small quantities of fungal DNA present in the specimen. DNA techniques (Box 6.1) offer the following advantages:

- A comprehensive analysis of DNA fragments to identify the causative fungal pathogen including genus and species
- Early initiation of appropriate antifungal after assessing susceptibility
- Avoid injudicious use of antifungal in case of negative results
- Monitor treatment response in cases of candidiasis, cryptococcosis, and aspergillosis
- Reclassification of some fungi which could not be classified appropriately in the past by conventional methods. Beginning in 2013, an effort is being made to simplify the fungal

---

Box 6.1: Molecular diagnostic techniques

- Conventional PCR
- Fluorescence *in situ* hybridization (FISH)
- DNA array hybridization
- Multiplex tandem PCR (MT-PCR)
- Real-time PCR (RT-PCR)
- PCR ELISA
- Random amplified polymorphic DNA (RAPD)
- Loop-mediated isothermal amplification (LAMP)

nomenclature as per the Amsterdam Declaration "One Fungus = One Name." Molecular diagnostics are making a significant contribution towards the same

- Rapidly identify the mechanisms of fungal resistance
- Molecular genotyping is vital in cluster outbreaks to support or refute an epidemiological hypothesis. Isolates from a common source outbreak should be identical on molecular typing.

Limitations of molecular diagnostic tests include the following:

- False-positive results due to colonization of patient's airways by conidia and/or hyphae
- Inability to distinguish colonization from true infection
- Environmental contamination of samples
- False-negative results in culture positive patients may occur if the specimen contains a single-copy gene since the molecular test may not be sensitive enough to detect the same.

The reasons for rapid advancement in molecular diagnostics include the following:

- Development of technologically advanced amplification platforms
- Development of probes like dual-labeled probes, light cycler probes, and molecular beacons
- Newer quantitative polymerase chain reaction (qPCR), reverse transcription quantitative PCR (RT-qPCR), and digital PCR (dPCR) detection technologies

GenBank

Sequence data from an unknown fungus can be identified by using a public database such as GenBank. It has a wide array of thousands of fungal sequences but the search needs to be done with caution as there are errors in the database.

Conventional PCR (Fig. 6.1)

PCR plays an integral role in many molecular identification methods and can be used for live cells, fixed tissues, and specimens contaminated with human tissue or fluids. It is the preliminary step for many diagnostic assays. This is the simplest technique in which fungal DNA from clinical specimens is amplified using species-specific primers based on existing sequence data. The readout displays the presence or absence of a specific band. The dimensions of the band also help in identification of a fungus. The assay can be completed in few hours. It can amplify one molecule of DNA into billions of copies in a short period of time. Since there have been wide variations in interpretation and lack of standardization, conventional PCR techniques for fungal identification have not been approved by the Food and Drug Association (FDA).

PCR utilizes a DNA polymerase called Taq polymerase. Taq DNA polymerase is a thermostable enzyme, which was originally isolated in 1976 from **Thermus aq**uaticus, a thermophilic bacterium found in hot springs.

A basic PCR involves a series of repeating cycles involving three main steps:

Step 1: Denaturation: The double-stranded DNA (dsDNA) is melted to single-stranded DNA (ssDNA). The reaction is carried out at a high temperature of 95°C which disrupts the hydrogen bonds holding the two complementary strands of the DNA helix together.

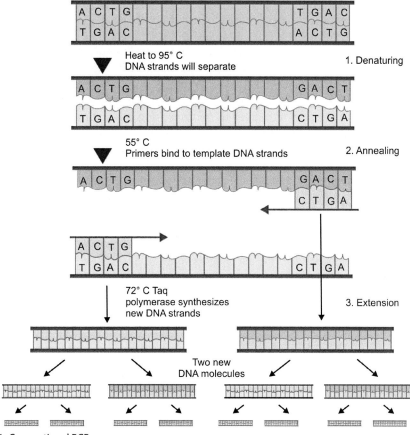

Fig. 6.1: Conventional PCR.

Step 2: Annealing: The temperature is lowered to approximately 45–60°C to promote the attachment/annealing of the oligonucleotide primers to the DNA template. Primers attach to the complementary sequences.

Step 3: Extension: At a temperature of 72°C, the DNA polymerase extends the primer sequences from the 3′ of each primer to the end of the amplicon to amplify the DNA sequences of interest.

Steps 1–3 are repeated in a cyclical manner.

Fluorescence In Situ Hybridization

Fluorescence in situ hybridization (FISH) is a novel molecular cytogenetic technique for the "in situ" detection of pathogens by using fluorescent probes. The first FISH probe for fungi was developed by Li et al. in 1996 for identification of *Aureobasidium pullulans*.

FISH allows location of specific DNA sequences on chromosomes in their natural position or "in situ." Since fluorescent probes are used for detection, the technique is called fluorescent in situ hybridization. Watson and Crick described the DNA double helix in 1953. The double helix is a stable structure due to the hydrogen bonds between the base pairs. Heat or chemicals denature and break these bonds. During favorable conditions, the DNA helix can renature or reform. This forms the basis of molecular hybridization.

The probe is a labeled DNA or RNA oligonucleotide containing 15–20 nucleotides sequence that is tagged with a fluorescent marker by incorporating dye-conjugated nucleotides or labeled directly using fluorochrome. It identifies the presence or absence of complementary counterpart sequences in a sample. There is no prior amplification required. The DNA sequences of fungi can be detected in a specimen.

The tissue specimen from the patient is chemically treated to increase cell permeability. The extracted chromosomal material is placed on a slide and denatured. The fluorescent probe complementary to the suspected pathogen's genetic code is denatured and added to the slide. The probe will specifically anneal with the complementary DNA sequences of the suspected pathogen. The fluorescent signals are observed using a fluorescent microscope, a charge-coupled device camera, and an imaging analysis software. The system allows the detection and localization of specific DNA sequences in chromosomes of fungal pathogens. The sites of hybridization are visualized.

Mitochondrial genes and ribosomal RNA are the most abundant sequences with each fungal cell containing multiple copies of these genes. The FISH probes generally target these genetic sequences.

The main advantage of FISH probes is that they can be applied to cultures as well as formaldehyde or ethanol-fixed samples. The success of the test depends on the specificity of probes. The limitations of FISH method include the following:
- Autofluorescence of substrate and fungi may produce false-positive results.
- Insufficient permeability of cell wall which can be improved by using specific enzymes such as glucanases and chitinases.
- Ribosome content in specimen being low will produce false-negative results.
- Nonspecific or low-stringency probes.

Peptide Nucleic Acid (PNA) Probes

These are synthetic probes with a neutral backbone in which the negatively charged phosphate–sugar–polynucleotide backbone of DNA is replaced with a non-charged flexible pseudopeptide polymer backbone to which nucleobases are linked. The neutral charge helps the probe to penetrate the cell wall more efficiently since it is not repelled by the electrostatic charges during hybridization. It improves the specificity and capacity of hybridization with complementary sequences. PNA probes-based technology has great potential for use in genetics and cytogenetics but these probes are more expensive than routine fluorescence probes.

DNA Array Hybridization/Reverse Dot-blot Hybridization

It is a microarray-based technique to detect the expression of numerous genes simultaneously. DNA arrays are microscope glass slides or other solid platforms such as a nylon membrane.

Thousands of synthesized oligonucleotides are printed or spotted in defined positions on the supporting platform. These can be printed manually or robotically. These are called DNA chips or gene chips. Reverse dot-blot hybridization works on the principle of hybridization of amplified and labeled genome regions from a clinical sample to these oligonucleotides spots. This reaction between the sample DNA and its PCR amplification product, that has been labeled with a fluorophore and a perfectly matched (PM) oligonucleotide, generates a signal which is chemiluminescent. The intensity of the hybridization signal can be visualized and quantified by a digital camera in a dark room. Captured images are then analyzed on a computer software.

DNA microarray technology enables detection and quantification of gene expression on a large scale compared with PCR-based methods since one membrane can accommodate large number of oligonucleotides. The membrane is reusable and more cost-effective compared to a southern dot-blot hybridization. It can identify genus, species, and subspecies of fungi.

Multiplex Tandem PCR

This technology allows the detection of multiple targets (multiplexed gene expression profiling) for the rapid identification of fungi. This platform consists of two rounds of amplification.

Step 1 consists of reverse transcription and first round of multiplexed pre-amplification. Single-tube amplification with highly multiplexed primers is carried out. Very little amount of sample is required. A multiplex PCR is performed for very few (10–15) cycles so that there is no competition between primers and the conditions favor enriching the target DNA. Each PCR is independent of other reactions. Nonspecific amplicons synthesized in Step 1 are discarded and not amplified in the next step.

Step 2 consists of real-time PCR and second round quantification amplification. The products generated in the first step are diluted and utilized as a template for the second round of amplification into a number of real-time PCRs (one PCR for each target). There are multiple individual quantitative PCRs with primers nested within those used in the multiplex PCR.

There is no competition as enriched samples from Step 1 are amplified in separate wells. It is highly specific as Step 2 primers are nested within Step 1 primers. Two sets of species-specific primers are incorporated for each target to increase the probability of correct amplification and detection of a fungal species. Up to 72 or more PCRs can be multiplexed and performed simultaneously. An automated software analysis determines the presence or absence of an organism.

Multiplex tandem PCR is better than traditional multiplex assays which inevitably get inhibited due to competition between primers. This competition is avoided in the MT-PCR as there are separate steps for multiplexing and quantification. Since the DNA is amplified for a limited number of cycles only (10–15 cycles) in the first step, there is no competition between the primers. During the second step, there is negligible carryover of primers from the first step since the products of first round are diluted 50-fold. Step 1 primers are prevented from taking part in Step 2 reactions and avoid the challenge of PCR inhibition. MT-PCR is a simple, rapid, and low-cost platform. Being sensitive and specific in identification of fungal pathogens from blood cultures, it helps in initiation of early targeted therapy to improve the patient outcomes.

Real-time PCR

Real-time PCR differs from conventional one since the process of amplification is monitored "real-time" with the help of a camera or a detector rather than looking for bands on a gel. The amplification of DNA is linked to the generation of fluorescence. As the number of gene copies increases, so does the fluorescence. The major advantage of this technique is that the efficiency of the process can be closely monitored. The main benefit is that this is a "quantitative" PCR for gene expression.

SYBR® Green or any other fluorescent intercalating dye intercalates with or binds to the DNA double helix. As the amount of generated DNA increases, it causes the dye to fluoresce more.

The other detection technique for real-time PCR is the hydrolysis probes (TaqMan® style). These are DNA oligonucleotides which are labeled fluorescently. They bind downstream on one of the primers. This generates a fluorescent signal during the PCR. A fluorescent "reporter" dye molecule with a fluorescein derivative is used to label the 5′ end of the probe. The common reporter molecules include FAM, ROX, and CY5. These emit light of different wavelengths. The 3′ end of the probe is labeled with a "quencher" molecule which quenches the output generated from the reporter.

The PCR process involves the binding of the probe downstream of the primer. The probe is then cleaved by the action of the polymerase enzyme. The cleavage of the probe causes the reporter and the quencher to separate and move apart. As the distance between the two increases, the quencher fails to influence the activity of the porter. As a result, the reporter dye fluorescence increases. As the number of PCR cycles increases, more probes are cleaved and the fluorescence correspondingly increases.

Hydrolysis probes are more expensive than intercalating dyes. However, the hydrolysis probes are more specific than the dyes. A post-run analysis is required to confirm the results of intercalating dyes since these can bind to and report on any DNA formed during the PCR irrespective of what it is. This analysis is in the form of a melt-curve or dissociation curve. If the target of interest is rare, it is preferable to use hydrolysis probes since these are more sensitive. If the target of interest is abundant, an intercalating dye may suffice.

RT-PCR is a very rapid technique since the results can be analyzed within minutes of completing the PCR. No post-amplification manipulation is required. This reduces the chances of laboratory contamination. It is commercially available for detection of *Candida* and *Aspergillus fumigatus.*

PCR ELISA

This analytical tool merges PCR and ELISA to detect genomic material in clinical specimens. It includes different procedures:
- A PCR amplification
- Hybridization of PCR amplicons with a complementary labeled probe
- Capture of labeled hybrids on microtiter plates
- The detection of specific PCR products by immunoassay. These are analyzed by calorimetric signal detection or fluorescent method.

Suitable primers are required to amplify the target DNA. The main advantage of this is a higher sensitivity than conventional ELISA, which only detects circulating antibodies in serum and requires purified monoclonal antibodies for the test. Low abundance sequences can also be detected due to amplification of the target DNA in the first step. Antibody cross-reactivity between closely related species is common in conventional ELISA. PCR-ELISA has higher specificity and can differentiate species based on the specific DNA sequences. PCR-ELISA has a faster throughput as 96/384 samples can be processed in 6–7 hours depending on which micrometer plate is used. It is potentially automatable and cost-effective. Conventional ELISA is not only cumbersome and time-consuming but also expensive since it requires a monoclonal antibody/purified antigen. It offers better sensitivity for *Candida* and *Aspergillus* than ethidium bromide staining does. Accurate diagnosis helps in choosing appropriate antifungal agent.

Random Amplified Polymorphic DNA

This differs from other PCR techniques since random fragments of genomic DNA are amplified. The primer may or may not amplify the DNA segment depending on the presence or absence of complementary base sequences. The PCR results are analyzed to develop a unique profile for identification of the fungus. This method has been utilized for differentiation of *Cryptococcus neoformans* and *Cryptococcus gattii*.

Loop-mediated Isothermal Amplification

Loop-mediated isothermal amplification (LAMP) is a low-cost alternative for nucleic acid amplification, which has been developed by Notomi et al. It has the advantage over other PCR techniques that a high-precision thermal cycler is not required, as the LAMP reaction is carried out at a constant temperature (Table 6.1). It has the ability to amplify a few copies of target DNA to millions of copies within a short span of 1 hour and that too under isothermal conditions. The key component is a DNA polymerase with high-strand displacement activity. There are two sets of four specifically designed primers—two inner and two outer primers, which identify six specific regions of the target gene. DNA synthesis involves autocycling strand displacement. The inner primers contain the sense and antisense sequences of the target DNA. The primers and DNA sample are heat denatured and then rapidly cooled on ice. The subsequent step involves the addition of DNA polymerase, carrying out the reaction at 64°C in a regular laboratory water bath for 1 hour. The inner primers hybridize with the target DNA and promote complementary strand synthesis whereas the outer primers are a few bases shorter and cause strand displacement DNA synthesis. This releases a complementary strand with a looped structure at one end. The reaction takes place in a single tube containing target DNA, primers, DNA polymerase, and buffer.

The advantages of LAMP include the following:

- Direct observation of products as a white precipitate or a yellow–green solution by adding SYBR®Green or by ultraviolet illumination
- Simple operation, rapid amplification, and easy and time-efficient detection of fungal species and no requirement of trained personnel or sophisticated equipment; can be ideal for developing countries.

LAMP assays have been used for detecting *Scedosporium* spp., *Cryptococcus* spp., *Penicillium marneffei* spp., and *Pseudallescheria* spp. in clinical samples.

Table 6.1: Comparison of LAMP and conventional PCR	
LAMP	*Conventional PCR*
Isothermal reaction	Cyclic reaction
Isothermal temperature	Variable temperature for denaturation, annealing, and polymerization
Does not require expensive thermocycler	Requires thermocycler
Visualization of DNA can be done directly or through gel electrophoresis	Visualization of DNA is done through gel electrophoresis
Greater detection limit	Lower detection limit
Amplification specificity is higher as 4–6 oligonucleotides are used	Amplification specificity is lower than that of LAMP

▦ OTHER TECHNIQUES

MALDI-TOF MS (Proteomics Profiling/Fingerprinting) (Fig. 6.2)

Matrix-assisted laser desorption/ionization time-of-flight mass spectrometry (MALDI-TOF MS) is an innovative ionization technique for identifying fungi. This Nobel Prize-winning

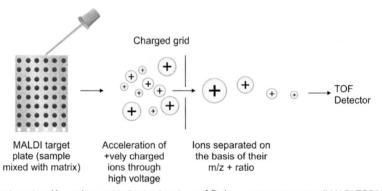

Fig. 6.2: Matrix-assisted laser desorption/ionization time-of-flight mass spectrometry (MALDI-TOF MS).

technology by Koichi Tanaka uses mass spectrometry to generate spectra that are a unique characteristic of each different species. It can identify most of the species of *Candida, Cryptococcus,* and *Aspergillus.*

The instrumentation for MALDI-TOF MS consists of the following:
- An ion source that causes desorption/ionization of sample
- A mass analyzer that analyzes mass-to-charge (m/z) ratio of ions
- A detector that detects the ions.

Technique

Step 1: Samples for analysis are mixed with a suitable solution of matrix and applied to a metal plate. The matrix is an organic compound, which is energy absorbent.

Step 2: When the matrix is dried, it crystallizes. The sample also crystallizes since it is entrapped in the matrix.

Step 3: The specimen undergoes ionization with the laser beam because of energy absorption by the matrix. Single protonated ions are generated from the analytes due to desorption and ionization.

Step 4: The TOF component of the equipment is a tube through which the protonated ions are accelerated at a fixed potential. The excited ions separate from each other on the basis of their mass to charge (m/z) ratio. The time-of-flight/transit time of individual ions is recorded.

Step 5: A mass analyzer records the time required for the ion to travel the length of the flight tube. An ion mirror at the rear end of the tube reflects back ions to a detector. Based on the TOF, peptide mass fingerprint (PMF) is obtained. Each fungus has a characteristic spectrum. This is matched to the library of spectra and the fungus is identified.

Advantages of MALDI-TOF

- The system is speedy and data can be analyzed within minutes.
- Downstream data manipulation is absent, which makes it accurate.

Limitations of MALDI-TOF

- Identification of unknown fungi is a challenge as the reference library would lack matching spectra.
- Variations in spectra may also occur if the fungi growth conditions including culture media and incubation time similar to those for the reference spectra in library are not replicated.
- There is a co-existence of different phenotypes in a fungus and the hyphal and/or conidia state may pose a challenge.
- Each instrument manufacturer maintains a library and since these are specific for an instrument proprietary, it may be difficult to modify by the end user.
- Lack of portability of instruments, advanced technical skills required, and capital investment.

▩ PRACTICAL UTILIZATION OF MOLECULAR TECHNIQUES

- *Direct detection of dermatophytes and cutaneous fungal DNA*: Since conventional techniques are cumbersome, PCR kits for dermatophytes give a rapid and reliable diagnosis.
- *Direct identification of Pnemocystis jirovecii nucleic acid*: P. jirovecii is difficult to culture. Molecular techniques are more sensitive than routine stains. The target regions for DNA amplification of *P. jirovecii* include mitochondrial large subunit rRNA (mt LSU rRNA) and the major surface glycoprotein gene family. Other targets are dehydrofolate reductase (DHFR) and heat shock protein 70 (HSP70). The mt LSU rRNA is an excellent target for BAL and sputum samples with sensitivity ranging from 90% to 100%. Quantitative RT-PCR

kits minimize the time required for detection and the quantitation helps in distinguishing asymptomatic carriers from clinical disease. Signal strength of PCR is usually stronger in HIV-positive patients, increasing the sensitivity of the test. Low-level positive signals are difficult to interpret as a cutoff for colonization versus infection has not been defined. Successful treatment entails a fall in the signal strength. The PCR can be performed on BAL, endotracheal aspirates, sputum, blood, and vitreous fluid. CDC has classified molecular technology as gold standard for *P. jirovecii* diagnosis.

- Direct detection of *Aspergillus* species nucleic acid: Aspergillum can be cultured from respiratory secretions and blood but has a very low yield. Galactomannan and other biomarkers fail to identify the species. Molecular diagnosis is not only a faster technique but also provides species information. The 18S rRNA, 28S rRNA, and ITS (internal transcribed) regions are multicopy genes most commonly detected as these provide natural amplification, thereby improving sensitivity. The challenge is developing a highly sensitive RT-PCR since environmental contamination of container or reagent by *Aspergillus* can cause false-positive reactions. *Penicillium* spp. may be confused for *Aspergillus*. PCR is a more sensitive technique for respiratory samples compared to culture. The samples in patients with cystic fibrosis are not only extremely viscus but also the host and fungal nucleic acid is simultaneously present. Liquefaction of the sample prior to processing improves yield.

- Direct detection of *Candida* species nucleic acid: Although three commercial PCR systems for *Candida* spp. are available, more data need to be analyzed for patients with candidemia. The sensitivity and specificity in blood are 99% and 94%, respectively.

- Direct detection of pan-fungal DNA: Using database from GenBank and other repositories, pan-fungal detection has been attempted. The specific fungus can be identified by sequencing the DNA targets in the second step. The issue remains that reagents tend to get contaminated from the environment and produce false-positive results.

- Drug inhibition of PCR: PCRs can be inhibited by the presence of certain drugs. An amplification control should be incorporated in all molecular diagnostic assays to rule out a false-negative result due to drug inhibition. Negative control assays are also provided in commercial kits to rule out environmental contamination resulting in false-positive results.

■ CONCLUSION

Molecular technology is vital in diagnosis of fungi and improving epidemiological data on fungi. The major challenges are the cost of tests, accuracy and specificity, frequency of testing, as well as identification of cryptic species. The issues preventing full implementation of molecular-based technology in the mycology laboratory are as follows:

- The number of disease-causing fungi being identified is rapidly expanding
- Laboratory staff lack training in identifying rare fungi based on morphology
- The nomenclature of fungi is confusing. Mycologists need a lot of experience to deal with this confusion
- Unlike systems for bacterial identification, there is no single assay for fungi. The equipment is expensive and needs specialized training to operate.

These methods need to be developed further to become an important part of diagnostic mycology.

■ SUGGESTED READING

1. Azab MM, Abo Taleb AF, Mohamed NAE, et al. Rapid diagnosis of invasive fungal infections. Int J Curr Microbiol Appl Sci. 2015;4(11):470-86.
2. Buchan BW, Ledeboer NA. Emerging technologies for the clinical microbiology laboratory. Clin Microbiol Rev. 2014;27:783-822.
3. Clark AE, Kaleta EJ, Arora A, et al. Matrix-assisted laser desorption ionization-time-of-flight mass spectrometry: a fundamental shift in the routine practice of clinical microbiology. Clin Microbiol Rev. 2013;26:547-603.
4. Patel R. Matrix-assisted laser desorption ionisation-time-of-flight mass spectrometry in clinical microbiology. Clin Infect Dis. 2013;57(4):564-72.

7

Radiodiagnosis of Systemic Fungal Infections: An Organ-based Approach

Monica Mahajan, Anandamoyee Dhar

INTRODUCTION

Fungal infections can involve almost every organ system in the body resulting in myriad conditions including pneumonitis, meningitis, sinusitis, and osteomyelitis. Imaging plays a vital role in invasive fungal infection (IFI) in the following:

- Diagnosis and evaluation of disease activity at an early stage
- Narrowing differential diagnosis
- Detecting associated complications
- Starting early targeted treatment, assessing therapeutic response in terms of treatment success or failure
- Guiding percutaneous tissue sampling.

Various imaging modalities including radiography, ultrasonography, computed tomography (CT), and magnetic resonance imaging (MRI) play an important role in an organ-based approach to diagnosing systemic fungal infections. Early detection will reduce mortality.

X-rays are easily available, low-cost, lower radiation exposure, and suitable for bedside imaging. Digital X-rays optimize the image quality and allow comparison of sequential radiographic images. Ground-glass opacities and diffuse miliary lesions can be missed on a chest X-ray. Positive findings on a chest X-ray should be corroborated by a CT scan. A CT scan should be ordered in the case of a negative X-ray if the index of suspicion is high. Ultrasonography is a bedside modality, especially useful in the ICU setting to detect pleural effusions, ascites, abscesses, and collections. It is useful in guiding percutaneous procedures and does not involve radiation exposure. Multidetector CT scanning is the best option for imaging the lungs and mediastinum. It can provide multiplanar reconstructed images and justify preemptive specific therapy. MRI plays a vital role in imaging central nervous system (CNS), paranasal sinuses, liver, bones, and joints. Motion and breathing artifacts in critically ill patients degrade image quality in MRI. Positron emission tomography imaging with F-18 fluorodeoxyglucose is more important in detecting metabolically active tumors and has a limited role in IFIs.

■ CENTRAL NERVOUS SYSTEM MANIFESTATIONS

Fungal infections of the CNS are encountered in immunocompromised patients including those with AIDS, solid-organ transplant, or uncontrolled longstanding diabetes. Cryptococcal meningoencephalitis is the most frequent infection followed by aspergillosis and candidiasis.

Meningitis

- Direct extension from contiguous structures or hematogenous spread with cerebrospinal fluid (CSF) seeding.
- Most common fungal pathogens are *Candida* species and *Cryptococcus neoformans.*
- Nonenhanced CT—communicating hydrocephalus due to impaired CSF absorption.
- Dural enhancement is adjacent to infected paranasal sinuses.
- Magnetic resonance imaging—leptomeningeal enhancement particularly at skull base is the most pronounced.
- Leptomeningeal enhancement can also extend to the spinal canal.
- Differential diagnoses—pyogenic meningitis, granulomatous meningitis, and leptomeningeal carcinomatosis.

Mycotic Aneurysm

- CT/MR angiogram—fusiform aneurysm involving the proximal vasculature, such as internal carotid artery and circle of Willis.
- Aspergillosis is the most common cause of mycotic aneurysm.

Intracranial Hemorrhage

- Complication of vasculitis or mycotic aneurysm
- Hyperattenuating on nonenhanced CT
- Variable appearance as per temporal window on MRI.

Ischemic Infarction

- Hypoattenuating areas involving the cortex and/or subcortical white matter, basal ganglia, thalamus, and internal capsule on CT are indicative of multiple areas of infarction.
- Restricted diffusion on diffusion-weighted MR images.
- Areas of hyperintensity on T2-weighted image (T2WI) develop 12–24 hours after the infarction and resolve within 2–3 weeks.
- Differential diagnoses include progressive multifocal leukoencephalopathy and neoplasm.
- Restricted diffusion can be the earliest detectable abnormality in acute, ischemic optic neuropathy.

Granuloma/Abscess Formation/Pseudocysts (Figs. 7.1A and B)

- Pathogens implicated are *Aspergillus* species, *Mucorales*, and *C. neoformans.*
- Nonenhanced CT—indistinct hypoattenuating areas due to surrounding vasogenic edema.

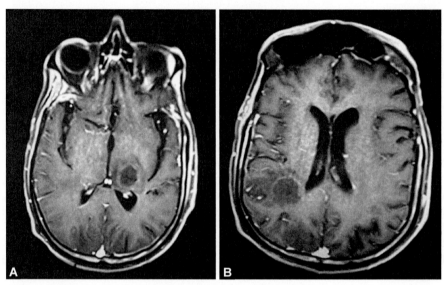

Figs. 7.1A and B: Postcontrast axial MRI scan of brain reveals hypointense lesions in left thalamus and right posterior parietal region with peripheral wall enhancement and perilesional edema in a case of disseminated aspergillosis with brain abscesses.

- Parenchymal abscesses are hypoattenuating with or without vasogenic edema on plain CT.
- Abscesses have peripheral rim enhancement on contrast CT.
- Magnetic resonance images show fungal abscesses as hypointense on T1-weighted image (T1WI) and hyperintense on T2WI with well-defined peripheral rim enhancement on contrast imaging, perilesional edema appearing indistinguishable from pyogenic abscesses.
- On proton MR spectroscopy (PMRS), fungal lesions show lipids, lactate, alanine, acetate, succinate, choline, and unidentified resonance at variable ppm. The identification of multiple signals seen between 3.6 ppm and 3.8 ppm assigned to trehalose sugars on PMRS improves diagnostic probability.
- A ring-enhancing T2-heterointense lesion with irregular walls and nonenhancing intra-cavitary projections having low apparent diffusion coefficient are more likely to be fungal rather than bacterial abscesses. These projections are directed centrally from the wall and are hypointense or isointense on T1WI and hypointense on T2WI.
- Gelatinous pseudocysts are intra-axial deep perivascular well-circumscribed, round, or oval low-density, and nonenhancing lesions in the basal ganglia due to cryptococcal infection. These are formed due to dilatation of Virchow–Robin spaces with mucoid gelatinous material produced by the capsule of the organism. Clusters of these cysts in the basal ganglia and thalami strongly suggest cryptococcal infection.
- Cryptococcomas and chronic granulomas lead to communicative or obstructive hydro-cephalus. Cryptococcomas show hypointensity in the central cavity on diffusion-weighted

imaging and mimic a necrotic brain tumor. Granulomas are focal white matter or deep gray matter enhancing lesions.

SINUS MANIFESTATIONS

- Sinus infections due to *Aspergillus* species are more common in neutropenic immuno-compromised patients, whereas patients with diabetes are more prone to sinusitis caused by Zygomycetes, including *Rhizopus* and *Mucor* species.
- There are five subtypes: Acute invasive fungal sinusitis, chronic invasive fungal sinusitis, and chronic granulomatous invasive fungal sinusitis comprise the invasive group, whereas noninvasive fungal sinusitis includes allergic fungal sinusitis and fungus ball/fungal mycetoma. These subtypes have distinct clinical and radiological features. In non-IFI, there is an absence of hyphae within the mucosa of the sinuses.
- In patients with acute invasive fungal sinusitis, mucosal thickening and bone erosion can be very subtle and insignificant to begin with. Severe unilateral soft tissue thickening in the sinuses is seen on CT scan. High index of suspicion is needed, and biopsy of the mucosa confirms the diagnosis.
- Fungal sinusitis is more locally invasive invading the pterygopalatine fossa, cavernous sinus, and intracranial cavity.
- Osseous destruction and hematogenous spread are known complications.
- CT scan shows mucosal thickening, hyperattenuating soft tissue collection in the sinuses, and osseous destruction (Fig. 7.2). Orbital invasion results in inflammatory changes in orbital fat and extraocular muscles with exophthalmos. It may mimic a malignant lesion.
- MRI is better at assessing infraorbital and intracranial extension. There is decreased signal intensity on T1WI and markedly increased signal intensity on T2WI. Findings include mucosal edema, osteomyelitis, carotid artery invasion or occlusion, vascular or cavernous sinus thrombosis, pseudoaneurysms, leptomeningeal enhancement, epidural abscess, cerebritis, and cerebral abscesses.

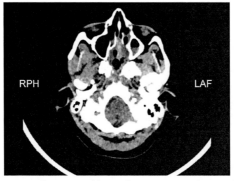

Fig. 7.2: Axial CT image showing soft tissue and bony destruction involving sphenoid sinus in a patient of mucormycosis.

- Allergic fungal sinusitis involves multiple sinuses. The sinuses show near-complete opacification and expansion of the sinuses. Noncontrast CT shows hyperattenuating mucin within the lumen of the sinuses.
- Fungal ball appears as a mass within the lumen of the paranasal sinus. It usually involves a single sinus. The maxillary sinus is most frequently involved, followed by the sphenoid sinus. It appears as hyperattenuating on noncontrast CT due to a dense ball of tangled fungal hyphae. There can be punctate calcification.

PULMONARY INFECTIONS

The lungs are the most frequent site of involvement of IFI since these are the portal of entry for most fungi. The spectrum of involvement ranges from pulmonary nodules to consolidation and invasion of contiguous structures.

The radiological features may include the following:
- Pulmonary nodules
- Bronchopneumonia with tree-in-bud appearance
- Lobar consolidation
- Ground-glass opacities
- Mediastinal lymphadenopathy
- Pleural effusions.

Pulmonary Nodules

- A pulmonary macronodule is defined as an ovoid nodular space occupying opacity of the lung ≥1-cm diameter that displaces rather than confirms to the shape of the preexisting aerated lung and completely obscures the background vasculature (Fig. 7.3). This is the most common finding in invasive pulmonary aspergillosis and is detected in >90% of patients. It results from angioinvasion of the airspaces by mycelia leading to a hemorrhagic

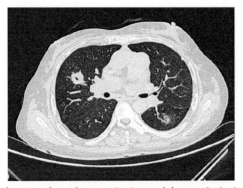

Fig. 7.3: Chest CT scan. Axial section shows large cavitating nodular opacity in right upper lobe and ground-glass opacity in left lower lobe in a case of aspergillosis.

nodule with infarction, and the absence of the macronodule on CT scan should suggest an alternative diagnosis. A high number of patients display pulmonary nodules in pulmonary zygomycosis.

- The differential diagnosis of macronodule includes the following:
  - Tuberculosis
  - Nocardiosis
  - Lung abscess
  - Lung cancer
  - Lung metastases
  - Lymphoproliferative disorder
  - Vasculitis
  - Pulmonary infarcts
- A nodule ≥3-cm diameter is called a mass.

The "Halo Sign"

- The halo sign is defined as a macronodule with a perimeter of ground-glass opacity or intermediate increased lung density between solid and air density. The lung vasculature should be visible through this intermediate density (Figs. 7.4 and 7.5). The halo results from coagulation necrosis and oozing hemorrhage at the perimeter of the macronodule (infarction). The halo sign is extremely transient and seen in about 60% patients of invasive aspergillosis. It may disappear on the subsequent scans conducted in the next few days. The differential diagnosis of the halo sign is mentioned in Box 7.1.
- The halo sign is regarded as a specific indicator of invasive mold disease in high-risk population, and preemptive antifungal therapy can be started based on finding a halo sign.

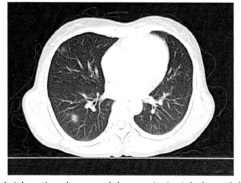

Fig. 7.4: Chest CT scan. Axial section shows nodular opacity in right lower lobe with surrounding halo in a case of candidiasis.

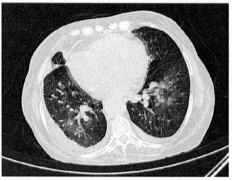

Fig. 7.5: Chest CT scan. Axial section shows patchy confluent nodular opacities in lower lobes with surrounding ground-glass haze in a case of aspergillosis.

Box 7.1: Differential diagnosis of "Halo sign."

Invasive pulmonary aspergillosis

Zygomycetes

- *Trichosporon* species
- *Fusarium* species
- *Penicillium* species
- *Coccidioides immitis*
- *Candida* species
- *Nocardia* species
- *Mycobacterium tuberculosis*
- *Cytomegalovirus*
- *Herpes simplex virus*
- *Pseudomonas aeruginosa*
- *Bronchioloalveolar cell carcinoma*
- *Lymphoproliferative disorders*
- Kaposi sarcoma
- Wegener granulomatosis
- Eosinophilic lung disease

Air Crescent Sign

- It is a sickle-shaped lucency, partially surrounding a soft tissue mass in a pulmonary cavity as seen on conventional radiography or CT scan (Figs. 7.6 and 7.7). This is a sign of late angioinvasive mild infection. Air crescent sign or *Monad's* sign is seen in angioinvasive pulmonary aspergillosis and pulmonary zygomycosis. It usually occurs after the recovery

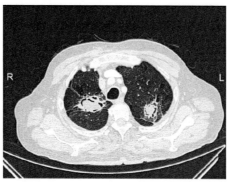

Fig. 7.6: Chest CT scan. Axial section shows bilateral apical cavitary lesions with crescent of air suggestive of fungal ball. Adjacent lung shows emphysematous changes and fibrosis.

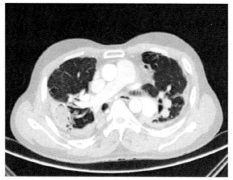

Fig. 7.7: Chest CT axial section. Case of aspergilloma shows cavitary lesion in right upper lobe with intracavitary soft tissue density and eccentric air.

of the neutrophil function. MRI reveals necrotic target lesions with a gadolinium-enhanced rim with T2-weighted hyperintensity.

- This sequestrum of devitalized lung in the air crescent cavity needs to be distinguished from the mobile fungal ball in aspergilloma, tuberculosis, nocardiosis, cavitary malignancy, and cavitary hematoma.

Reverse Halo Sign

The reversed halo sign or the *atoll* sign or the *fairy-ring* sign are defined as a central ground-glass opacity surrounded by a halo or crescent of consolidation and are features of pulmonary mucormycosis.

Parenchymal Consolidation

- Imaging findings in IFI may include parenchymal consolidations and consolidative infarcts with air bronchograms. Centrilobular opacities include subcentimeter nodular opacities

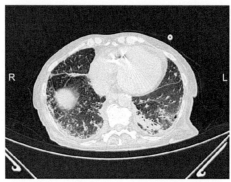

Fig. 7.8: Chest CT scan. Axial section shows patchy interstitial infiltrates in bilateral lower lobes and confluent parenchymal opacities and collapse consolidation in aspergillosis.

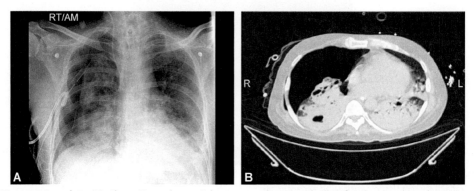

Figs. 7.9A and B: (A) Chest X-ray shows right pneumothorax with ill-defined parenchymal opacities and consolidation in bilateral lungs, predominantly lower zone (*Aspergillus* infection); (B) Chest CT scan (axial section) of the same patient showing bilateral lung consolidation with cavitations and right-sided pneumothorax (*Aspergillus* infection).

located in the center of secondary lobules in conjunction with opacified segments of small branching bronchi and bronchioli called *tree-in-bud opacities* (Figs. 7.8 to 7.11). These findings are also noted in tuberculosis, cryptococcal infection, and bacterial and viral infections (Fig. 7.11).

♦ Consolidation due to mucormycosis tends to develop cavities. Similarly, *Actinomyces* and *Nocardia* species also produce consolidation with cavitation. Empyema necessitans or empyema necessitasis refers to extension of a pleural infection out of the thorax and into the neighboring chest wall and soft tissues.

♦ Blastomycosis, histoplasmosis, coccidioidomycosis, mucormycosis, and cryptococcosis result in parenchymal consolidation. Histoplasmosis may result in consolidation and lymphadenopathy in the acute phase. Chronic histoplasmosis is associated with calcified

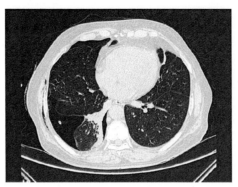

Fig. 7.10: Chest CT scan. Axial section shows occlusion right lower lobe bronchus with associated right pneumothorax (*Aspergillosis*).

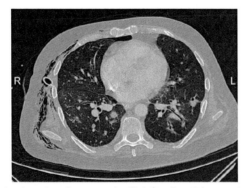

Fig. 7.11: Chest CT scan. Axial section shows patchy ill-defined nodular opacities in bilateral lower lobes with surrounding ground-glass haze in *Cryptococcus* infection. Right-sided ICD with pneumothorax with subcutaneous emphysema is also present (ICD, intercostal tube drain).

granulomas. Disseminated progressive disease appears as miliary lesions. Calcified pulmonary nodules and mediastinal lymphadenopathy indicate previous exposure in residents in an endemic area. Pleural effusion is rare. Consolidation due to blastomycosis is more central and abuts the mediastinum with focal or patchy consolidations and noncalcifying nodules.

♦ *Phantom consolidations* are transient areas of consolidation that resolve in one area and are recurring in another. These fleeting consolidations are a feature of coccidioidomycosis. Frank consolidations in coccidioidomycosis are generally multilobar. Patients may have pleural effusion and lymphadenopathy. Disseminated coccidioidomycosis resembles disseminated histoplasmosis and features include miliary nodules and lymphadenopathy.

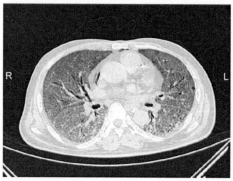

Fig. 7.12: Axial CT scan showing diffuse ground-glass haze with septal thickening in entire lung. Small cystic areas are noted—Case of PJP (PJP, *pneumocystis jirovecii* pneumonia).

Ground-glass Opacity

Uncommon radiological finding in IFI classically seen in *Pneumocystis jirovecii* in patients who are HIV positive. There is a scattered or diffuse ground-glass opacity with superimposed interlobular septal line thickening (Fig. 7.12). This pattern is called *crazy-paving*. The differential diagnosis includes acute respiratory distress syndrome, alveolar proteinosis, sarcoidosis, nonspecific interstitial pneumonia, and bronchoalveolar carcinoma. The patients with *P. jirovecii* may subsequently develop irregular lung cysts and tendency to develop pneumothorax. Pleural effusion is rare.

▓ BONE AND JOINT INFECTIONS

- Fungal osteomyelitis and articular infections are rare and have a much lower incidence than bacterial osteomyelitis. They have an indolent course.
- The incidence is increasing in immunocompromised patients. These pose a diagnostic dilemma leading to ineffective treatment and resolution.
- Bones and joints get involved as a direct inoculation, locoregional spread from the contiguous structures, or from hematogenous dissemination.
- The presenting complaints are generally subacute and include pain at the involved site, fever, malaise, and night sweats.
- Patient with fungal spondylodiscitis has lower back pain which is insidious, intermittent, and progressive. The course of the illness can be indolent. It may result in bony destruction and deformities. The radiographic findings are nonspecific.
- The fungi causing osteoarticular involvement include *Candida, Aspergillus, Cryptococcus, Mucor, Blastomyces, Coccidioides, Sporothrix*, and *Histoplasma* species.
- The radiological findings are similar for both bacterial and fungal osteomyelitis. CT scans may reveal a combination of lytic and sclerotic lesions, osseous destruction, narrowing of joint space, synovitis, and joint effusion.

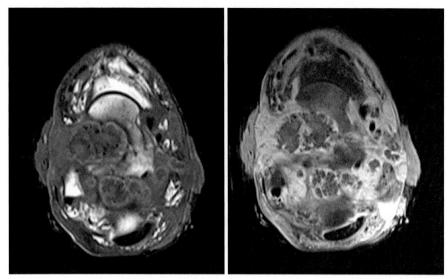

Fig. 7.13: MRI scan of "Madura foot" T1W and postcontrast images of ankle reveal extensive destruction of multiple bones of foot with marrow signal alteration and extensive adjoining collections and soft tissue thickening.

- In fungal osteomyelitis, there is osteolysis with discrete or permeated margins, surrounding sclerosis that is less florid than in bacterial infection, and variable amounts of periosteal reaction. Extensive bone sclerosis and sequestra are unusual.
- Magnetic resonance imaging is better at delineating the soft tissue involvement (Fig. 7.13). Maxillary fungal osteomyelitis may occur secondary to sinusitis. Osteomyelitis of facial bones needs to be investigated thoroughly as there is no difference in clinical presentation of bacterial and fungal osteomyelitis.
- Fungal involvement of the spine resembles caries spine due to *Mycobacterium tuberculosis*. The vertebral body, posterior bony vertebral elements, epidural space, and perispinal soft tissues may be involved. Features include discitis and osteomyelitis at multiple vertebral levels with sparing of intervertebral disc space. It may result in gibbus formation.
- Contrast-enhanced MRI is a better imaging modality since it detects marrow involvement, epidural inflammation, and paravertebral extension. Marrow edema is T1-hypointense or T2-hyperintense that enhances on contrast-enhanced T1WIs. Hyperintensity on T2WIs within the intervertebral discs is typical of pyogenic infections. However, in fungal infections, there is an absence of hyperintensity within the disc, and the intranuclear cleft is preserved in all discs in which the disc height is maintained. These findings are nonspecific and seen in other nonpyogenic infections including *Nocardia*, *Actinomycosis*, and tuberculosis. The pathogenesis for this absence of hyperintensity is multifactorial and includes an absence of fungal invasion, blunted immune response in immunocompromised individuals, and paramagnetic substances within fungi. Endoscopic biopsy accompanied by discectomy and drainage can be performed.

- Recognition of MR characteristics of fungal osteomyelitis should prompt biopsy and early treatment.
- Nuclear medicine detection of osteomyelitis is performed utilizing technetium-99m methylene diphosphonate, either alone or in conjunction with Gallium-67- or Indium-111-labeled leukocytes.
- Scintigraphy is more sensitive than radiography and CT for early osteomyelitis and affords imaging of the entire skeleton. In osteomyelitis, scintigraphy shows abnormal increased uptake on all three phases, with increasing activity on the delayed images.
- Gallium and indium scanning are adjunct techniques that are particularly useful when there is an underlying disorder (e.g. trauma, tumor, surgery) that produces bone remodeling.
- Endoscopic biopsy can be performed to confirm diagnosis accompanied with discectomy and drainage.

■ CARDIAC AND PERICARDIAL INFECTION

- Isolated cardiac fungal infection is extremely rare and has an overall survival rate of less than 25%. It accounts for 3–4% of all cases of infective endocarditis.
- Major surgery, antibiotic therapy, indwelling catheters for nutritional, therapeutic, or diagnostic purposes, pericatheter sleeve thrombi contaminated with environmental fungi, gut surgery, abortions, gynecological procedures, intravenous drug use, congenital heart disease, cardiac surgeries including vascular grafts, complex intracardiac repair, and prosthetic valves predispose to fungal endocarditis.
- Cardiac involvement is a component of fungemia in immunocompromised patients with disseminated disease.
- The most common fungal pathogens causing cardiac involvement are *Candida* and *Aspergillus* species. Other fungi known to cause cardiac involvement include *Histoplasma*, *Blastomyces*, *Cryptococcus*, *Coccidioides*, and *Scedosporium* species.
- Apart from systemic symptoms including fever and malaise, distal septic embolization produces symptoms due to end-organ damage. Fungal infections can cause endocarditis, myocarditis, or pericarditis.

Endocarditis

- The fungal vegetations are generally larger than the bacterial vegetations and have a higher potential for embolization.
- The vegetations on mitral and aortic valves cause arterial embolization, resulting in stroke and visceral involvement.
- Vegetations on the tricuspid and pulmonary valves can cause septic pulmonary emboli.
- Echocardiography, especially transesophageal echocardiography, is the best modality to visualize these vegetations. These are seen as mobile nodules attached to a valve.
- Chest radiography may reveal cardiomegaly, embolic pulmonary infiltrates, and pleural effusion.
- Computed tomography and MR imaging are better at detecting cerebral and visceral infarction consequent to the infection rather than the actual vegetation.

- Gated cardiac examination and use of β-blockers to decrease heart rate may improve yield of detecting vegetations on the valves.

Myocarditis

- It is rare and part of disseminated IFI.
- The features have not been well delineated.
- Computed tomography scan reveals myocardial hypoattenuation.
- Magnetic resonance imaging findings are nonspecific and include hyperemia on T1WI.
- Cine cardiac MR imaging shows reduced cardiac contractility.
- There can be left ventricular enlargement.

Pericarditis

- Fungal pericarditis presents with chest pain and pericardial effusion.
- There is enhancement of parietal and visceral pericardium with "split-pericardial" sign.
- Later on, constrictive pericarditis may develop with dilated atria and cavae, flattening of interventricular septum, and isovolumic ventricles.

GASTROINTESTINAL INFECTIONS

- Invasive fungal infection involving the bowel are rare and seen in immunocompromised host. The patients present with fever, abdominal pain, distension, vomiting, and diarrhea. Imaging findings include bowel wall thickening, perforation, and peritonitis. Patients on peritoneal dialysis are more prone to fungal peritonitis. Imaging patterns may include omental stranding, nodularity, ascites, peritoneal enhancement, and thickening.
- The most common IFI involving the liver are *Candida albicans, C. neoformans,* and *Histoplasma capsulatum.* The patients present with fever, anorexia, and abdominal pain. The imaging of liver reveals multiple microabscesses that are subcentimeter in size. These appear as hypoechoic foci on ultrasonography and hypoattenuating foci on CT scan. Larger abscesses may resemble pyogenic abscesses.
- Ultrasonography features of hepatosplenic candidiasis have been summarized into four distinct patterns:
  1. "Wheel-within-wheel" pattern, which consists of a hypoechoic nidus representing necrotic fungal debris, an inner hyperechoic ring composed of inflammatory cells, and a peripheral hypoechoic ring secondary to fibrosis.
  2. "Bull's-eye" appearance, similar to the wheel-within-wheel pattern but lacking the hypoechoic nidus and consisting of only two rings—the inner hyperechoic inflammatory lesion and the outer hypoechoic halo/ring of fibrosis.
  3. *Hypoechoic homogeneous nodule* is the most common but least specific pattern and results from fibrosis in a region of prior inflammation.
  4. *Echogenic focus of scar* or calcification which results in variable posterior acoustic shadowing. This occurs in later stages of infection and generally indicates early resolution.

Computed tomography usually reveals small, hypoattenuating hepatic and splenic lesions. Tiny foci with increased attenuation can be detected in the center of the inflammatory nodules, presumably representing the presence of pseudohyphae. This feature helps to distinguish these lesions from benign liver cysts.

- Arterial phase CT depicts significantly more hepatic lesions than does CT performed during other phases. Rim enhancement can be noted.
- MR imaging is 100% sensitive and 96% specific for the diagnosis of fungal disease involving liver and spleen. Lesions appear hypointense on T1WI and markedly hyperintense on T2WI. Intense ring enhancement can be seen on early gadolinium-enhanced arterial phase images. Fungal abscesses may also show restriction on diffusion-weighted images.
- Imaging findings of hepatic histoplasmosis are similar to those seen in candidiasis or other disseminated fungal diseases, with multiple small lesions seen throughout the liver and splenic parenchyma. Lymph nodes, adrenals, and bone marrow are also involved. Chronic microabscesses develop calcification.

GENITOURINARY INFECTIONS

- Majority of the genitourinary fungal infections are due to *C. albicans*. Other fungi involving the genitourinary system are *Aspergillus*, *Mucor*, *Cryptococcus*, *P. jirovecii*, and *Histoplasma*. The patients present with fever, chills, dysuria, hematuria, and acute kidney injury. Lower urinary tract infections are confined to the bladder and urethra. Renal involvement may result from an ascending infection or as a consequence of hematogenous spread.
- Microabscesses develop in the kidneys. Fungal concretions may result in obstructive uropathy. Renal abscesses appear as hypoechoic on ultrasound, hypoattenuating on CT scans, and hyperintense on T2WI. Larger renal abscesses appear heterogeneous on ultrasound. CT images define the extent of involvement with hypoattenuating parenchymal collections and hydronephrosis. Renal infarction appears as hypoenhancing on CT/MRI. Emphysematous pyelonephritis is a rare but serious complication.
- Renal fungal ball or fungal bezoar is the saprophytic colonization of the renal collecting system by a conglomerate of fungal mycelia without the invasion of the adjacent tissue. Fungal bezoar is commonly seen in the immunocompromised state, prolonged bladder catheterization, and antibiotic use for a longer duration. The fungal ball appears as a heterogeneous hypoechoic mass within dilated calyces. It is isointense on T1WI and hyperintense on T2WI. The differential diagnosis includes a mass lesion, blood clot, debris, or calculus. The invasion of local vasculature leads to thrombosis. Chronic parenchymal infections cause calcification.
- Adrenal involvement by IFI can be asymptomatic or may result in Addison disease in half of the patients. Imaging of the adrenals shows circumscribed, homogeneous masses on ultrasonography. Necrosis and calcification result in heterogeneous lesions. CT scan shows homogeneous hypoattenuating masses to heterogeneous masses with areas of hypoenhancement or calcification. On MRI, masses are hypointense on T1 and hyperintense on T2 imaging.

Fungal involvement of the female reproductive tract results in hydrosalpinx, pyosalpinx, tubo-ovarian masses, local invasion, adhesions, abscess, tubal pregnancy, or peritonitis. *Fitz–Hugh–Curtis* syndrome is a rare disorder characterized by inflammation of the peritoneum and liver capsule secondary to pelvic inflammatory disease (PID). *Actinomyces* species cause PID associated with intrauterine devices. *Candida* species cause balanitis and prostatitis.

CLINICAL PEARLS

- With increasing incidence of IFI in immunocompromised patients, clinicians and radiologists need to have a low threshold for suspecting fungal infections.
- Various radiological patterns and signs can be able to offer a possible etiological diagnosis, and empiric antifungal therapy can be instituted.

SUGGESTED READING

1. Boiselle PM, Tocino I, Hooley RJ, et al. Chest radiograph interpretation of *Pneumocystis carinii* pneumonia, bacterial pneumonia, and pulmonary tuberculosis in HIV-positive patients: accuracy, distinguishing features, and mimics. J Thorac Imaging. 1997;12(1):47-53.
2. Chinen K, Tokuda Y, Sakamoto A, et al. Fungal infections of the heart: a clinicopathologic study of 50 autopsy cases. Pathol Res Pract. 2007;203(10):705-15.
3. Erden A, Fitoz S, Karagülle T, et al. Radiological findings in the diagnosis of genitourinary candidiasis. Pediatr Radiol. 2000;30(12):875-7.
4. Fisher JF, Kavanagh K, Sobel JD, et al. *Candida* urinary tract infection: pathogenesis. Clin Infect Dis. 2011;52(Suppl 6):S437-51.
5. Georgiadou SP, Sipsas NV, Marom EM, et al. The diagnostic value of halo and reversed halo signs for invasive mold infections in compromised hosts. Clin Infect Dis. 2011;52(9):1144-55.
6. Hoey ET, Gulati GS, Ganeshan A, et al. Cardiovascular MRI for assessment of infectious and inflammatory conditions of the heart. Am J Roentgenol. 2011;197(1):103-12.
7. Katragkou A, Fisher BT, Groll AH, et al. Diagnostic imaging and invasive fungal diseases in children. J Paediatr Infect Dis Soc. 2017;6(Suppl_1):S22-31.
8. Kumar N, Singh S, Govil S. Adrenal histoplasmosis: clinical presentation and imaging features in nine cases. Abdom Imaging. 2003;28(5):703-8.
9. Mathur M, Johnson CE, Sze G. Fungal infections of the central nervous system. Neuroimaging Clin N Am. 2012;22(4):609-32.
10. McAdams HP, Rosado de Christenson M, Strollo DC, et al. Pulmonary mucormycosis: radiologic findings in 32 cases. Am J Roentgenol. 1997;168(6):1541-8.
11. Murthy JM, Sundaram C. Fungal infections of the central nervous system. Handb Clin Neurol. 2014;121:1383-401.
12. Payne SJ, Mitzner R, Kunchala S, et al. Acute invasive fungal rhinosinusitis: a 15-year experience with 41 patients. Otolaryngol Head Neck Surg. 2016;154(4):759-64.
13. Starkey J, Moritani T, Kirby P. MRI of CNS fungal infections: review of aspergillosis to histoplasmosis and everything in between. Clin Neuroradiol. 2014;24(3):217-30.
14. Symeonidou C, Standish R, Sahdev A, et al. Imaging and histopathologic features of HIV-related renal disease. Radio Graphics. 2008;28(5):1339-54.
15. Walker CM, Abbot GF, Greene RE, et al. Imaging pulmonary infection: classic signs and patterns. Am J Roentgenol. 2014;202(3):479-92.

ANTIFUNGAL DRUGS

8

Antifungal Agents: Classification

Monica Mahajan

INTRODUCTION

The development of antifungals has lagged behind the advances in antibacterial therapies since mycology has come into focus much later in the realm of microbiology.

MILESTONES IN THE DEVELOPMENT OF ANTIFUNGAL THERAPY

- Amphotericin B deoxycholate was introduced in 1958 but was associated with renal toxicity.
- Flucytosine was introduced in 1973 but had major toxicities and development of drug resistance if used as monotherapy.
- Lipid-based amphotericin formulations introduced in 1990s.
- Triazole drug class (fluconazole, 1990; itraconazole, 1992) was good drug for yeast but had CYP 450-mediated drug interactions.
- Second-generation azoles (voriconazole, 2002; posaconazole, 2006) show activity against yeast and filamentous fungi.
- Echinocandins introduced in 2001 with caspofungin being the first to be approved. Micafungin and anidulafungin follow. Have excellent efficacy against *Candida* but only available as parenteral preparations.
- Newest azole isavuconazole released in 2015.

CLASSIFICATION OF ANTIFUNGAL AGENTS

- Based on mechanism of action
- Based on class of drugs
- Based on treatment indications.

Classification of Antifungals Based on Mechanism of Action (Fig. 8.1)

- *Cell wall inhibitors (inhibit cell wall synthesis)*: Caspofungin, micafungin and anidulafungin
- *Cell membrane disruption (binds to cell membrane ergosterol)*: Amphotericin B and nystatin

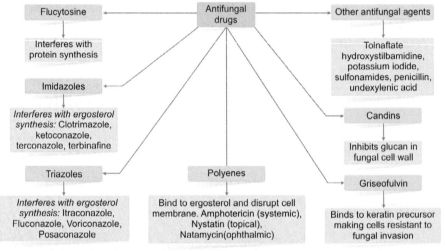

Fig. 8.1: Classification of antifungals based on mechanism of action.

- *Ergosterol biosynthesis inhibitors—azoles*: Fluconazole, itraconazole, voriconazole, posaconazole, and isavuconazole
- *Inhibition of ergosterol and lanosterol synthesis*: Terbinafine and naftifine
- *Inhibition of nucleic acid synthesis*: Flucytosine
- *Disruption of mitotic spindle and inhibition of fungal mitosis*: Griseofulvin
- *Miscellaneous*: Tolnaftate, ciclopirox, and undecylenic acid

Classification of Antifungals Based on Drug Class (Fig. 8.2)

- *Antibiotics*:
  - *Polyenes*: Amphotericin B, nystatin, natamycin and hamycin
  - *Heterocyclic benzofurans*: Griseofulvin
- *Azoles*:
  - *Imidazoles*: Ketoconazole, miconazole, clotrimazole, econazole, tioconazole and enilconazole
  - *Triazoles*: Fluconazole, itraconazole, voriconazole, posaconazole, ravuconazole and isavuconazole
- *Antimetabolites*: 5-flucytosine
- *Echinocandins*: Caspofungin, micafungin and anidulafungin
- *Allylamines*: Terbinafine, butenafine and naftifine
- *Others/topical*: Ciclopirox, tolnaftate, undecylenic acid and quindochlor.

Classification of Antifungals Based on Treatment Indications

- Drugs for systemic fungal infections:
  - Amphotericin B

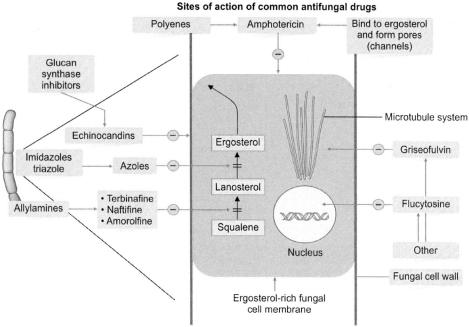

Fig. 8.2: Classification of antifungals based on structures.

- ♦ Triazoles
- ♦ Ketoconazole
- ♦ Echinocandins
- ♦ Flucytosine
- *Drugs given systemically for treating superficial infections*:
  - ♦ Griseofulvin
  - ♦ Terbinafine.
- *Topically used antifungal drugs*:
  - ♦ Nystatin
  - ♦ Clotrimazole, miconazole, butoconazole, sertaconazole and oxiconazole
  - ♦ Ciclopirox
  - ♦ Benzoic acid and sodium thiosulphate.

■ SUGGESTED READING

1. Elewski BE. Mechanisms of action of systemic antifungal agents. J Am Acad Dermatol. 1993; 28(5):S28-34.
2. Groll AH, Gea-Bancloche JC, Glasmacher A, et al. Clinical pharmacology of antifungal compounds. Infect Dis Clin North Am. 2003;17:159-91.
3. Zonios DI, Bennett JE. Update on azole antifungals. Semin Respir Crit Care Med. 2008;29:198.

9

Azoles

Monica Mahajan

INTRODUCTION

Azoles are a class of five-membered heterocyclic compounds containing a nitrogen atom and at least one more non-carbon atom as part of the ring. They are classified into two groups—imidazole and triazoles (Table 9.1). Imidazoles have two nitrogens in the azole ring. They include clotrimazole, econazole, ketoconazole, miconazole, and tioconazole. The imidazoles are mainly applied topically because they have poor water solubility, limited oral bioavailability, and unacceptable side effects if administered orally. The triazoles have three nitrogens in the azole ring. They have a broader spectrum of activity, better bioavailability, and improved safety profile. This is the most widely used group of antifungal agents. Itraconazole use is limited due to inconsistent bioavailability. Fluconazole lacks activity against molds and a number of *Candida* species are developing resistance to it. Voriconazole has excellent spectrum of activity against *Aspergillus*. Posaconazole and isavuconazole have the broadest spectrum of activity among the azoles.

MECHANISM OF ACTION

The azoles work primarily by inhibiting cytochrome P450 from family CYP51-dependent enzyme lanosterol 14-α-demethylase. This enzyme is necessary for conversion of lanosterol to ergosterol, an integral part of the cell membrane of fungi. Inhibition of fungal CYP51 leads to blockage of biosynthesis of ergosterol, depletion of ergosterol, and accumulation of 14-α-methylated precursors. Changes in the membrane sterol composition alter the integrity and fluidity of the fungal membranes. These ultimately lead to cell lysis and death. The triazoles are considered fungistatic against *Candida* species while voriconazole has fungicidal activity against *Aspergillus* species.

Table 9.1: Classification of azoles

Group	Drugs
Imidazoles	Clotrimazole, econazole, ketoconazole, miconazole
Triazoles	Fluconazole, itraconazole, voriconazole, posaconazole, isavuconazole

CYP51 is present not only in fungi but also in humans. This enzyme is involved in the biosynthesis of cholesterol, the major sterol of mammalian membranes. Azoles inhibit some of the host P450s (e.g. human CYP3A4, CYP2C9, and CYP2C19). These P450 isoforms play an important role in humans in the metabolism of endogenous and exogenous compounds. Inhibition of these causes undesired drug–drug interactions. Administration with drugs that are metabolized by these enzymes can result in increased concentrations of the azoles, the interacting drug, or both.

■ MICROBIOLOGICAL ACTIVITY

Every azole has a unique spectrum of activity.

Fluconazole

- Fungistatic with relatively narrow spectrum of activity
- Activity limited to yeasts and some endemic fungi (*Histoplasma, Blastomyces, Coccidioides,* and *Paracoccidioides* species)
- Excellent activity against *Candida* species but has less activity against *C. glabrata* and *C. guilliermondii.*
- *C. krusei* is inherently resistant to fluconazole
- It has excellent activity against *Cryptococcus neoformans* and *Coccidioides immitis.*
- It has no activity against *Aspergillus* species, *Fusarium* species, and zygomycosis.

Itraconazole

- Active against fluconazole-sensitive and fluconazole-resistant *Candida* species except *C. glabrata*
- It also has activity against the dimorphic or endemic fungi including *C. immitis, H. capsulatum, B. dermatitidis,* and *S. schenckii.*
- Fungicidal activity against filamentous fungi and some strains of *C. neoformans*
- Good activity against *Aspergillus* species
- Variable activity against *Fusarium* species
- Limited activity against zygomycosis.

Voriconazole

- Broader spectrum of activity than fluconazole against yeasts and molds
- Highly active against *Aspergillus* species
- Active against *Candida* species including *C. albicans, C. glabrata, C. krusei, Cryptococcus* species, and *Trichosporon* species
- Active against amphotericin-resistant molds including *Scedosporium* and *Fusarium* species
- Active against dimorphic fungi including *B. dermatitidis, H. capsulatum, P. marneffei,* and *Coccidioides* species
- No activity against zygomycosis.

Posaconazole and Isavuconazole

- They have expanded the spectrum to include the mucorales while maintaining activity against yeasts and molds.
- Fungicidal against non-albicans *Candida* species including *C. krusei, C. lusitaniae, C. glabrata, C. guilliermondii,* and *C. parapsilosis*
- Fungicidal against *Aspergillus* species and *C. neoformans*
- Very potent against dimorphic fungi including *C. immitis, H. capsulatum, B. dermatitidis,* and *S. schenckii*
- Variable activity against *Scedosporium* species and zygomycosis
- No activity against *Fusarium* species

Ketoconazole

Active against the recalcitrant dermatophytes, Candida species and endemic mycosis including blastomycosis, histoplasmosis, coccidioidomycosis, and paracoccidioidomycosis.

▓ PHARMACOKINETICS (TABLE 9.2)

All azoles are lipophilic weak bases with good oral bioavailability. However, no two triazoles have the same pharmacokinetic profiles.
- Capsule form of itraconazole has variable bioavailability.
- Dissolution of ketoconazole and itraconazole is significantly affected by the elevation of gastric pH.
- Unlike other azoles, posaconazole does not require extensive CYP metabolism, it undergoes glucuronidation.

Pharmacologic Properties of Systemic Azoles (Table 9.2)

Table 9.2: Pharmacokinetics of azoles			
Drug	Oral bioavailability (%)	Half-life (hours)	Metabolism
Fluconazole	>90%, unaltered by food	24 hours, prolonged in renal impairment	80% renal clearance as unchanged drug, 11% hepatic metabolism
Itraconazole	55%, increased by food and acidic beverages, reduced by PPIs	25–50 hours	Hepatic-CYP3A4
Voriconazole	>90%, food reduces absorption by almost 30%	Variable due to CYP2C19 polymorphism	Hepatic-CYP2C19
Posaconazole	54%, preferably with fatty food	Suspension-31 hours, tablet-26–31 hours, IV 24.6 hours	Minimally metabolized, 77% cleared unchanged in feces, 15% undergoes hepatic UGT glucuronidation
Isavuconazole	98%, unaltered by food	130 hours	Hepatic-CYP3A4 and UGT glucuronidation

CYP, *cytochrome P450 metabolism; IV, intravenous; PPI, proton pump inhibitor; UGT:* uridine 5'-diphospho-glucuronosyltransferase (i.e. phase II {non-CYP} hepatic metabolism)

Fluconazole

- Highly hydrophilic (less lipophilic) and is almost completely absorbed following oral administration
- Oral bioavailability above 90%, not affected by food
- Widely distributed in tissues as only 10–12% protein bound. Good penetration into CSF, urine, sputum, skin, eye, and peritoneal fluid
- Levels in CSF 50–90% in normal meninges and 70–80% in inflamed meninges
- Vitreous body 20–70% of serum levels
- Long half-life (20–50 hours), therefore can be used as a single daily dose
- Similar serum concentrations attained by oral and parenteral administration indicating absence of first-pass metabolism of the drug.
- Patients with renal impairment need dose adjustment as 80% renal clearance as unchanged drug. Drug is removed during hemodialysis; a 3-hour session reduces the serum concentration by about 50%.
- Available as 10 mg/mL suspension, and 50, 100, 150, and 200 mg of tablets.

Itraconazole

- Different formulations cannot be used interchangeably as capsule and oral solution have major variability in bioavailability.
- Capsules require an acidic gastric pH and should be taken with food; absorption increased by cola or cranberry juice. Proton pump inhibitors should not be co-administered as these impair absorption.
- Liquid formulation increases bioavailability which is not altered by gastric pH. Optimal absorption is on empty stomach but can be given in the presence of food. Oral solution is swished in mouth for several seconds and then swallowed.
- Intravenous preparation has to be used with caution in renal impairment patients as cyclodextrin used in IV formulation accumulates in these patients and is nephrotoxic.
- Long half-life (25–50 hours) allows once daily dosing if using up to 200 mg daily. Split into two divided doses when 400 mg is required.
- Approximately 99.8% protein bound.
- Very high penetration in skin, nails, liver, adipose tissue and bone and levels are three times the corresponding serum levels
- Only traces are detected in CSF and the eye. Very little active drug reaches urine, hence no role in the treatment of urinary infections.
- Metabolized in liver and excreted in urine and feces.
- 10 mg/mL suspension, 100 and 200 mg tab/cap.

Voriconazole

- Oral tablet formulation has a bioavailability of almost 96%. Fatty meals reduce bioavailability by 30%, so drug is administered empty stomach or 1 hour before or after meal.
- Approximately 58% protein bound.
- CSF levels are 30–60% of corresponding blood concentration.
- Intravenous voriconazole contains a cyclodextrin vehicle sulfobutylether-β-cyclodextrin (SBECD), which accumulates in patients with impaired renal function, thus use limited

to patients with creatinine clearance (CrCl) > 50 mL/min. In patients with CrCl <50%, use oral formulation only.

- Metabolizes by cytochrome P450 enzyme system. In Child–Pugh classes A and B, use full loading dose but reduce maintenance dose by 50%. No data available in Child–Pugh C.
- CYP 2 C19 gene polymorphisms: As a consequence of a point mutation in the gene encoding the CYP 2C19 enzyme, this plays an important role in the interindividual variability observed with voriconazole. Slow metabolizers via CYP 2 C19 (15–20% Asians and 3–5% Caucasians) have elevated levels and greater dose-related side-effects such as hepatotoxicity.
- Voriconazole is an inhibitor of cytochrome P450 3A4 and hence shows drug interactions.
- Less than 2% of a given dose of voriconazole is excreted in the urine as unchanged drug. Thus, it should not be used to treat urinary tract infections. Well distributed throughout the rest of the body and penetrates CSF.
- Exhibits nonlinear pharmacokinetic profile, which complicates dosing in different populations and different conditions; increasing the dose of voriconazole by 50% can lead to 150% increase in serum concentration and a significant increase in serum half-life. There are interpatient and intrapatient variabilities of serum concentrations associated with decreased efficacy and increased side effects. Hence, serum concentrations need to be monitored in selected patients.
- Higher dose of voriconazole increases toxicities without improving clinical outcomes. The drug is not removed by hemodialysis.
- Infuse IV over 1–2 hours.
- Available as 200 mg/mL suspension, 50 mg and 200 mg of tab, and 200 mg IV lyophilized form.

Posaconazole

- This was initially available only as an oral suspension.
- In 2013, the FDA-approved delayed release tablets for prophylaxis of invasive *Aspergillus* and *Candida* infections in patients at high risk, e.g. hematologic malignancies, GVHD, and hematopoietic stem cell transplant recipients.
- In 2014, the FDA approved an IV formulation of posaconazole for prophylaxis of invasive *Aspergillus* and *Candida* infections in patients aged 18 years and older at high risk for these infections.
- IV is used when oral administration is not viable.
- Absorption improved by intake with fatty foods.
- The delayed release tablets are more useful in patients who cannot eat a full meal.
- Tablets and suspension cannot be used interchangeably.
- Patients on delayed release tablets achieve higher serum concentration than patients taking the oral suspension.
- Serum concentrations of suspension increase with more frequent administration.
- Half-life: About 35 hours (oral suspension), 26–31 hours (tab), and 24.6 hours (IV).
- About 15% of drug undergoes non-cytochrome P450 (CYP) hepatic metabolism by glucuronide conjugation.

- Mostly eliminated through the feces as unchanged drug
- Minimal amounts are recovered in the urine and the drug cannot be relied upon to treat urinary tract infections.
- Available as oral suspension 200 mg/5 mL, 100 mg delayed release tablet, and 300 mg/vial IV.

Isavuconazole

- Approved by FDA in March 2015
- Formulated as prodrug, isavuconazonium sulfate, which is rapidly hydrolyzed in blood to isavuconazole by esterases, predominantly butylcholinesterases.
- Available as IV and oral capsules
- Prolonged half-life of 130 hours, which enables once daily dosing.
- Oral capsule can be taken with or without food.
- Switching between IV and oral formulations is acceptable as bioequivalence is demonstrated.
- Excreted equally through faces and urine
- Strong CYP 3A4 inhibitor
- No dose adjustment required for renal impairment or in mild-to-moderate hepatic impairment.
- Prodrug converts completely (>99%) to active drug and an inactive cleavage product. Inactive cleavage product is not nephrotoxic unlike cyclodextrin in voriconazole.
- The 186 mg of isavuconazonium sulfate oral capsule provides 100 mg of isavuconazole.
- 372 mg injection of isavuconazonium sulfate injection provides 200 mg of isavuconazole.

Ketoconazole

- Usually used as an oral formulation, as 200–400 mg/day, and as cream, gel, foam, and shampoo.
- Taken with food as gastric acid is essential for its dissolution, absorption can be increased with juices and carbonated beverages. Proton pump inhibitors reduce absorption.
- Poorly absorbed on an empty stomach in patients of AIDS with gastric atrophy or on antacids.
- Majority of the drug is excreted by biliary system.
- Potent inhibitor of CYP3A4.

■ ADVERSE EFFECTS OF AZOLES

Gastrointestinal Symptoms

Frequent including nausea, dysgeusia, vomiting, diarrhea, and abdominal pain. The latter is most notable with intraconazole oral solution.

Hepatotoxicity

All azoles cause variable degrees of hepatotoxicity ranging from mild rise in transaminases to severe hepatic derangement such as hepatitis, cholestasis, hepatic necrosis, fulminant hepatic failure. Fatal hepatotoxicity is known with all azoles. The toxicity is usually hepatocellular but may be cholestatic or a combination of both. Early discontinuation of therapy may normalize LFT over weeks.

Drug-specific Adverse Effects

Fluconazole

Reversible alopecia, chapped lips, anorexia, dizziness, headache, eosinophilia, pruritus, rash, anaphylaxis, Stevens–Johnson syndrome, hypokalemia, and fever.

Itraconazole

Triad of hypertension, hypokalemia, and peripheral edema due to accumulation of corticosteroids and an aldosterone-like activity. It can precipitate congestive heart failure especially in elderly patients or those on calcium channel blockers.

Voriconazole

Visual side effects: Visual side effects occur within 30 minutes of oral or intravenous administration. These include transient vision changes including photopsia, photophobia, and color vision-related changes. These generally subside with continued therapy; counseling the patients helps. Visual disturbances are produced in approximately 20–30% of subjects in clinical trials. In case, voriconazole is continued for longer than 4 weeks, visual acuity, fields, and color vision should be monitored.

Neurologic side effects: Visual and auditory hallucinations, confusion, agitation, myoclonic movements, and peripheral demyelinating neuropathy of lower limbs in transplant patients on tacrolimus.

Dermatological side effects: Skin rashes in 7% patients including photosensitivity. Rarely, Stevens–Johnson syndrome and association with skin cancers, alopecia, and nail changes on prolonged use.

Skeletal side effects: Periostitis due to excess of fluoride on long-term use. Stop drug if patient has skeletal pain and radiologic findings of periostitis.

Cardiac side effects: Prolonged QTc interval, torsades de pointes, and sudden death.

Nephrotoxicity: IV formulation causes nephrotoxicity due to cyclodextrin.

Posaconazole

Less side effects than other azoles. It causes gastrointestinal symptoms including liver dysfunction, headache, prolonged QTc interval and torsades de pointes, rhabdomyolysis when co-administered with statins, and increase in concentration of calcineurin inhibitors including cyclosporine and tacrolimus. IV formulation nephrotoxic due to cyclodextrin.

Isavuconazole

Nausea, vomiting, diarrhea, headache, insomnia, confusion, hallucinations, encephalopathy, migraine, back pain, elevated transaminases, hypokalemia, constipation, dyspnea, cough, peripheral edema, and infusion reactions.

It causes shortening of QTc interval unlike other azoles. In patients with familial short QTc syndrome, it shortens the QTc interval in a dose-related manner.

IV formulation does not contain cyclodextrin and does not cause renal dysfunction.

Ketoconazole

In 2013, the FDA warned against the use of ketoconazole tablets as first-line therapy for any fungal infection including *Candida* and dermatophytes due to risk of fatal liver injury associated with the use of this drug. Ketoconazole tablets were withdrawn from the European market at the same time. It can cause adrenal insufficiency.

Topical preparations including creams, shampoos, foams, and gels can cause irritation and pruritus.

Pregnancy

Total fluconazole dose >300 mg is considered teratogenic and remains contraindicated throughout pregnancy, with FDA designation category D.

A single low dose of fluconazole of 150 mg for vaginal candidiasis does not increase the risk of congenital disorders and can be considered in the absence of a topical alternative after the first trimester—Category C.

Prolonged use of fluconazole in pregnancy causes craniofacial abnormalities including craniosynostosis, cleft lip with or without cleft palate, limb defects, polydactyly, syndactyly, and cardiac defects including hypoplastic left heart and tetralogy of Fallot.

FDA labels itraconazole category C. The manufacturers recommend that effective contraception should be continued throughout the treatment and for 2 months thereafter.

Nystatin is poorly absorbed and classifieds category A. Topical antifungals have limited systemic absorption and may be used in pregnancy except for potassium iodide, which was shown to be associated with fetal goiter.

No major studies of other triazoles in pregnant women are available. Therefore, avoid the use of azoles in first trimester.

▓ DOSING

Dosing of triazoles depends on the indication and severity of infection as well as the formulation of the drug being used.

Fluconazole

A loading dose of fluconazole is twice that of the maintenance dose. Since fluconazole has excellent bioavailability, equivalent doses of the oral and intravenous formulations are used.

In patients with renal impairment, dose remains unchanged during the first 48 hours of treatment.

    Creatinine clearance—21–40 mL/min—dosage interval doubled to 48 hours or dose halved

    Creatinine clearance—10–20 mL/min-72—hour interval between doses

    Hemodialysis—full dose given after each dialysis session

- Oropharyngeal candidiasis—200 mg of loading dose, then 100–200 mg daily for 7–14 days
- Esophageal candidiasis—400 mg of loading dose, then 200–400 mg daily for 14–21 days
- Vaginal candidiasis—150 mg of stat dose
- Candidal UTI—200 mg daily for 10 days
- Cryptococcal meningitis (IV or oral)—following induction therapy, 400 mg daily as consolidation dose, then 200 mg daily as maintenance dose
- Histoplasmosis/blastomycosis/coccidioidomycosis—400–800 mg orally daily
- Candidemia/invasive candidiasis—800 mg loading followed by 400 mg daily.

Itraconazole

If the total dose of itraconazole is 400 mg or greater, it should be given in divided doses. Dose modification is not required in renal insufficiency as it is metabolized in the liver. Dosing with liquid formulation should be decided keeping in consideration that it achieves approximately 30% higher concentration than capsules. IV preparation is discontinued.

- Oropharyngeal or esophageal candidiasis—200 mg of the solution daily
- Histoplasmosis/blastomycosis—200–400 mg daily
- Coccidioidomycosis—200 mg two or three times daily
- Allergic bronchopulmonary aspergillosis—200 mg twice daily
- Onychomycosis (toenails)—200 mg daily for 12 weeks or pulse therapy
- Onychomycosis (fingernails)—200 mg twice daily for 1 week (repeat course after 3-week drug holiday)

Voriconazole

Loading dose: Both oral and intravenous preparations of voriconazole require a loading dose.

    Oral: 400 mg every 12 hours for two doses

    Intravenous: 6 mg/kg every 12 hours for two doses

Maintenance dose:

    Oral: 200 mg every 12 hours

    Intravenous: 3–4 mg/kg every 12 hours.

    Note: Oral medication should be given empty stomach as fatty meals hamper absorption. Dosing in patients with obesity has not been determined.

For more resistant pathogens, the oral dose may be increased to 300 mg every 12 hours.

Intravenous therapy should be avoided in patients with renal insufficiency with CrCl <50 mL/min due to accumulation of the intravenous carrier, sulfobutyl ether-β-cyclodextrin.

In patients with mild-to-moderate hepatic derangement, standard loading dose should be used whereas maintenance dose should be halved. It should not be used in patients with severe hepatic insufficiency.

Posaconazole

The dosage of posaconazole depends upon the formulation used and the indication. The IV formulation is avoided in patients with moderate-to-severe renal impairment due to the presence of cyclodextrin.

Delayed Release Tablets

Loading dose: 300 mg (3 × 100 mg tablets) every 12 hours on the first day

Maintenance dose: 300 mg (3 × 100 mg tablets) daily starting on the second day onward

Oral suspension: Effective absorption of the oral suspension of the drug requires oral intake optimally with a fatty meal or a carbonated beverage.

200 mg three times daily.

IV Formulation

Loading dose: 300 mg IV every 12 hours on the first day

Maintenance dose: 300 mg IV every 24 hours

Oral suspension and delayed release tablet are indicated for prophylaxis of invasive aspergillosis and candidiasis in immunocompromised patients. Oral suspension is used for oropharyngeal candidiasis as a loading dose on first day followed by maintenance dose for 13 days. Suspension and tablets are not interchangeable due to differences in dosing.

Isavuconazole

Oral isavuconazole can be taken with or without food. IV administration requires an in-line filter as particulate matter has been seen in reconstituted solutions. The drug is avoided in severe hepatic impairment whereas no dose adjustment is needed in renal impairment.

Loading dose: 200 mg of isavuconazole (equivalent to 372 mg of isavuconazonium sulfate) given every 8 hours for six doses (48 hours) via oral (two 100 mg capsules) or IV administration.

Maintenance dose: 200 mg once daily orally or IV starting 12–24 hours after the last loading dose.

Ketoconazole

Its use has been replaced by other triazoles due to significant hepatotoxicity and drug interactions.

Topical Imidazoles (Table 9.3)

Table 9.3: Topical Imidazoles	
Drug	*Uses*
Bifonazole	For dermatophytosis and pityriasis versicolor
Butoconazole	Pessaries for vaginal candidiasis
Clotrimazole	Dermatophytosis, oral, cutaneous, and genital candidiasis as oral troches, ointments, and pessaries
Econazole	Dermatophytosis, oral, cutaneous, corneal, and vaginal infections
Fenticonazole	Pessaries for vaginal candidiasis
Isoconazole	Dermatophytosis, oral, and vaginal candidiasis
Miconazole	Dermatophytosis, pityriasis versicolor, oral, cutaneous, and genital candidiasis
Oxiconazole	Dermatophytosis and cutaneous candidiasis
Sertaconazole	Dermatophytosis and vaginal candidiasis
Terconazole	Dermatophytosis, cutaneous, and genital candidiasis
Tioconazole	Dermatophytoses including nail infections, cutaneous, and genital candidiasis

■ SERUM DRUG CONCENTRATION MONITORING

Serum drug concentrations are measured for itraconazole, voriconazole, and posaconazole to ensure adequate drug levels assuring efficacy and avoiding toxicity.

Voriconazole trough concentration should be checked 4–7 days after initiation of therapy.

■ DRUG INTERACTIONS

Azoles have numerous drug–drug interactions due to involvement of cytochrome P450 system. Medications that induce hepatic CYP enzymes accelerate the metabolism of azoles, e.g. rifampicin, rifabutin, phenobarbital, phenytoin, and carbamazepine.

Important/Serious Drug Interactions

- Rhabdomyolysis when concomitant use with statins such as simvastatin, atorvastatin, and lovastatin. There are other statins including rosuvastatin and pravastatin, which are not metabolized by CYP3A4 and are, therefore, preferred in patients on azoles.
- Long QT syndrome, torsades de pointes, and sudden cardiac death are documented on use with amiodarone, quinidine, and haloperidol.
- Interaction with immunosuppressive agents including cyclosporine, sirolimus, and tacrolimus alters drug levels and these need to be monitored.
- Use of warfarin with fluconazole prolongs prothrombin time and increases INR resulting in increased chances of bleed.

- Use of azoles concomitantly with midazolam and triazolam causes excessive sedation. The same is not observed with lorazepam since it is not metabolized by CYP3A4.

CLINICAL PEARLS

- Azoles are generally considered fungistatic against *Candida*; voriconazole is fungicidal against *Aspergillus*.
- Azoles should be avoided during pregnancy.
- Drug interactions happen through cytochrome P450 enzyme.
- Monitor serum concentrations of itraconazole, voriconazole, and posaconazole.

SUGGESTED READING

1. CRESEMBA (isavuconazonium sulfate) prescribing information. [online] Available from <http://www.accessdata.fda.gov/drugsatfda_docs/label/2015/207500Orig1s000lbl.pdf>.
2. Cumpston A, Caddell R, Shillingburg A, et al. Superior serum concentrations with posaconazole delayed-release tablets compared to suspension formulation in hematological malignancies. Antimicrob Agents Chemother. 2015;59:4424.
3. Dolton MJ, Ray JE, Chen SC, et al. Multicenter study of posaconazole therapeutic drug monitoring: exposure–response relationship and factors affecting concentration. Antimicrob Agents Chemother. 2012;56:5503.
4. FDA Center for Drug Evaluation and Research (CDER). VFEND (voriconazole) tablets, IV for infusion and oral suspension. Safety labeling changes approved by FDA Center for Drug Evaluation and Research (CDER). [online] Available from <http://www.fda.gov/Safety/MedWatch/SafetyInformation/ucm283035.htm>; November 2011.
5. Koselke E, Kraft S, Smith J, et al. Evaluation of the effect of obesity on voriconazole serum concentrations. J Antimicrob Chemother. 2012;67:2957.
6. Krishna G, Moton A, Ma L, et al. Effects of oral posaconazole on the pharmacokinetics of atazanavir alone and with ritonavir or with efavirenz in healthy adult volunteers. J Acquir Immune Defic Syndr. 2009;51:437.
7. Luong ML, Al-Dabbagh M, Groll AH, et al. Utility of voriconazole therapeutic drug monitoring: a meta-analysis. J Antimicrob Chemother. 2016;71:1786.
8. Maertens JA, Raad II, Marr KA, et al. Isavuconazole versus voriconazole for primary treatment of invasive mould disease caused by *Aspergillus* and other filamentous fungi (SECURE): a phase 3, randomised-controlled, non-inferiority trial. Lancet. 2016;387:760.
9. Miceli MH, Kauffman CA. Isavuconazole: a new broad-spectrum triazole antifungal agent. Clin Infect Dis. 2015;61:1558.
10. Nicolau DP, Crowe HM, Nightingale CH, et al. Rifampin–fluconazole interaction in critically ill patients. Ann Pharmacother. 1995;29:994.
11. Nivoix Y, Levêque D, Herbrecht R, et al. The enzymatic basis of drug–drug interactions with systemic triazole antifungals. Clin Pharmacokinet. 2008;47:779.
12. Ordaya EE, Alangaden GJ. Real-life use of isavuconazole in patients intolerant to other azoles. Clin Infect Dis. 2016;63:1529.
13. Rachwalski EJ, Wieczorkiewicz JT, Scheetz MH. Posaconazole: an oral triazole with an extended spectrum of activity. Ann Pharmacother. 2008;42(10):1429-38.

14. Singer JP, Boker A, Metchnikoff C, et al. High cumulative dose exposure to voriconazole is associated with cutaneous squamous cell carcinoma in lung transplant recipients. J Heart Lung Transplant. 2012;31:694.

15. Walsh TJ, Raad I, Patterson TF, et al. Treatment of invasive aspergillosis with posaconazole in patients who are refractory to or intolerant of conventional therapy: an externally controlled trial. Clin Infect Dis. 2007;44:2.

16. Wingard JR, Carter SL, Walsh TJ, et al. Randomized, double-blind trial of fluconazole versus voriconazole for prevention of invasive fungal infection after allogeneic hematopoietic cell transplantation. Blood. 2010;116(24):5111-8.

10

Amphotericin B

Monica Mahajan

■ INTRODUCTION

Amphotericin B is a polyene antibiotic produced by *Streptomyces nodosus*. This polyene antifungal binds to ergosterol, thereby disrupting the cell membrane of the fungus. It is the preferred antifungal drug for treatment of life-threatening invasive fungal infections.

■ MECHANISM OF ACTION (FIG. 10.1, TABLE 10.1)

Amphotericin B is a lipophilic compound that is fungistatic or fungicidal depending on the drug levels achieved in the various tissues and the fungal susceptibility. It binds with sterols, primarily ergosterol. This leads to the formation of transmembrane channels or pores that increase cell membrane permeability. Important intracellular components and monovalent ions including sodium, potassium, hydrogen, and chloride ions leak through the pore causing cell rupture and eventually cell death. The drug may also induce oxidative damage in fungal cells. It also activates the host immune response through the endothelial cells. Since amphotericin B also binds to cholesterol in humans, this leads to cytotoxicity.

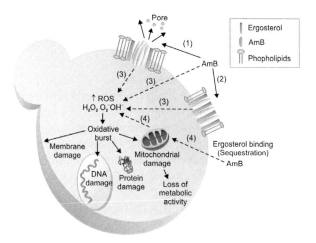

Fig. 10.1: Mechanism of action of amphotericin B.

> **Table 10.1:** Mechanisms of action of amphotericin B
>
> Amphotericin B exerts its action at different levels on the on fungal cell: on membrane and intracellularly.
> - *Cell membrane effect of Amphotericin B (Fig. 10.1):*
> Binding to ergosterol forming pores (1) or
> Ergosterol sequestration and membrane disruption (2)
> - *Intracellular effect of Amphotericin B (Fig. 10.1):*
> Pro-oxidant activity with accumulation of reactive oxygen species (ROS) (3)
> ROS influence the mitochondrial activity in the respiratory chain (4) Oxidative burst damaging cell components and causing cell death.

SPECTRUM OF ACTIVITY

Amphotericin B demonstrates activity against *Histoplasma capsulatum, Coccidioides immitis, Candida* species, *Blastomyces dermatitidis, Cryptococcus neoformans, Sporothrix schenckii, Mucormyces,* and *Aspergillus fumigatus.* It is also active against leishmania species.

AMPHOTERICIN B RESISTANCE

Resistance to amphotericin B is secondary to reduction in ergosterol biosynthesis as well as synthesis of alternative sterols. This lessens the disruptive ability of the drug on the fungal cell membrane. Moreover, oxidant scavengers may also be produced.

Primary drug resistance to amphotericin B is noted in the following:
- *Scedosporium* spp.
- *Trichosporon* spp.
- *Pseudallescheria boydii*

FORMULATIONS OF AMPHOTERICIN B

Four commercially available formulations are as follows:
1. Amphotericin B deoxycholate (AmBd)
2. Amphotericin B colloidal dispersion (ABCD)
3. Amphotericin B lipid complex (ABLC)
4. Liposomal amphotericin B (LAmB)

The last three are lipid-associated formulations.

The pharmacokinetics of amphotericin B gets modified as per the formulation used. Since the drug has poor absorption from the gastrointestinal tract, it is administered parenterally. In attempts to produce less expensive lipid-associated formulations, amphotericin B deoxycholate (AmBd) has been mixed with a parenteral fat emulsion. The use of this preparation in patients is discouraged since it does not achieve adequate serum concentrations.

All formulations of amphotericin B must only be administered in 5% dextrose.

AMPHOTERICIN B DEOXYCHOLATE (AmBD)

Since AmBd is a colloidal suspension, it becomes cloudy on addition of electrolytes due to aggregation the colloids. This is to be strictly avoided.

Pharmacokinetics

On administration, the drug has a multicompartmental distribution. The highest concentrations of the drug are in the liver, spleen, and kidney. From there, it reenters the circulation slowly. The drug concentrations achieved in the inflamed pleura, peritoneal cavity, synovial fluid, and aqueous humor are about 60% of the corresponding plasma concentration. The drug has poor penetration into vitreous humor, pericardial and pleural fluid, bronchial secretions, muscle, and bone. CSF concentrations are extremely low with only 3% of the peak serum concentrations being attained. Despite this low penetration into the inflamed and uninflamed meninges, the drug shows efficacy in central nervous infections including cryptococcal meningitis. Low concentrations are attained in the amniotic fluid. Urine concentrations are equivalent to serum concentrations.

The drug is 95% protein bound, mainly to lipoproteins. It does not have any active metabolites. Serum concentration with conventional AmBd doses has ranged from 1 μg/mL to 2 μg/mL. The plasma $t_{1/2}$ is 24 hours and the elimination terminal $t_{1/2}$ of the drug is up to 15 days. AmBd has a prolonged renal elimination over weeks to months. The drug is present in blood for up to a month and in urine for up to 1–2 months after discontinuation of the therapy. Since the drug is released from the peripheral compartment at a very slow rate, it results in the long elimination half-life. A single dose of AmBd will have an approximate 40% cumulative urinary excretion. There is minimal biliary excretion. The drug is not dialysable.

Binding of the drug to cholesterol and other sterols in human cells such as renal cells and RBC may explain some of the toxicities associated with AmBd.

Pregnancy and Lactation

Pregnancy category B
Lactation: Excretion of the drug in milk is unknown.

Dosage

Daily AmBd dose for invasive fungal infections (IFIs) is 0.5–1 mg/kg per day. Doses exceeding 1 mg/kg per day are generally reserved for mucormycosis, invasive aspergillosis, or azole-refractory invasive coccidioidomycosis meningitis.

Daily dose should not exceed 1.5 mg/kg per day.
The dose of AmBd does not need to be adjusted for renal dysfunction.

Administration Technique

- Intravenous infusions are prepared by combining AmBd with 5% dextrose.
- A test dose of 1 mg is given as an aliquot of the initial infusion. However, tolerance of the test dose is mainly to assess allergic response and does not exclude other toxicities associated with the drug.
- Infusion time should be 2–6 hours; continuous infusion is not recommended.
- Premedication should be considered to prevent infusion-related reactions.

- Local instillation of AmBd into CSF, joints, or pleural space is not routinely indicated. *C. immitis*-related meningitis is an exception since intrathecal AmBd shows higher clinical efficacy compared to systemic azole therapy. It can be given through a ventricular Ommaya or Rickham reservoir. It moves from the CSF to the extracellular compartment by the arachnoid villi, gets stored there, and acts as a drug reservoir. Adverse effects include nausea, vomiting, headache, back pain, loss of bowel and/or bladder control, nerve palsies, arachnoiditis, and bacterial infection of the reservoir.
- Intraocular administration of AmBd is occasionally required for fungal endophthalmitis. Corneal baths in sterile water with 1 mg/mL concentration of the drug are useful for fungal keratitis but can cause corneal irritation.
- Aerosolized or nebulized amphotericin B has been used both as adjunctive therapy as well as a preventive measure for management of invasive fungal infections.
- Bladder irrigation with amphotericin B has been rarely used in symptomatic cystitis with azole-resistant species of *C. glabrata* and *C. krusei*.

Adverse Effects

Acute infusion-related reactions: Amphotericin B can cause anaphylaxis and reexposure to the drug should be strictly avoided in these cases. Infusion-related reactions due to AmBd are maximum within 15–30 minutes of initiation of drug and then slowly subside over 2–4 hours. These include nausea, vomiting, chills, rigors, tachypnea, dyspnea, back pain, chest tightness, hypertension, hypotension, and hypoxemia. Subsequent infusion of the same dose causes progressively milder reactions especially if the infusion rate is slowed.

Premedication with acetaminophen and hydrocortisone diminish the acute reaction. Promethazine, prochlorperazine, or ondansetron reduce nausea and vomiting. Meperidine reduces rigors but worsens nausea and vomiting.

Thrombophlebitis is common in patients receiving the infusions via a small peripheral vein. Ways to reduce phlebitis include using a central line, alternating infusion sites and ensuring infusion time of at least four hours.

Nephrotoxicity: Amphotericin B is associated with dose-dependent decline in glomerular filtration rate (GFR), which is transient and reversible. AmBd is more toxic than all the lipid-based formulations. Renal functions recover fully on discontinuation of drug although some patients may experience chronic decline in eGFR if high cumulative doses were used. Patients with high low-density lipoprotein (LDL) levels are more prone to nephrotoxicity.

Amphotericin B causes vasoconstriction of the renal arterioles that reduces blood flow to the glomeruli and tubules. The other effects of the drug include potassium, magnesium, and bicarbonate wasting. Many patients require significant amounts of potassium and/or magnesium supplementation during therapy to compensate for urinary losses. Hypokalemia will not correct unless hypomagnesemia is corrected. RTA due to bicarbonate wasting does not need to be corrected by base replacement. The drug decreases the production of erythropoietin by the kidney. False elevations in serum phosphate may occur.

Other etiologies include damage to renal tubular cells and cholesterol-rich lysosomal tubular basement membrane by lytic action of the drug. There is a loss of functioning nephrons.

Attempts to give AmBd without a resultant azotemia generally implies inadequate response to therapy. Other factors precipitating nephrotoxicity include preexisting renal disease, hypotension, and intravascular volume depletion. Saline loading prior to administration of the drug reduces nephrotoxicity.

Important Drug Interactions

The concurrent or sequential use of AmBd and other nephrotoxic drugs is avoided. These include aminoglycosides, cisplatin, cyclosporine, polymyxin B, colistin, and vancomycin.

Corticosteroids may worsen hypokalemia caused by amphotericin B. Restrict steroid use to control adverse effects of the drug.

Since amphotericin B use results in hypokalemia, it may increase probability of cardiac glycoside-induced toxicity. The neuromuscular blocking effect of drugs such as tubocurarine get enhanced because of the same reason.

When amphotericin B and flucytosine are concurrently used, toxicity of flucytosine increases due to higher cellular uptake and/or impaired renal excretion.

Combination of amphotericin B with azoles may result in fungal resistance to amphotericin B.

It is important that renal, hepatic, and hematopoietic functions and serum electrolytes including potassium and magnesium levels are closely monitored.

Other Chronic Toxicity

Reversible normocytic normochromic anemia occurs gradually up to 10 weeks after initiation of therapy due to bone marrow depression. Moderate-to-severe leukopenia, thrombocytopenia, and coagulopathy have been documented with the use of the drug. Mild and transient elevations in liver enzymes are seen in up to 20% of the patients. Other side effects include arrhythmias, encephalopathy, seizures, vertigo, tinnitus, and enteritis.

Renal function, serum electrolytes, and complete blood count need to be routinely monitored throughout the therapy. The drug may be used in pregnancy if the advantages outweigh the risks involved.

▇ LIPID-ASSOCIATED FORMULATIONS OF AMPHOTERICIN B

Lipid formulations of amphotericin B include the following:
- Liposomal amphotericin B (LAmB, AmBisome)
- Amphotericin B lipid complex (ABLC, Abelcet)
- Amphotericin B cholesteryl sulfate complex (amphotericin B colloidal dispersion, ABCD, amphotec)

▇ LIPOSOMAL AMPHOTERICIN B

Encapsulating a drug into the lipid bilayer of a liposome protects it from enzymatic degradation and immunological neutralization. The liposomes prevent the drug from getting metabolized before it reaches the target tissue. It also reduces the toxicity of the drug since it remains encapsulated during its circulation in the blood. So liposomal drugs have a better therapeutic index. LAmB consists of closed, spherical liposomes with a mean diameter of <100 nm. These vesicles are composed of cholesterol, hydrogenated soy phosphatidylcholine, and phosphatidylglycerol with amphotericin B in the center of the liposome. These are arranged as multiple concentric bilayer membranes. Microemulsification using a homogenizer forms single bilayer liposomes of the drug.

Pharmacokinetics

LAmB has nonlinear pharmacokinetics. There is a variable increase in serum concentrations when dose is increased from 1 mg/kg/day to 5 mg/kg/day. Serum levels achieved after 3 mg/kg dose are 10–35 mg/L, whereas serum levels after 5 mg/kg dose are 25–60 mg/L. Maximum drug levels are found in hepatic tissue and spleen while low levels are present in kidneys. Terminal half-life is 100–153 hours. The drug attains a steady-state concentrations within 4 days.

Dosage

The typical cumulative dosage of LAmB may be 1–3 g over 3–4 weeks but maximum tolerated dose of the drug has not been conclusively determined. Cumulative dosages of up to 30 g have been studied without a significant increase in toxic potential. The recommended initial dose of LAmB is as in Table 10.2.

It is used in patients who have experienced side effects to AmBd or in whom AmBd is contraindicated due to impaired kidney function.

Off-label use of LAmB is recommended by CDC for treatment of *Candida auris.*

Doses of LAmB recommended for visceral leishmaniasis are as in Table 10.3. If parasitic clearance is not achieved, a repeat course with the drug is advocated. Most immunocompetent individuals do not experience a relapse during follow-up periods of 6 months or longer. Relapse rates are high in immunocompromised host following initial clearance of the parasite.

Table 10.2: Dosage of liposomal amphotericin B in systemic fungal infections

Indication	Dose (mg/kg/day)
Empirical therapy	3 mg/kg/day
Systemic fungal infections: *Aspergillus, Candida,* and *Cryptococcus*	3–5 mg/kg/day
Cryptococcal meningitis in HIV-infected patients	6 mg/kg/day

Table 10.3: Dosage of liposomal amphotericin B In visceral leishmaniasis

Visceral leishmaniasis	Dose (mg/kg/day)
Immunocompetent patients	3 mg/kg/day (days 1–5) and 3 mg/kg/day on days 14, 21
Immunocompromised patients	4 mg/kg/day (days 1–5) and 4 mg/kg/day on days 10, 17, 24, 31, 38

Administration

Liposomal amphotericin B is reconstituted using sterile water. It is further diluted with 5% dextrose injection to achieve a final concentration of 1–2 mg/mL. It may be infused through an in-line filter with a pore diameter of >1 μm. It is administered over 120 minutes. It should not be reconstituted with saline to avoid precipitation of the drug. Any existing intravenous line being used for administering other drugs in the patient must be flushed with 5% dextrose prior to infusing amphotericin B. If unfeasible, insert a separate line to administer the drug. Each injection is equivalent to 50 mg of amphotericin B.

Adverse Effects

The adverse effects with LAmB are significantly less than that due to conventional AmBd. Renal impairment defined as twice baseline serum creatinine concentration is much lower with LAmB. Drug interactions are similar to AmBd. It is contraindicated in those who have a history of hypersensitivity to amphotericin B.

AMPHOTERICIN B LIPID COMPLEX (ABLC)

ABLC structure consists of amphotericin B complexed with two phospholipids in a drug:lipid ratio of 1:1. The recommended adult daily dose is 5 mg/kg/day. Each vial contains 100 mg of amphotericin B, which is reconstituted with 5% dextrose to achieve a final concentration of 1–2 mg/mL. The most commonly reported adverse effects are infusion-related chills and/or fever, which generally diminish with subsequent doses. The pharmacokinetics are nonlinear. The nephrotoxicity is significantly less than that for AmBd.

AMPHOTERICIN B COLLOIDAL DISPERSION (ABCD)

ABCD is a colloidal dispersion of amphotericin B with cholesterol sulfate in a ratio of 1:1 to form disk-shaped particles. Initial dose of 1 mg/kg is increased to 3–4 mg/kg infused at a rate of 1–2 mg/kg/day. Dosages up to 6 mg/kg have been used. It is available as 50 mg and 100 mg per vial of amphotericin B. It is rapidly taken up by reticuloendothelial system and distributed in tissues with maximum drug levels achieved in liver and spleen, high tissue distribution, and lower serum concentration. Nephrotoxicity is markedly reduced compared with AmBd. Infusion-related adverse effects are more frequent with ABCD than in patients receiving LAmB. It is to be used in patients where renal toxicity precludes the use of AmBd or in patients with invasive aspergillosis where prior therapy with AmBD has failed.

COMPARATIVE EFFICACY

With the lipid formulations, there is a reduction in both the frequency and intensity of acute infusion reactions and chronic nephrotoxicity. An exception is ABCD, which induces more infusion-related reactions.

Although the lipid-associated formulations are more expensive, they compensate well for the cost involved in treating the AmBd-associated nephrotoxicity.

A trial comparing LAmB with AmBd for empiric therapy in patients with persistent fever and neutropenia found the overall clinical success rates to be "equivalent" as evidenced by resolution of fever, the absence of an emergent fungal infection, patient survival for at least 7 days post therapy, and no discontinuation of therapy due to toxicity or lack of efficacy. The main advantage associated was a reduction in infusion-related adverse effects and nephrotoxicity when LAmB was used.

Infusion-related intolerance to one formulation may not necessarily result in similar reactions to other amphotericin B formulations.

CLINICAL PEARLS

- Polyene antifungals are treatment of choice for many life-threatening fungal infections. These disrupt the fungal cell wall synthesis by binding to ergosterol.
- To avoid precipitation, do not reconstitute with saline, electrolytes, or other drugs.
- Monitor renal function, potassium, and magnesium levels.
- In patients on renal dialysis, amphotericin B should be administered at the end of each dialysis session.
- Avoid concurrent or sequential use of nephrotoxic drugs.

SUGGESTED READING

1. Alexander BD, Wingard JR. Study of renal safety in amphotericin B lipid complex-treated patients. Clin Infect Dis. 2005; 40(Suppl 6):S414.
2. Bicanic T, Bottomley C, Loyse A, et al. Toxicity of Amphotericin B Deoxycholate-based induction therapy in patients with HIV-associated cryptococcal meningitis. Antimicrob Agents Chemother 2015; 59:7224.
3. Bowden R, Chandrasekar P, White MH, et al. A double-blind, randomized, controlled trial of amphotericin B colloidal dispersion versus amphotericin B for treatment of invasive aspergillosis in immunocompromised patients. Clin Infect Dis. 2002;35:359-66.
4. Falci DR, da Rosa FB, Pasqualotto AC. Hematological toxicities associated with amphotericin B formulations. Leuk Lymphoma. 2015;56:2889.
5. Farmakiotis D, Tverdek FP, Kontoyiannis DP. The safety of amphotericin B lipid complex in patients with prior severe intolerance to liposomal amphotericin B. Clin Infect Dis. 2013;56:701.
6. Gallis HA, Drew RH, Pickard WW. Amphotericin B: 30 years of clinical experience. Rev Infect Dis. 1990;12:308.
7. Hayes D Jr, Murphy BS, Lynch JE, Feola DJ. Aerosolized amphotericin for the treatment of allergic bronchopulmonary aspergillosis. Pediatr Pulmonol. 2010;45:1145.
8. Kneale M, Bartholomew JS, Davies E, Denning DW. Global access to antifungal therapy and its variable cost. J Antimicrob Chemother. 2016;71:3599.
9. Mistro S, Maciel Ide M, de Menezes RG, et al. Does lipid emulsion reduce amphotericin B nephrotoxicity? A systematic review and meta-analysis. Clin Infect Dis. 2012;54:1774.
10. Seibel NL, Shad AT, Bekersky I, et al. Safety, tolerability, and pharmacokinetics of liposomal amphotericin B in immunocompromised pediatric patients. Antimicrob Agents Chemother. 2017; 61.

11. Steimbach LM, Tonin FS, Virtuoso S, et al. Efficacy and safety of amphotericin B lipid-based formulations: a systematic review and meta-analysis. Mycoses. 2017;60:146.

12. Stevens DA, Shatsky SA. Intrathecal amphotericin in the management of coccidioidal meningitis. Semin Respir Infect. 2001;16:263.

13. Wingard JR, White MH, Anaissie E, et al. A randomized, double-blind comparative trial evaluating the safety of liposomal amphotericin B versus amphotericin B lipid complex in the empirical treatment of febrile neutropenia. L Amph/ABLC Collaborative Study Group. Clin Infect Dis. 2000; 31:1155.

11

Echinocandins

Monica Mahajan

INTRODUCTION

The echinocandins are a new and exciting armamentarium in the world of mycology. They were accidentally discovered while screening for new antibiotics. They inhibit the synthesis of $(1,3)$-β-D-glucan that is necessary to maintain integrity of the fungal cell wall. The main advantages of this class of antifungals are as follows:

- Rapid fungicidal (for yeast)/fungistatic (for molds) activity
- Low-toxicity potential
- Fewer drug–drug interactions
- Favorable kinetics permitting once-daily dosing.

However, cost is a limiting factor for their use in patients with severe invasive fungal infections.

Caspofungin was the first molecule of this class approved by the Food and Drug Administration (FDA) in 2002 having the maximum approved indications. Subsequently, two other semisynthetic echinocandins, namely micafungin and anidulafungin, were approved for use in 2005 and 2006, respectively. The molecular weight of all three echinocandins is large. Therefore, all the three compounds are given intravenously.

MECHANISM OF ACTION (FIG. 11.1)

The echinocandins are semisynthetic compounds that are large, cyclic lipopeptides. They were derived from the fermentation broth of various fungi. For example, anidulafungin is the fermentation product of *Aspergillus nidulans*. This group was initially named pneumocandins since they demonstrated in vitro activity against *Pneumocystis jirovecii* (formerly *P. carinii*) and *Candida* species.

Echinocandins are unique in their action as they target the glucan synthesis. They noncompetitively inhibit the $(1,3)$-β-D-glucan synthase enzyme responsible for the synthesis of a major polysaccharide $(1,3)$-β-D-glucan, a vital component of the fungal cell wall. It is absent in mammalian cells. Inability of the organism to synthesize $(1,3)$-β-D-glucan results in osmotic instability and cell death. The $(1,3)$-β-D-glucan synthase complex is composed of two subunits:

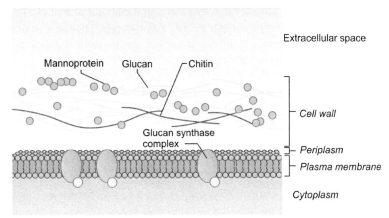

Fig. 11.1: Mechanism of action of echinocandins.

- *FKS* (encoded by *FKS1*, *FKS2*, and *FKS3* genes): A plasma membrane–bound *catalytic subunit* of (1,3)-β-D-glucan synthase
- *Rho1*: A guanosine triphosphate–binding protein which regulates the activity of glucan synthase. This activating subunit *activates* the catalytic subunit.

The (1,3)-β-D-glucans are an important structural component to maintain integrity of cell wall by cross-linking with chitin and mannoproteins. Echinocandins target the gene *FKS1* that encodes for the internal membrane components that make up the catalytic subunit of glucan synthase. Decreased (1,3)-β-D-glucans cause osmotic ballooning of the cell, which results in cell lysis.

Echinocandins have *fungicidal* activity against *Candida* species since 30–60% cell wall mass in yeasts is β-glucans. In filamentous fungi, such as *Aspergillus fumigatus*, the β-glucan is concentrated mainly in the apical tips and branching points of growing hyphae. Echinocandins block these and result in dysmorphic, highly branched, short, stubby, and swollen hyphae. Hence, this causes a *fungistatic* rather than a fungicidal effect.

Organisms that do not rely on (1,3)-β-D-glucans for cell wall integrity are less susceptible to echinocandins, which include *Cryptococcus neoformans*. Echinocandins have no activity against *Blastomyces dermatitidis*, *Rhizopus* spp., and *Fusarium* spp.

Since (1,3)-β-D-glucans are not present in mammalian cells, echinocandins cause less toxicity compared to azoles and amphotericin B.

Echinocandins may also work through immunomodulatory mechanisms in the host.

SPECTRUM OF ACTIVITY

- The echinocandins have fungicidal activity against yeasts, including *Candida albicans*, *Candida parapsilosis*, *Candida guilliermondii*, and *Candida glabrata*. Echinocandins are fungistatic against *Aspergillus* species unlike amphotericin B and triazoles that are fungicidal.

- These drugs are not active against fungi that lack significant amount of (1,3)-β-D-glucan, such as *C. neoformans*, *Trichosporon* species, and zygomycetes. They have minimal activity against dimorphic fungi. *Fusarium* and *Scedosporium* species show significant variation in susceptibility between different species.
- Traditional susceptibility testing methods—minimal inhibitory concentration (MIC)—may not be adequate for measuring the susceptibility of molds, such as *Aspergillus* to echinocandins. The minimal effective concentration (MEC) might be a more accurate way of testing this susceptibility.

ECHINOCANDIN RESISTANCE

Organisms, such as *B. dermatitidis*, *Fusarium* spp., *Rhizopus* spp., *Histoplasma capsulatum*, are inherently resistant to echinocandins as they do not depend on (1,3)-β-D-glucan for the integrity of their cell wall. Compensatory cell wall mechanisms, melanin, and drug degradation pathways contribute to the inherent resistance.

"Acquired" echinocandin resistance in certain susceptible fungal species has been reported. Resistance to echinocandins and elevated MICs are associated with single amino acid substitutions in two "hotspot" regions of well-conserved target genes—*FKS1* for all *Candida* species and *FKS2* specifically for *C. glabrata*. The nature and position of the substitution determines the degree of MIC elevation in an isolate. These point mutations are genetically dominant. They result in cross-resistance to all echinocandins. These decrease the drug sensitivity of glucan synthase by 1,000-fold or more. *FKS1* mutations occur in both yeasts and molds.

However, there can be a lack of correlation between therapeutic failure and elevated MIC values for echinocandins. *C. parapsilosis* and *C. guilliermondii* have much higher MIC values for echinocandins. *C. parapsilosis* harbors a naturally occurring *FKS1* polymorphism that confers diminished susceptibility to echinocandins. It is unclear whether this intrinsic reduced susceptibility has any relevance in the clinical scenario since these infections can be managed with echinocandins administered in regular doses. Of note, resistance rates for *C. glabrata* are increasing and are now reported at 8–18% at some high-risk centers.

Unlike azoles, drug efflux transporters do not play any role in echinocandin resistance.

Paradoxical Effect

The "paradoxical effect" (Fig 11.2) refers to the breakthrough growth of echinocandin-susceptible organisms at highly elevated drug concentrations way above the MIC. This was observed as a turbid growth of *C. albicans* at higher concentrations of caspofungin. These strains demonstrated a normal susceptibility at a typical low MIC of caspofungin but then paradoxically showed a breakthrough growth when the concentration of the drug was increased. Biochemical analysis of these strains revealed a significant increase in chitin which compensated for the corresponding decrease in (1,3)-β-D-glucan, following the activity of caspofungin. It is unclear whether the paradoxical effect has a clinical relevance in vivo.

Candida Biofilms

Candida albicans has a unique property of forming biofilms by increasing secretion of polysaccharides, including (1,3)-β-D-glucan. The activity of azoles and amphotericin B gets

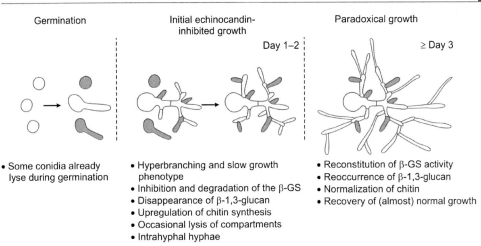

| Germination | Initial echinocandin-inhibited growth | Paradoxical growth |

Fig. 11.2: Paradoxical effect of *C. albicans* at a higher concentration of echinocandins.

inhibited by this biofilm. On the other hand, echinocandins are the only antifungals, which have displayed significant activity against this biofilm embedded inoculum of *C. albicans*. Therefore, echinocandins work in candidemia associated with catheters and prosthetic devices where the other antifungals may fail.

PHARMACOKINETICS (TABLE 11.1)

Echinocandins have poor bioavailability due to large molecular weight and can be used only in intravenous (IV) formulations. All echinocandins bind extensively to plasma. Due to their large structure, they penetrate minimally in cerebrospinal fluid (CSF), urine, and

Table 11.1: Pharmacokinetics of echinocandins.

Drug	Metabolism	Half-life (h)	Hepatic dose modification	Renal dose modification
Caspofungin	Hepatic hydrolysis and *N*-acetylation, some spontaneous degradation to form an open-ring peptide	27–50	▪ Mild (Child-Pugh 5–6): None ▪ Moderate (Child-Pugh 7–9): Maintenance dose 35 mg/day ▪ Severe (Child-Pugh > 9): No data	No modification
Micafungin	Hepatic: COMT	15	▪ Mild-to-moderate (Child-Pugh 5–9): None ▪ Severe (Child-Pugh > 9): No data	No modification
Anidulafungin	Not metabolized, undergoes spontaneous degradation	30–50	No modification of dose	No modification
COMT, Catechol-O-methyltransferase.				

eyes. Therefore echinocandins are not ideal agents for fungal meningitis, endophthalmitis, or urine infections. Echinocandins do not have primary interactions with cytochrome P450 (CYP450) or *P*-glycoprotein pumps, thus displaying minimal drug interactions. Caspofungin has triphasic nonlinear pharmacokinetics, while micafungin undergoes hepatic metabolism by arylsulfatase, catechol *O*-methyl-transferase, and hydroxylation in a linear fashion. Anidulafungin is spontaneously degraded in the system.

Echinocandins are not excreted significantly in the urine as they are highly protein bound. They are not dialyzable. *No dose adjustment is required in patients with renal impairment.*

Caspofungin maintenance dose is reduced to 35 mg once daily in moderate hepatic insufficiency with Child-Turcotte–Pugh score 7–9. The loading dose is not reduced. However, the dose of micafungin does not require reduction in mild-to-moderate hepatic insufficiency. There is insufficient data to support the use of caspofungin and micafungin in severe hepatic insufficiency. Anidulafungin does not undergo hepatic metabolism. Since the serum levels of anidulafungin do not increase in hepatic insufficiency, dose adjustment is not needed.

◼ DOSAGE

The dosing of each echinocandin depends on the following indication:
- *Esophageal candidiasis:*
  - Caspofungin—50 mg IV daily; no loading dose.
  - Micafungin—150 mg IV daily; no loading dose.
  - Anidulafungin—100 mg IV loading on day 1, followed by 50 mg IV daily thereafter.
  - Treatment is continued for a minimum of 2 weeks, and for at least 1 week, following resolution of symptoms.
- *Invasive candidiasis/candidemia* (including intra-abdominal abscesses, peritonitis, and pleural space infections):
  - Caspofungin—70 mg IV loading dose on day 1, followed by 50 mg IV daily.
  - Micafungin—100 mg IV daily, no loading dose is required.
  - Anidulafungin—200 mg IV loading dose on day 1, followed by 100 mg IV daily thereafter.
  - Treatment is continued for at least 2 weeks after the last positive culture.
- *Candida prophylaxis for hematopoietic stem cell transplant recipients:*
  - Micafungin—50 mg IV daily (only approved echinocandin for this indication).
- *Neutropenic fever* (*empiric therapy*) (adults and pediatric patients ≥3 months of age):
  - Caspofungin—70 mg IV loading on day 1, followed by 50 mg IV daily.
- *Salvage therapy for invasive aspergillosis* (in patients who are refractory to or intolerant to other therapies):
  - Caspofungin—70 mg IV on day 1, followed by 50 mg IV daily (FDA approved).
  - Micafungin—100 mg to 150 mg IV daily, no loading dose.
  - Anidulafungin—200 mg IV loading dose on day 1, followed by 100 mg IV daily.

Dose Adjustment in Obesity

A daily dose increase of 25–50% in patients weighing more than 75 kg with severe infection.

Pediatric Dosing

Caspofungin and micafungin are approved by FDA for use in pediatric age-group; doses are as per body surface area and body weight, respectively. The efficacy as well as safety of anidulafungin has not been adequately documented in pediatric patients.

ADVERSE EFFECTS

Generally, well-tolerated groups of antifungals with tolerability profile comparable to that of fluconazole and are better than that of amphotericin B.

- *Histamine-mediated symptoms:* Histamine release during rapid infusions causes rash, angioedema, pruritus, and bronchospasm. Anaphylaxis and shock have been reported. These symptoms are managed by decreasing the rate of infusion and using antihistaminics, including diphenhydramine. The cases of Stevens–Johnson syndrome and toxic epidermal necrolysis have been reported with caspofungin.
- *Hepatotoxicity:* Asymptomatic mild derangement in transaminases can happen. Hepatic failure occurs rarely. Isolated cases of hepatitis and hepatic failure have been reported with caspofungin. It is prudent that liver functions are monitored, especially in the case of caspofungin.
- *Other adverse effects:* These include fever, thrombophlebitis, vomiting, hypokalemia, chills, diarrhea, and abdominal pain.
- *Pregnancy:* Category class C.

DRUG INTERACTIONS

Echinocandins demonstrate very few drug–drug interactions because they are not metabolized through the CYP450 enzymatic pathway.

- *Caspofungin* uses the Organic anion-transporting polypeptide B (OATP-B) transporter. This can be responsible for its drug interactions.
  - *Rifampin* is an inhibitor of OATP-B. It causes reduction in caspofungin level. Consequently the daily maintenance dose of caspofungin should be increased from 50 mg to 70 mg for patients who are on rifampin. A similar dose increase may be required with concomitant use with *efavirenz, nevirapine, phenytoin, carbamazepine,* and *dexamethasone.*
  - Caspofungin decreases *tacrolimus* serum concentration by approximately 20%. Therefore, regular monitoring of tacrolimus blood levels is required to avoid graft rejection
  - *Cyclosporine* is a substrate of OATP-B transporters. It increases caspofungin total plasma concentration exposure (area under the curve) by approximately 35%. Conversely, caspofungin does not alter the cyclosporine time versus plasma concentration profile. Coadministration of these two drugs may increase liver enzymes that need to be monitored.
- *Micafungin:* This has lesser drug–drug interactions compared to caspofungin. It does not affect tacrolimus levels. It modestly reduces the clearance of *cyclosporine, sirolimus,* and *nifedipine.*
- *Anidulafungin:* This is neither an inducer nor an inhibitor or substrate for CYP450. Therefore it has no interaction with drugs metabolized by CYPP450 isoenzymes. Anidulafungin may be coadministered with cyclosporine, voriconazole, tacrolimus, amphotericin B, and rifampin without any dose adjustment for either drug. It is the best echinocandin to use in case of liver failure.

FORMULATIONS

- Caspofungin—70-mg or 50-mg single-dose vial
- Micafungin—50-mg single-dose vial
- Anidulafungin—50-mg,100-mg single-dose vial.

Echinocandins are the best option for multidrug-resistant fungal infections where azoles or amphotericin B fail. Considering the cost of therapy involved vis-à-vis the azoles, these drugs are used as reserve drugs for azole-resistant invasive *Candida* or as salvage therapy for invasive aspergillosis. They can be a more logical and economical option than liposomal amphotericin B, especially in patients with renal impairment. Voriconazole is more cost-effective than echinocandins in invasive aspergillosis.

CLINICAL PEARLS

- Antifungals of choice in invasive candidiasis. Moreover, it is useful in empiric antifungal therapy in febrile neutropenia patients and salvage therapy for invasive aspergillosis.
- Similar spectrum of activity, so interchangeable. However, drug interactions, although few, need to be considered.
- Serious adverse effects requiring drug discontinuation are rare. Liver functions may need to be monitored. Safe in renal impairment.
- Poor penetration in CSF, eyes, and urine.

SUGGESTED READING

1. Chandrasekar PH, Sobel JD. Micafungin: a new echinocandin. Clin Infect Dis. 2006;42:1171-8.
2. Denning DW. Echinocandin antifungal drugs. Lancet. 2003;362:1142.
3. Deresinski SC, Stevens DA. Caspofungin. Clin Infect Dis. 2003;36:1445-57.
4. Heresi GP, Gerstmann DR, Reed MD, et al. The pharmacokinetics and safety of micafungin, a novel echinocandin, in premature infants. Pediatr Infect Dis J. 2006;25:1110-5.
5. Kofteridis DP, Lewis RE, Kontoyiannis DP. Caspofungin-non-susceptible *Candida* isolates in cancer patients. J Antimicrob Chemother. 2010;65:293.
6. Mora-Duarte J, Betts R, Rotstein C, et al. Comparison of caspofungin and amphotericin B for invasive candidiasis. N Eng J Med. 2002;347:2020-9.
7. Pfaller MA, Boyken L, Hollis RJ, et al. In vitro susceptibility of invasive isolates of *Candida* spp. to anidulafungin, caspofungin, and micafungin: six years of global surveillance. J Clin Microbiol. 2008;46:150.
8. Pham CD, Iqbal N, Bolden CB, et al. Role of FKS mutations in *Candida glabrata*: MIC values, echinocandin resistance, and multidrug resistance. Antimicrob Agents Chemother. 2014;58:4690.
9. Seibel NL, Schwartz C, Arrieta A, et al. Safety, tolerability, and pharmacokinetics of Micafungin (FK463) in febrile neutropenic pediatric patients. Antimicrob Agents Chemother. 2005;49:3317-24.
10. Walsh TJ, Teppler H, Donowitz GR, et al. Caspofungin versus liposomal amphotericin B for empirical antifungal therapy in patients with persistent fever and neutropenia. N Eng J Med. 2004;351:1391-402.
11. Zimbeck AJ, Iqbal N, Ahlquist AM, et al. FKS mutations and elevated echinocandin MIC values among *Candida glabrata* isolates from U.S. population-based surveillance. Antimicrob Agents Chemother. 2010;54:5042.

12

Flucytosine

Monica Mahajan

INTRODUCTION

Flucytosine is also known as 5-fluorocytosine (5-FC). It is a thymidylate synthase inhibitor. It is used in the treatment of *C. neoformans*, susceptible strains of *Candida* and chromoblastomycosis. It figures in the World Health Organization's List of Essential Medicines.

Flucytosine is the fluorinated pyrimidine analog of cytosine (Fig. 12.1). It was synthesized in 1957 by Roche Laboratories as an antitumor agent, but it was discovered to have antifungal activity. It is mostly used in combination therapy and not as a monotherapy due to the following two reasons:

1. Lower efficacy than other antifungals
2. Early development of secondary drug resistance on use as monotherapy.

MECHANISM OF ACTION (FIG. 12.2)

Flucytosine is a fluorinated pyrimidine (5-fluorocytosine) that interferes with protein synthesis by incorporation into fungal ribonucleic acid. After transporting into the fungal cell by fungal cytosine permease, it is converted to 5-fluorouracil (5-FU) by the protein cytosine deaminase. The subsequent metabolites of 5-FU inhibit the enzyme thymidylate synthetase. Reduced thymidine results in reduced DNA synthesis, ultimately interfering with protein synthesis. Mammalian cells do not contain cytosine deaminase.

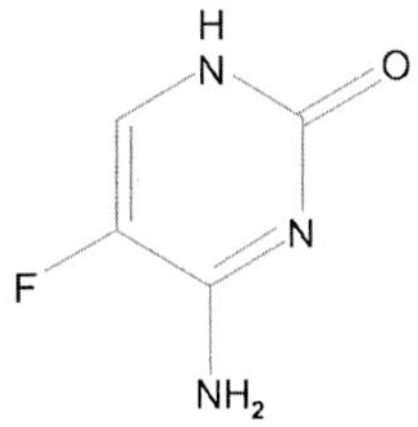

Fig. 12.1: Structure of flucytosine.

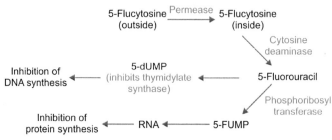

Fig. 12.2: Mechanism of action of flucytosine.

▰ SPECTRUM OF ACTIVITY

- Flucytosine is used in combination with amphotericin B in the treatment of *Cryptococcus* species.
- It is also used for candidiasis and chromoblastomycosis (*Phialophora* spp., *Cladosporium* spp., *Exophiala* spp.). It can be used as monotherapy as an exception in candiduria without systemic infections.
- It is not active against the dimorphic and filamentous fungi.

▰ FLUCYTOSINE RESISTANCE

- *Primary drug resistance*: *Candida* spp. may demonstrate primary resistance, and up to 10% of *Candida albicans* may be resistant to flucytosine.
- *Secondary drug resistance*: It may be common in cryptococcosis and chromoblastomycosis due to the loss of the cytosine permease that permits flucytosine to cross the fungal cell membrane. Moreover, mutations in enzymes converting flucytosine to the toxic metabolites of 5FU may also be responsible for secondary drug resistance.

▰ PHARMACOKINETICS

Flucytosine is available as an oral formulation which is 75–90% absorbed. It undergoes minimal metabolism and has high bioavailability. Protein binding is only 2–4%. Due to its short half-life of 2.5–6 hours, it is dosed four times daily. Most of the drug (90%) is excreted unchanged in the urine. It has excellent antifungal activity in urine since it is majorly excreted by glomerular filtration. Unabsorbed drug is excreted in feces. Due to high water solubility, significant levels are also achieved in cerebrospinal fluid (CSF) (74% of serum concentrations). It is widely distributed in aqueous and vitreous humor, bronchial secretions, peritoneal fluid, bile, cardiac vegetations, liver, spleen, bones, and joints.

Patients with renal insufficiency have impaired drug clearance, with a half-life up to 250 hours in patients with end-stage renal disease. No data on dosing in patients with hepatic impairment is available, and usual dose may be used.

The serum flucytosine concentration needs to be monitored to target peak concentration of 30–100 ng/mL. The levels of the drug should be monitored for patients with renal insufficiency.

Creatinine clearance (mL/min)	Dosage of flucytosine
>40	Standard dosage
20–40	Standard dosage given 12 hourly
<20	Once daily 37.5 mg/kg
Hemodialysis	Single dose of 37.5 mg/kg postdialysis

Table 12.1: Renal dose modification of flucytosine based on creatinine clearance.

The levels >100 ng/mL for more than 2 weeks are associated with increased risk of toxicity. The levels <25 ng/mL have been associated with the emergence of resistance in vitro. The drug is readily cleared by hemodialysis. Neonates demonstrate higher levels than adults on administration of standard doses.

DOSAGE

The oral dose ranges from 100 mg/kg/day to 150 mg/kg/day in four divided doses (i.e. 37.5 mg/kg 6 hourly) unless there is a reduced renal function (Table 12.1).

- *Cryptococcal meningitis:*
  - Used in the induction phase in combination with amphotericin B. Combination therapy with flucytosine results in more rapid CSF sterilization and reduced mortality when compared with monotherapy with amphotericin B. When compared with a combination of amphotericin B and fluconazole, this combination does not offer a better survival benefit but results in faster CSF clearance.
  - NON-HIV INFECTED: A 25 mg/kg/dose every 6 hours along with amphotericin B for at least 1 month. If clinical improvement is achieved, then both may be discontinued and start on an extended course of fluconazole.
  - HIV INFECTED: A 25 mg/kg/dose every 6 hours along with liposomal amphotericin B for at least 2 weeks to be extended further till CSF sterilization is achieved.
- *Candidiasis:*
  - *Meningitis:* 25 mg/kg/dose every 6 hours along with amphotericin B.
  - *Endocarditis* (native or prosthetic valve) or *infected implantable cardiac device:* 25 mg/kg/dose 6 hourly with amphotericin B lipid formulation for 4–6 weeks (along with surgery).
  - *Cystitis:* 25 mg/kg/dose 6 hourly for 7 to 10 days for fluconazole-resistant *Candida glabrata.*
  - *Endophthalmitis:* For fluconazole or voriconazole-resistant isolates. 25 mg/kg/dose 6 hourly with liposomal amphotericin B. An intravitreal injection of voriconazole or amphotericin B is also recommended.

ADVERSE EFFECTS

Oral flucytosine is generally well tolerated.
- *Bone marrow suppression:* Bone marrow suppression is reported in 6–22% of patients. Myelosuppression is more likely if flucytosine levels are elevated above 125 ng/mL.

The toxic metabolites cause agranulocytosis, leukopenia, anemia, aplastic anemia, thrombocytopenia, and pancytopenia. The drug has to be used cautiously in patients with hematologic disease or those receiving chemotherapy or radiotherapy. Bone marrow suppression can be irreversible.

- *Hepatic toxicity*: Transient hepatomegaly and acute liver injury along with elevated transaminases, jaundice, and hepatic necrosis have been noted. Monitor liver function tests regularly in patients on flucytosine.
- *Renal toxicity*: The US black box warning has been issued for the use of flucytosine with caution in patients with renal insufficiency due to renal dysfunction/failure associated with flucytosine.
- *Other toxicities*: Flucytosine administration may cause fever, rash, photosensitivity, gastrointestinal upset, including nausea and diarrhea, enterocolitis, abdominal pain, taste perversion, hearing loss, headache, ataxia, hallucinations, peripheral neuropathy, cardiotoxicity, and hypoglycemia.
- Teratogenic and contraindicated in pregnancy (Pregnancy Category C).

DRUG INTERACTIONS

There are few clinically relevant drug interactions with flucytosine since it is not a substrate of the cytochrome P450 enzymes. Drugs that impair glomerular filtration will decrease the elimination of flucytosine. Amphotericin B may enhance the adverse effects of flucytosine due to renal impairment, so drug levels of flucytosine need to be monitored. Drugs, such as azidothymidine, ganciclovir, and interferon, increase probability of bone marrow suppression. Aluminium hydroxide and magnesium hydroxide suspension delay the absorption of flucytosine.

FORMULATIONS

Oral capsules—250/500 mg.

CLINICAL PEARLS

- Avoid the use of monotherapy as resistance develops rapidly.
- First-line therapy along with amphotericin B in induction phase of cryptococcal meningitis.
- It may be used in *Candida* cystitis due to its high urinary concentration.

SUGGESTED READING

1. Charlier C, El Sissy C, Bachelier-Bassi S, et al. Acquired flucytosine resistance during combination therapy with caspofungin and flucytosine for *Candida glabrata* cystitis. Antimicrob Agents Chemother. 2015;60:662.
2. DHHS. DHHS panel on opportunistic infections (OI) in HIV-infected adults and adolescents: guidelines for prevention and treatment of opportunistic infections in HIV-infected adults and adolescents. Recommendations from the Centers for Disease Control and Prevention (CDC), the

National Institutes of Health (NIH), and the HIV Medicine Association (HIVMA) of the Infectious Diseases Society of America (IDSA). [online] Available from <http: //aidsinfo.nih.gov/contentfiles/lvguidelines/adult_oi.pdf>; May 7, 2013.

3. Merry M, Boulware DR. Cryptococcal meningitis treatment strategies affected by the explosive cost of flucytosine in the United States: a cost-effectiveness analysis. Clin Infect Dis. 2016;62:1564.

4. Pfaller MA, Messer SA, Boyken L, et al. In vitro activities of 5-fluorocytosine against 8,803 clinical isolates of *Candida* spp.: global assessment of primary resistance using National Committee for Clinical Laboratory Standards susceptibility testing methods. Antimicrob Agents Chemother. 2002;46:3518.

5. Vermes A, Guchelaar HJ, Dankert J. Flucytosine: a review of its pharmacology, clinical indications, pharmacokinetics, toxicity and drug interactions. J Antimicrob Chemother. 2000;46:171.

13

Antifungal Susceptibility Testing

Monica Mahajan

INTRODUCTION

As the spectrum of systemic fungal infections and the array of antifungal medication increase, we need antifungal susceptibility testing and resistance patterns to choose the appropriate treatment. The decision is made more difficult with the increase in drug resistance of fungi to a single or multiple antifungal agents. The consensus documents on antifungal susceptibility have been generated by the efforts of the "Clinical and Laboratory Standards Institute" (CLSI) and "European Committee on Antibiotic Susceptibility Testing" (EUCAST). Both CLSI and EUCAST have defined breakpoints (BPs) of certain antifungal drugs to *Candida* and *Aspergillus* species. These are used to identify resistant strains. Both CLSI and EUCAST lack specific BPs for dimorphic fungi as they exist in both mold and yeast form.

Antifungal susceptibility testing aids choosing of appropriate antifungal drugs for therapeutic purposes. The main advantages of antifungal susceptibility testing include the following:

- To correlate the in vivo and in vitro activity of the existing as well as investigational antifungal drugs.
- To compare various therapeutic options against a particular fungal pathogen and compare minimum inhibitory concentration (MIC) of the antifungals available.
- To study the emerging resistance patterns among fungi which would be normally susceptible to a particular antifungal.
- To study the changes in epidemiology of fungal infections.

DEFINITIONS

- *Minimum inhibitory concentration (MIC)*: The lowest concentration of an antifungal that inhibits the growth of fungi, as established by a standardized end point.

  MIC_{50}—concentration of an antimicrobial agent at which 50% of the organisms tested are inhibited.

  MIC_{90}—concentration of an antimicrobial agent at which 90% of the organisms tested are inhibited.

- *Minimum effective concentration (MEC):* Echinocandin sensitivity cannot be read in the same manner as the other antifungal drugs. The MEC applies to mold testing.
  The MEC is defined as the lowest concentration of an echinocandin that results in conspicuously aberrant growth in molds. This is characterized as small, round, and compact microcolonies in contrast to the matt of hyphal growth in the control well that lacks an antifungal agent. The MEC of the echinocandin is the lowest concentration where aberrant growth is first noted.
- *Clinical BPs:* Clinical interpretive MIC BPs for in vitro susceptibility testing are used to indicate the isolates that are likely to respond to treatment with a given antimicrobial agent administered using the approved dosing regimen for that agent.

As per CLSI, the clinical BPs sort isolates into the following categories:
- Susceptible (S)
- Susceptible dose-dependent (SDD)
- Intermediate (I)
- Resistant (R).

With the echinocandins, only two categories are considered—susceptible and non-susceptible. Nonsusceptible is used to categorize isolates that do not fall within the susceptible range for a drug but where resistance has not yet been defined.

Since the BPs for rare fungi are absent, epidemiological cutoff values help define the upper limit of the wild-type population.

INDICATIONS FOR SUSCEPTIBILITY TESTING OF ANTIFUNGALS

- *Candida glabrata* isolated from blood or deep site (e.g. normally sterile fluids, tissues, abscesses) should be tested for susceptibility to azoles or echinocandins as susceptibility testing can be problematic and unreliable for this fungus.
- Mucosal candidiasis unresponsive to usual antifungal therapy
- Invasive fungal infections unresponsive to the initial antifungal regimen
- Clinical failure in invasive fungal disease due to acquired resistance in the fungal species initially sensitive to a particular antifungal
- Invasive disease by unusual fungal species where the antifungal susceptibility patterns have not been well established or are unpredictable.

INTRINSIC RESISTANCE (TABLE 13.1)

Some fungi are intrinsically resistant to certain class of antifungals. Susceptibility testing is not necessary for agents where intrinsic resistance is known.

For mold infections, routine susceptibility testing is not recommended, and clinical interpretive criteria have not been well established.

Table 13.1: Intrinsic resistance to antifungals.	
Species	Intrinsic resistance
Candida krusei	Fluconazole, flucytosine
Aspergillus terreus	Amphotericin B
Cryptococcus	Echinocandins
Trichosporon	Echinocandins
Mucorales	Voriconazole, echinocandins

Note:
1. *Susceptibility testing is not necessary for species, such as C. krusei where intrinsic resistance is known; the patient should be treated empirically with antifungal agents known to have activity against the species.*
2. For mold infections, routine susceptibility testing is not recommended and clinical interpretive criteria have not been well established.

METHODS OF SUSCEPTIBILITY TESTING

The methods for susceptibility testing of antifungal agents include:
- *Standardized methods*: Broth dilution testing, disk diffusion testing
- *Commercial MIC methods*: Epsilometer (E) test, Sensititre YeastOne panel, VITEK 2 yeast susceptibility test.

STANDARDIZED METHODS

The broth dilution and disk diffusion testings of yeasts are more accurate and reproducible but require further study for filamentous fungi.

Broth Dilution Methods

This includes the following two methods:
1. Broth macrodilution
2. Broth microdilution.

Tubes contain broth inoculated with serial dilutions of concentrated antifungal solution in serial twofold dilution (Fig. 13.1). Specified amount of fungal suspension of interest is added and incubated. Development of turbidity in the tube represents fungal growth. The MIC is the first well that is clear or shows a significant diminution in turbidity relative to the control well.

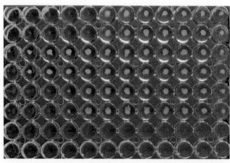

Fig. 13.1: Broth dilution method.

The microdilution technique is better than macrodilution as multiple tests can be performed simultaneously in the 96-well plate.

The microdilution method employs a 24-hour incubation at 35°C. It provides a MIC end point of ≥50% inhibition (100% inhibition for amphotericin B) relative to the "control well" that has no antifungal added.

Clinical Breakpoints for Yeasts

- *Fluconazole:*
  - Clinical BPs are the same for *Candida albicans, Candida tropicalis*, and *Candida parapsilosis* but are higher for *C. glabrata*.
- *Voriconazole:*
  - Same clinical BPs for *C. albicans, C. parapsilosis*, and *C. tropicalis* but slightly higher BPs for *Candida krusei*. However, *C. glabrata* BPs are not set as it has low clinical response to voriconazole.
- *Echinocandins:*
  - Clinical BPs are similar for *C. albicans, C. tropicalis*, and *C. krusei*. Clinical BPs are higher for *C. parapsilosis* and *Candida guilliermondii*. For *C. glabrata*, clinical BPs vary for each echinocandin.

Clinical Breakpoints for Filamentous Fungi

These are applicable for testing rapidly growing molds—*Aspergillus, Fusarium, Paecilomyces, Scedosporium*, and *Mucorales*. The MIC end point criterion for molds is the lowest drug concentration that shows "complete growth inhibition" when testing amphotericin B, itraconazole, posaconazole, isavuconazole, and voriconazole. The antifungal end point for the echinocandins while testing *Aspergillus* and the other molds is MEC and not MIC.

Disk Diffusion Methods

Disk diffusion method is a convenient method for the determination of antifungal susceptibility. Suspension of the inoculum is prepared and inoculated onto Mueller–Hinton agar medium. A filter paper disk impregnated with the antifungal drug is placed on the culture plate. The concentration of the drug is maximum nearest to disk and decreases as the distance increases. After incubation for 24 hours at 35°C, the zone of inhibition is measured in millimeter using a dial caliper. The zone of inhibition is inversely proportional to the MIC value. It is compared to a database of zone standards determined by the CLSI. This test has been validated for *Candida* species for the azole and echinocandin groups of drugs. The susceptibility testing for *Cryptococcus neoformans* by this technique is under investigation. For filamentous fungi, the clinical BPs have not been clearly defined.

- Zone of inhibition ≥ standard zone: Sensitive strain
- Zone of inhibition < standard zone: Resistant strain.

The main advantage of this test is the ease of performing the test and the low cost involved. Certain factors which affect the results include the density of the inoculum, incubation time and temperature, depth of agar, and spacing of disks.

■ COMMERCIAL MINIMUM INHIBITORY CONCENTRATION TECHNIQUES

A number of commercial techniques to determine MIC and susceptibility are now available for use by clinical laboratories. These include the following tests:

- Epsilometer test (bioMerieux)
- Sensititre YeastOne calorimetric plate (TREK diagnostic systems)
- VITEK 2 yeast susceptibility test (bioMerieux).

Epsilometer Test (Fig. 13.2)

It is an exponential gradient-based commercial test utilizing the principles of dilution and diffusion of drug into the medium to determine antimicrobial susceptibility or resistance. The technique comprises a predetermined, stable, and exponential concentration gradient of antifungal drug immobilized along a 5 × 60-mm plastic strip on one side and an MIC scale on the other side. The preformed and stable concentration gradient in E-test gives more precise values than the discontinuous twofold serial dilutions in conventional procedures. The MIC is not impacted by molecular weight, aqueous solubility, and diffusion characteristics of the drug. The MIC values are calibrated in µg/mL on one side of the nonporous strip, whereas the other side has a two-letter code inscribed on it to designate a particular antifungal drug. The technique involves applying the strip on an inoculated agar surface. This results in the antifungal agent being transferred immediately from the plastic surface onto the agar matrix and an antimicrobial concentration gradient being established in the agar medium. A symmetrical inhibition ellipse centered along the strip is formed after incubating for 24–48 hours. The MIC results are read

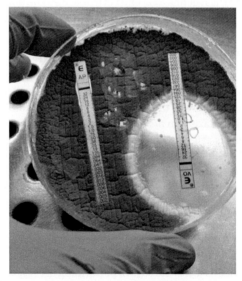

Fig. 13.2: Epsilometer test.

directly from the numeric scale on the strip at the point where the edge of the ellipse intersects the graded test strip. The confounding factors are the formulation of the medium and the depth of the agar which may alter MIC values. It is important to follow the manufacturer's instruction manual to avoid technical errors. It is important to verify that the entire length of the strip is in complete contact with the surface of agar. Once applied, the strip cannot be removed because of the instantaneous release of drug into the agar. A forceps or E-test applicator is used to place the strip. Four to six different test strips can be applied onto a 150-mm agar plate. The plates are incubated at 37°C for 24 hours. If growth occurs along the entire length of the strip and there is the absence of an inhibition ellipse, the MIC is reported as more than the highest value on the MIC scale. If the MIC value is seen between two twofold dilutions, the higher value is considered the MIC. If the intersect differs on either side of the strip, the higher value is reported as the MIC. E-test method is applicable to antifungal susceptibility testing of yeasts, such as *Candida* and *C. neoformans*. Since *C. krusei* is intrinsically resistant to fluconazole, the result should not be interpreted. MIC distribution based on the National Committee for Clinical Laboratory Standards M27-A interpretive guidelines are tightly clustered between 0.25 µg/mL and 1 µg/mL. The results are reported as susceptible, intermediate, or resistant.

The advantages of E-test include the following:
- Easy to perform and does not require extensive training of laboratory personnel
- Useful for even a small number of clinical isolates
- Easy to recognize contamination.

Sensititre YeastOne Calorimetric Antifungal Panel (Table 13.2)

It is a Food and Drug Administration–approved plate to report echinocandin sensitivities. It is an in vitro diagnostic disposable plate which uses a calorimetric microdilution panel in a 96-well microtiter tray. It tests for nine antifungals, including the echinocandins, anidulafungin, and micafungin. Alamar Blue is a calorimetric agent used as an indicator. Various antifungal drugs are serially diluted so that the individual wells are dried in serial twofold dilution of the drug. It also contains the indicator. The plates are inoculated with a multichannel pipette. Nephelometer is used to standardize the amount of inoculum. After inoculation the plates are sealed and inoculated at 35°C for 24 hours.

The "first well" which shows a change in the color of indicator to red indicates growth. Purple color denotes inhibition of growth, whereas the indicator continues to remain blue if there is no fungal growth in the well. Quality control strains, e.g. *C. parapsilosis* ATCC22019, are run in parallel with every run. In low-volume laboratories the test plates can be read manually with a mirrored view box using normal laboratory lighting. Larger laboratories can operate using a fully automated bench-top incubating and reading system.

Table 13.2: Calorimetric alamar Blue test result color.	
Red	Growth
Purple	Inhibition of growth
Blue	No growth

Table 13.3: Interpretation of Sensititre YeastOne Calorimetric Test Results and MIC.

Growth	Indicator color	Interpretation	MIC
No growth	No change in indicator color (blue)	Fungus is *susceptible* to lowest concentration of antifungal	MIC is the lowest concentration of antifungal in first blue well that substantially inhibits growth
Growth in all wells	Indicator color changes to red	Fungus is *resistant* to highest concentration of antifungal	MIC > highest concentration of the antifungal in the wells

This technique is based on the calorimetric determination of REDOX state produced by the fungal pathogen. It is more accurate than the disk diffusion method as it does not rely on measuring turbidity in the test medium. It gives actual MIC results rather than extrapolated values. The MIC for azoles and 5-fluorocytosine is the lowest concentration of antifungal solution changing from red to purple (growth inhibition) or blue (no growth) after 24–72 hours of incubation (Table 13.3). MIC for amphotericin B is the lowest concentration of the antifungal solution changing from red to blue after 48 h of incubation.

▦ INTERPRETATION OF MINIMUM INHIBITORY CONCENTRATION

Advantages of Sensititre YeastOne are as follows:
- Reduced turnaround time as results are available within 24 hours.
- Easy-to-read end points with a consolidated fungal testing platform with visual read option.
- More sensitive, reports susceptibilities for caspofungin and micafungin which promote early initiation of treatment recommended for candidemia.
- Improves decision-making regarding step-down therapy, reduces treatment cost and average length of stay.
- Advantageous in monitoring antimicrobial resistance.
- Gives actual rather than extrapolated MIC values meeting BP requirements of CLSI and EUCAST.
- More accurate than disk diffusion technique, easy to set up, and needs minimal personnel training.

VITEK® 2 Yeast Susceptibility Test (Fig. 13.3)

It is a fully automated system (bioMerieux) using a fluorescence-based technique for spectrophotometric species identification and susceptibility testing for pathogenic yeasts. It is based on the principle of using visible light to directly measure the growth of the organism. The transmittance optics measure the initial light reading of the well before the growth of the pathogen has begun. Subsequently, it measures how much light is prevented from going through the well by the organism's growth.

It uses disposable VITEK® 2 identity (ID) cards which are ready-to-use disposable miniaturized version of the doubling dilution technique for determining MIC. It can identify 50 yeast species, including *Candida, Cryptococcus, Malassezia,* and *Trichosporon* species.

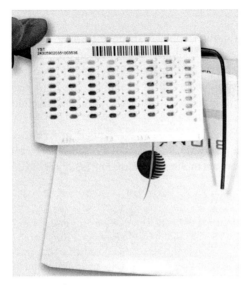

Fig. 13.3: VITEK® 2 card for yeast identification.

The card consists of 64 microwells with 47 fluorescent biochemical tests. These tests measure the carbohydrate assimilation and carbon source utilization, substrates for the detection of oxidases, arylamidases, and other enzymatic activities. Each well contains a measured quantity of specific antimicrobial agent in a culture medium base. The control well contains only the culture medium.

There is an option of automatic pipetting by a vacuum-filling process, dilution, sealing, and placement of card into incubator. Once the cards have been inoculated, they are loaded into a carousel incubator. Every card is automatically removed from the carousel incubator every 15 minutes subjecting to a fluorescence measurement. After an incubation cycle of 15 h the profile result obtained is a quantitative value which is compared to the ID-YST database for proximity to each of the database taxa. The unique identification pattern can give "unequivocal identification" in the majority of the cases. In a few cases, it may give a list of possible organisms (low discrimination). If the strain is determined to be outside the scope of the database, the unknown biopattern results in no identification. Rarely, there can be erroneous misidentification. Based on the growth characteristics, discriminate analysis provides susceptibility and MIC values.

The advantages of the system include the following:
- Results comparable to the E-test with a shorter turnaround time
- Rapid; identifies up to 50 yeast species
- Convenient, automated, and ready-to-use disposable card system
- High accuracy with results consistent with CLSI BPs.

CLINICAL PEARLS

- The recent increase in antimicrobial resistance leading to clinical failure of antifungals necessitates antifungal susceptibility testing. Moreover, the activity of two or more antifungals against a particular fungal pathogen needs to be estimated.
- Several automated techniques are now available. These are based on agar diffusion or the use of calorimetric indicators, accurate with reproducible results and shortened turnaround time.
- The limitation of susceptibility testing is the limited in vivo–in vitro correlation. In vitro susceptibility may not always result in successful therapy, and resistance may not always result in treatment failure. There are multiple confounding factors as well.

SUGGESTED READING

1. Ashbee HR, Barnes RA, Johnson EM, et al. Therapeutic drug monitoring (TDM) of antifungal agents: guidelines from the British Society for Medical Mycology. J Antimicrob Chemother. 2014;69:1162.
2. Clinical and Laboratory Standards Institute. CLSI document M27. In: Reference method for broth dilution antifungal susceptibility testing of yeasts; approved standard, 4th edition. Wayne, PA: Clinical and Laboratory Standards Institute; 2017.
3. Clinical and Laboratory Standards Institute. CLSI document M38. In: Reference method for broth dilution antifungal susceptibility testing of filamentous fungi; approved standard, 3rd edition. Wayne, PA: Clinical and Laboratory Standards Institute; 2017.
4. Clinical and Laboratory Standards Institute. CLSI document M44. In: Method for antifungal disk diffusion susceptibility testing of yeasts, 2nd ed. Wayne, PA: Clinical and Laboratory Standards Institute; 2009.
5. Clinical and Laboratory Standards Institute. CLSI document M51. In: Method for antifungal disk diffusion susceptibility testing of nondermatophyte filamentous fungi, 1st edition. Wayne, PA: Clinical and Laboratory Standards Institute; 2010.
6. Clinical and Laboratory Standards Institute. CLSI document M60. In: Performance standards for antifungal susceptibility testing of yeasts, 1st edition. Wayne, PA: Clinical and Laboratory Standards Institute; 2017.
7. Gupta P, Khare V, Kumar D, et al. Comparative evaluation of disc diffusion and e-test with broth micro-dilution in susceptibility testing of amphotericin B, voriconazole and caspofungin against clinical *Aspergillus* isolates. J Clin Diagn Res. 2015;9(1):DC04-7.
8. Johnson EM. Issues in antifungal susceptibility testing. J Antimicrob Chemother. 2008;61(Suppl 1):i13.
9. Pfaller MA. Antifungal drug resistance: mechanisms, epidemiology, and consequences for treatment. Am J Med. 2012;125:S3.
10. Sanguinetti M, Posteraro B. Susceptibility testing of fungi to antifungal drugs. J Fungi (Basel). 2018;4(3). doi: 10.3390/jof4030110.

14

Antifungal Resistance

Monica Mahajan

▓ INTRODUCTION

Management of invasive fungal infections (IFIs) relies on early diagnosis and treatment with only four major classes of currently available antifungal drugs—triazoles, polyenes, echinocandins and pyrimidine analogs. These drugs have an expanded role and are being used for prophylaxis, empirical, and directed therapy in high-risk patients which has led to selective pressure towards drug-resistant strains. There is an emerging resistance not just to a single drug class but also a multidrug resistance which is posing a major challenge for successful patient outcomes. *Candida* and *Aspergillus* species are showing increasing resistance to azoles. *Candida glabrata* is resistant to multiple drugs including echinocandins. *Candida auris* is multidrug resistant. Antifungals are being increasingly used in agriculture which has created reservoirs of drug-resistant opportunistic fungi in the environment. Agriculturally derived *Aspergillus fumigatus* is azole resistant. About 90% of mortality due to IFI can be attributed to *Cryptococcus*, *Candida*, and *Aspergillus* species.

The mechanism of azole resistance involves four distinct gene expression pathways. There is an increased interest in evaluating the role of heat-shock protein 90 (Hsp90 in antifungal drug resistance). Mechanisms for echinocandins and polyene drug resistance have not been completely deciphered. An active surveillance for antifungal drug resistance and a robust antifungal stewardship (AFS) program is the urgent need of the hour.

Clinical Resistance

Clinical resistance refers to "therapeutic failure" of an antifungal drug with in vitro activity to eradicate a fungus following administration of a standard dose. The patient fails to respond or no longer responds to the drug.

Microbiological Resistance

It refers to the nonsusceptibility of a fungus to an antifungal drug by in vitro susceptibility testing. The minimum inhibitory concentration (MIC) of the drug exceeds the susceptibility breakpoint for that fungus.

Intrinsic Resistance

The absence of drug activity in a fungal species that was not preexposed to a specific antifungal agent being tested is known as intrinsic resistance. These are inherently resistant fungi demonstrating a "primary" resistance by natural mechanisms. For example, *A. fumigatus* and *Candida krusei* are intrinsically resistant to fluconazole. *C. krusei* is intrinsically multidrug resistant.

Acquired Resistance

Acquired resistance is acquired in vitro during therapy following drug exposure, which results in elevated MICs as compared to those of a wild-type strain. There is a "secondary" resistance with a resistant subpopulation of the normally susceptible fungus. The fungi develop adaptation mechanisms on drug exposure.

■ ASSESSMENT OF ANTIFUNGAL RESISTANCE

European Committee on Antimicrobial Susceptibility Testing (EUCAST) and Clinical Laboratory Standards Institute (CLSI) have standardized in vitro antifungal susceptibility testing (AST) for yeasts and molds to define MICs and a clinical breakpoint (CBP). MIC values expressed as microgram per milliliter measure the antifungal activity of a drug against a particular fungus. For rare yeasts and molds, epidemiological cutoff values are used in the absence of CBPs. AST is unreliable for certain fungi including *C. glabrata* and certain drugs, including caspofungin. The Infectious Diseases Society of America recommends drug-susceptibility testing for yeasts but not for *Aspergillus*. Specialist laboratories utilize EUCAST and CLSI reference methods for yeast-susceptibility testing. Routine microbiology laboratories use commercial techniques such as *Epsilometer test, Sensititre YeastOne,* or *VITEK.*

■ MECHANISMS FOR DRUG RESISTANCE

Host, drug, and microbial factors contribute to drug resistance. There is a complex interplay between multiple host and microbial factors (Table 14.1).

Host Factors

- Immunosuppressed host is less likely to respond to therapy due to lack of immune response to fight the IFI.
- Poor compliance to drug regimen may be responsible for subtherapeutic levels in patients suffering from chronic fungal infections.
- Indwelling catheters, surgical implants, and prosthetic valves may contribute to refractory infections due to the development of biofilms on their surfaces.
- Site of infection effects the drug penetration and the concentration of the drug resulting in subclinical reservoirs. These are responsible for seeding new infection.

Table 14.1: Factors for clinical resistance.

Host factors:
- Immune status
- Severity of IFI
- Site of infection
- Indwelling catheters, devices, and implants
- Noncompliance with drug regimen
- Wrong diagnosis ± IRIS

Microbial factors:
- Yeast or mold—morphology, cell types, serotypes
- Genomic stability of a strain
- Biofilm formation
- Initial MIC
- Size of population and population bottlenecks

Drug factors:
- Fungistatic or fungicidal
- Pharmacokinetics and pharmacodynamics—absorption, distribution, metabolism
- Drug–drug interactions
- Dosing frequency, quantity, cumulative dose
- Drug toxicity

IFI, invasive fungal infections; IRIS, immune reconstitution inflammatory syndrome; MIC, minimum inhibitory concentration.

AZOLE RESISTANCE (TABLE 14.2)

ERG11/Cyp51A Substitutions

Azoles target the ergosterol biosynthesis. Ergosterol is a vital component of fungal cell membrane. These drugs prevent the cytochrome P450-dependent enzyme lanosterol 14α-demethylase from converting lanosterol to ergosterol. The genes responsible for encoding for this are as follows:

1. *ERG11* in yeasts
2. *Cyp51* in molds.

Amino acid substitutions in the drug target inhibit drug binding. This is frequently responsible for drug resistance in *Candida* species with over 140 substitutions having been documented in resistant strains. Some of these amino acid substitutions may have an additive effect. Two common enzyme alterations in *C. albicans* are R467K and G464S. Mutations in genes are less often responsible for drug resistance compared to drug efflux pumps. These mutations have a greater importance in haploid organisms—*C. glabrata*—than in diploid organisms, such as *C. albicans*. Mutations documented in *Cryptococcus neoformans* include Y145F and G484S. Mutations identified in *A. fumigatus* involve Cyp51A substitutions at codons 54 and 220. These result in acquired resistance.

Table 14.2: Mechanisms of antifungal resistance.

Drug class	Mechanisms of resistance
Triazoles	• *ERG11/Cyp51A* substitutions inhibiting drug binding • Overexpression of *ERG11*-target abundance • Drug efflux pumps—ABC superfamily, MFS • Chromosomal abnormalities and genomic plasticity • Mitochondrial defects • Biofilm formation • Hsp90 cellular stress-response mechanisms
Echinocandins	• *FKS* gene point mutations • Biofilm formation • Adaptive cellular responses
Polyenes	• Reduced ergosterol concentration • Genetic mutations • Catalase activity
Flucytosine	• Cytosine permease defect • Deregulation of pyrimidine biosynthetic pathway

ABC, adenosine triphosphate-binding cassette; Hsp90, heat shock protein; MFS, major facilitator superfamily.

Proximity to heme-binding site: Azoles bind to the ferric iron moiety of the heme-binding site, thereby blocking the enzymes' natural substrate lanosterol. The nature of the alteration within the protein structure and its proximity to the heme-binding site influences the binding of an azole to its target-binding site. Voriconazole and posaconazole are affected by specific modifications, whereas itraconazole resistance develops with all mutations.

Agricultural use of azoles: Rampant use of antifungals in agriculture has resulted in environmentally derived drug resistance in azole-naive patients in certain regions of Europe, including the Netherlands. These can be due to overexpression as a consequence of two changes—Cyp51A substitution at position 98 from leucine to histidine and a 34-base tandem repeat in the Cyp51A promoter. The mutation has a potential to transfer via the sexual cycle so that the resistant isolates outnumber the susceptible isolates. A high number of azole-resistant isolates have been reported in azole-naive patients as a consequence of agricultural azoles use.

Alterations in Ergosterol Biosynthetic Enzymes

Overexpression of *ERG11* causes target abundance. Therefore, more quantity of the drug would be required for inhibition, resulting in reduced drug susceptibility. Exposure to fluconazole and other azoles causes point mutations in ERG11. Mechanisms for the amplification of the *ERG11* gene and overexpression include the following:

- Formation of an isochromosome with two copies of the left arm of chromosome 5[i(5L)] in which *ERG11* resides
- Duplication of the entire chromosome

- Mutations in the gene encoding the transcription factor *UPC2* upregulate all the genes regulating ergosterol biosynthesis, resulting in azole resistance.

Azole resistance is also mediated through loss of function of the sterol $\Delta^{5,6}$-desaturase gene (*ERG3*). Inhibition of *ERG3* results in the depletion of ergosterol and accumulation of 14α-methylfecosterol, which permits continued growth of the fungus in the presence of an azole due to alterations in the cell membrane composition. ERG3 mutations also cause cross-resistance with polyenes due to the depletion of the target ergosterol.

Overexpression of *ERG11* has been reported in azole-resistant *C. albicans*, *C. glabrata*, *C. tropicalis*, *Candida parapsilosis*, and *C. krusei*. Overexpression of *Cyp51A* in *A. fumigatus* has been observed.

Drug Efflux

Membrane-associated efflux pumps are responsible for multidrug resistance. Once the efflux pumps get induced, these decrease the concentration of the drug inside the cell resulting in drug resistance. The genes encoding the drug efflux pumps in fungi belong to two superfamilies:
1. Adenosine triphosphate (ATP)-binding cassette (ABC) superfamily
2. Major facilitator superfamily (MFS).

Adenosine triphosphate-binding cassette superfamily: ATP-dependent transporters comprise two transmembrane span (TMS) domains and two cytoplasmic nucleotide-binding domains (NBD) that are catalysts for ATP hydrolysis. Variable numbers of ABC proteins are present in different fungal species. For example, *C. albicans* contains 28 ABC proteins. Although there are different classes of ABC transporters, the pleiotropic drug resistance (PDR) class is the most important for azole resistance. The PDR class for *C. albicans* includes CDR1 (*Candida* drug resistance 1) and CDR2, which get upregulated resulting in increased drug efflux and reduced drug concentration. TAC1 (transcriptional activator of *CDR* genes) is critical for upregulation of CDR1 and CDR2 in response to a drug. The other important regulator of multidrug resistance in *C. albicans* is the transcription factor Mrr1 (multidrug-resistance regulator 1). ABC transporters in *C. glabrata* include CgCdr1, CgCdr2, and CgSnq2. ABC transporters for azole resistance in *C. neoformans* is Afr1. *A. fumigatus* azole resistance is due to upregulation of AfuMDR1 (CDR1B).

Major facilitator superfamily transporters: These have multiple TMS domains. MFS efflux pumps leading to increased azole efflux are MDR1 in *C. albicans* and AfuMDR3 in *A. fumigatus*.

Chromosomal Abnormalities and Genomic Plasticity

There is a high genomic plasticity among *C. albicans* and *C. neoformans*. This causes the following:
- Loss of heterozygosity of specific genomic regions, especially for resistance determinants, including *ERG11*, *TAC1*, or *MRR1*.
- Increased chromosomal copy number—*ERG11* and *TAC1* are located on the left arm of chromosome 5. Isochromosome formation i(5L) results in azole resistance.
- Segmental or chromosomal aneuploidy.

Mitochondrial Defects

Candida glabrata and *Saccharomyces cerevisiae* may undergo partial or complete loss of mitochondrial deoxyribonucleic acid (DNA) and form "petite" mutants. These petite mitochondrial mutants are intrinsically resistant to azoles due to the upregulation of transcriptional activators. *C. albicans* cannot survive the loss of mitochondrial DNA and is considered "petite negative."

Biofilm Formation

Biofilms are produced by both yeasts and molds, the most important etiologic agent being *Candida*. Biofilms develop on the surface of indwelling catheters, implants, prosthetic valves, and on epithelial surfaces. These comprise a complex three-dimensional architecture with heterogeneous yeast and filamentous cell types enmeshed in an extracellular matrix of carbohydrates, proteins, and nucleic acids. The drug gets sequestered in the glucan-rich matrix polymer, and effective concentration of the drug reduces. *Candida* biofilms are intrinsically azole resistant. Processes have been studied to genetically or chemically modulate the $(1,3)$-β-glucan synthase to prevent sequestration of the drug in the biofilm and to make the biofilm susceptible to the antifungal agent.

Heat Shock Protein 90

Fungi have a cellular stress response mechanism enabling them to survive stress on the cell membrane on exposure to azoles. Heat shock protein 90 (Hsp90) is the molecular chaperone essential to regulate signal transducers. Inhibition of Hsp90 blocks the development of azole resistance. Hsp90 also regulates azole resistance of *Candida* biofilms, and depletion of Hsp90 reduces azole resistance by reducing matrix gluten levels.

Clinical Relevance of Azole Resistance

There has been a recent increase in resistance among *Candida* and *Aspergillus* species, whereas *Cryptococcus* has low resistance to triazoles. This is an acquired resistance due to epidemiological shift to less susceptible strains. *C. krusei* has intrinsic azole resistance. *C. glabrata* has high azole resistance.

The ARTEMIS Antifungal Surveillance Program and the Prospective Population Study on candidemia in Spain study have shown an increase in *C. glabrata* as well as an increase in fluconazole resistance in the past three decades. According to ARTEMIS data, *C. glabrata* increased as a cause of invasive candidiasis from 18% of all blood stream infection isolates in 1992–2001 to 25% in 2001–2007. During the same periods, fluconazole resistance increased from 9% to 14% in *C. glabrata* isolates. *Candida haemulonii* and *C. auris* are multidrug resistant which results in high mortality.

The use of azoles for prophylaxis and long-term use has resulted in *Aspergillus* resistance. Increasing use of azoles as crop fungicides has promoted resistance in *Aspergillus* species. *Aspergillus* has several cryptic species which are indistinguishable from the common *Aspergillus* species by conventional methods. About 10–15% of aspergillosis is caused by cryptic species. These species show high MICs and lack CBPs or epidemiological cutoff values. Some *A. fumigatus* complex species, such as *Aspergillus lentulus*, *Aspergillus fumigatiaffinis*, *Aspergillus viridinutans*, and *Aspergillus pseudofischeri*, show high MICs to azoles, and some to amphotericin B. Azole resistance in the *Aspergillus niger* complex is more common in the cryptic species, *Aspergillus tubingensis*. Some species, such as *Aspergillus ustus* complex, are multidrug-resistant species and show high MIC to azoles and other drugs.

Fusarium, Scedosporium, and mucorales show resistance to azoles. *Fusarium* is resistant to all azoles and amphotericin B. *Scedosporium apiospermum* shows high MICs to azoles and also to echinocandins. *Scedosporium prolificans* is multidrug resistant. Since mucorales are resistant to itraconazole and have high MICs to voriconazole; posaconazole remains the only alternative for the treatment of mucorales.

MECHANISMS OF ECHINOCANDIN RESISTANCE (TABLE 14.2)

- *FKS gene mutations*: The echinocandins block the catalytic subunit of the (1,3)-β-glucan synthase enzyme involved in cell wall biosynthesis for fungal cell integrity. The formation of defective cell leads to cell rupture or aberrant hyphal growth. Mutations in the *FKS* genes encoding the catalytic subunits of glucan synthase result in echinocandin resistance in *Candida* species. There is amino acid substitution in two highly conserved "hotspot" regions in *FKS1* for *C. albicans* and most *Candida* species. It is more frequent in the equivalent regions of *FKS2* in *C. glabrata*. The most significant amino acid substitution occurs at Ser-641 or Ser-645 and is responsible for 90% resistance in *C. albicans*. In *C. glabrata*, changes in Ser-663 in *FKS2* are the most important substitution. These substitutions result in decreased sensitivity of gluten synthase to drug by 50- to 3,000-fold leading to the development of resistance and breakthrough infections during therapy. The presence or absence of FKS mutation is better at predicting clinical outcomes compared with MICs. *FKS* resistance is dependent on both the frequency as well as the duration of exposure. *FKS2* expression is calcineurin dependent and can be reversed by treatment with calcineurin inhibitor FK506. However, resistance conferred by *FKS1* cannot be reversed. There is no cross-resistance between azoles and echinocandins since the latter are unaffected by multidrug transporters.
- *Biofilms*: The glucan matrix of biofilms sequesters echinocandins and prevents them from reaching the cell membrane.
- *Adaptive cellular responses and clinical reservoirs enhancing echinocandin resistance.*

On exposure to echinocandins, fungal cells may develop various adaptive cellular responses. These make the cells tolerate the drug and cause elevated in vitro MIC values. The adaptive or compensatory mechanisms involve the following:
- Cell wall integrity pathway
- High-osmolarity glycerol pathway
- Upregulation of chitin biosynthesis by chitin synthases, Chs2, and Chs8

These strains of the fungus are not drug resistant but are "drug tolerant" and produce high MICs in vitro. Drug tolerance can be an intermediate stage for the development of drug resistance. These responses of resistance and tolerance coexist since the drug still inhibits glucan synthase but the treated cells are attenuated. The fungal cells get enough time to mutate and form *FKS* stable mutants. High levels of drug may cause "paradoxical growth effect"—increase in the growth of the susceptible fungi at highly elevated drug concentrations. The paradoxical growth effect may be countered by chitin synthase inhibitor nikkomycin Z and calcineurin inhibitors.

Heat shock protein 90 stabilizes enzymes during stress and promotes survival of fungal cell despite drug exposure. It also impacts echinocandin resistance akin to azole resistance. Therefore, inhibitors of Hsp90 will reduce echinocandin resistance induced by mutations in the drug targets. There is major therapeutic potential in developing these inhibitors as they will address the problem of resistance for both classes of antifungals.

Candida glabrata may have defects in DNA repair, produce strains which hypermutate, and result in multidrug resistance.

Clinical Relevance of Echinocandin Resistance

Echinocandins are recommended for the therapy of candidiasis. However, echinocandins have lower efficacy and higher MIC values against *C. parapsilosis* complex (*C. parapsilosis* sensu stricto, *Candida orthopsilosis,* and *Candida metapsilosis*) and *Candida guilliermondii* compared to other susceptible species. These drugs are inactive against *Cryptococcus, Fusarium, Scedosporium,* and *Trichosporon* species.

European Committee on Antimicrobial Susceptibility Testing and CLSI have defined drug-specific and species-specific breakpoints for most echinocandins. Most *Candida* species have less than 1% resistance, whereas *C. glabrata* has 4–10% resistance to echinocandins in various studies. Echinocandin resistance has been reported to be lower in Europe than in America. It is debatable whether this is because of strain type or prescription patterns, or both. A major concern is the development of *C. glabrata* strains which are resistant to both echinocandins and azoles. In the SENTRY study, 11% of bloodstream isolates which were resistant to fluconazole were additionally resistant to echinocandins.

Candida auris was first described in 2009 for an isolate from the external ear canal of a patient; *C. auris* has spread to several continents and become a significant clinical challenge due to its multidrug-resistant nature. Antifungal therapy may be limited, as up to 90% of the isolates may be resistant to fluconazole, and 50% have elevated voriconazole MICs, which is secondary to point mutations in *ERG11* and *ERG3*. Posaconazole and isavuconazole appear to have clinically insignificant in vitro potency. Echinocandins are recommended for the treatment of *C. auris* infections but the fungus rapidly develops secondary resistance due to *FKS* mutations.

▓ POLYENE RESISTANCE (TABLE 14.2)

- *Reduced ergosterol concentration*: Amphotericin B binds to the ergosterol in the plasma membrane and causes the formation of concentration-dependent channels permitting cellular components and ions to escape out of the cell thereby killing the cell. It works as a sterol sponge and destabilizes the membrane function and integrity. The possible mechanism of amphotericin B resistance can be a reduced concentration of ergosterol in the fungal plasma membrane or accumulation of other sterols in the fungal membrane. Polyene-resistant *Cryptococcus* and *Candida* have relatively lower content of ergosterol in their plasma membrane compared with polyene susceptible isolates of the same species. Moreover, the use of azoles may reduce the sterol concentration thereby reducing susceptibility of the strain to amphotericin B.

- *Genetic mutations*: Genetic mutations involving *ERG1, ERG2, ERG3, ERG4, ERG6*, and *ERG11* may result in polyene resistance.
- *Catalase activity*: Increased catalase activity may also decrease susceptibility of fungi to amphotericin B-mediated oxidative damage to cells.

Some fungi can be inherently resistant to amphotericin B and include *Aspergillus nidulans, Aspergillus terreus, Aspergillus flavus, Aspergillus calidoustus, A. lentulus, Trichosporon* species, *Sporothrix schenckii, Scedosporium* species, and *Fusarium* species. Acquired resistance to amphotericin B has been reported for *C. neoformans, C. auris, C. krusei, Candida rugosa, Candida lusitaniae, C. glabrata*, and some *C. albicans* isolates.

FLUCYTOSINE RESISTANCE (TABLE 14.2)

5-Flucytosine is a prodrug which can be poorly converted to an active drug, and the fluorinated pyrimidine analogs inhibit nucleic acid and protein synthesis.

- *Cytosine permease mutations*: Flucytosine is a pyrimidine analog that inhibits synthesis of cellular DNA and ribonucleic acid. Some fungi can be intrinsically resistant to flucytosine due to mutations in cytosine permease.
- *Acquired resistance*: Acquired resistance develops due to mutations in cytosine deaminase or uracil phosphoribosyl transferase. Since acquired resistance develops very rapidly when flucytosine is used as monotherapy, it is preferable to use it in combination with other antifungal drugs (Table 14.1).

ANTIFUNGAL STEWARDSHIP

Antifungal stewardship entails the coordinated efforts toward the judicious use of available antifungal agents so that the future effectiveness of these agents is preserved. It aims at best clinical outcomes while minimizing both adverse events as well as the development of resistant strains. The challenges specific to management of IFIs is the financial implications due to high cost of therapy, emerging antifungal resistance, and high case-fatality rates especially if there is a delay in the initiation of therapy. Patients may be immunocompromised and need early, appropriate, and aggressive therapy. An increase in empirical or prophylactic antifungals may result in overuse or inappropriate antifungal use. Prior antifungal use and suboptimal dosing may result in the development of resistance.

There is an increasing consumption of antifungals. Despite introduction of newer triazoles and echinocandins, fluconazole remains the most frequently prescribed antifungal. Fluconazole-resistant *Candida* species is a serious threat. The main consumers as per defined daily dose/1,000 patient-days are medical and surgical intensive care units, transplant units, and hemato-oncology services. Pharmacoepidemiological data regarding drug utilization will be useful in improving outcomes in adults and pediatric patients.

Antifungal stewardship team adopts a multipronged approach. It involves postprescription review, feedback, education, and development of clinical guidelines. An audit team reviews the patient's chart for the appropriateness of the choice of antifungal, dose of drug, and duration of therapy. The spectrum of activity, pharmacokinetics and pharmacodynamics, duration and drug interactions are taken into account. Drug–drug interactions are a major concern when prescribing antifungals. This is especially important in transplant patients on immunosuppressive drugs. A clinical pharmacist plays a vital role in managing these interactions based on the pharmacokinetics of the drugs. A feedback is provided to the clinician regarding any change in drug or its dose. Various means of communication include meetings, telephonic conversation, or electronic patient record system. Clinical microbiologists can adopt rapid diagnostic techniques and therapeutic drug monitoring for drugs, such as voriconazole, to rationalize use of the drugs. Rapid identification methods for *Candida* include MALDI-TOF, multiplex polymerase chain reaction, peptide nucleic acid fluorescence in situ hybridization, and T2 magnetic resonance. Stewardship interventions may be based on the reports of these tests. At present, very few hospitals report fungal susceptibilities in their antibiograms. Various institutions can develop their own guidelines based on local and regional epidemiology to direct treatment including dosing, duration, therapeutic drug monitoring, shift from intravenous to oral medication, early de-escalation, and implementing formulary restriction. Infection control practices can be standardized. It reduces healthcare costs. AFS has a role in the development of a multidisciplinary care bundle, diagnosis, management, and prevention of IFI. It is important in reducing drug resistance (Box 14.1).

CLINICAL PEARLS

- Azole resistance may result from the modification of the drug target or by overexpression of drug efflux pumps.

Box 14.1: Scope of antifungal stewardship program—process and outcome metrics.

- Monitor antifungal drug consumption
- Compliance with guidelines regarding drug, dose, TDM, intravenous-to-oral conversion, de-escalation
- Use of appropriate diagnostic tests
- Source control in IFI
- Develop preventive strategies in high-risk patients
- Monitor treatment outcomes in IFI
- Study resistance patterns
- Monitor cost of therapy
- IFI, invasive fungal infections; TDM, therapeutic drug monitoring.

- *Candida glabrata* can acquire drug resistance to echinocandins and azoles.
- Echinocandin resistance develops from hotspot amino acid substitutions.
- Agricultural antifungal use has resulted in drug-resistant *Aspergillus* species.
- *Candida auris* is multidrug resistant.
- Antifungal stewardship program is vital in reducing drug resistance.

SUGGESTED READING

1. Ananda-Rajah MR, Slavin MA, Thursky KT. The case for antifungal stewardship. Curr Opin Infect Dis. 2012;25:107-15.
2. Berger S, El Chazil Y, Babu AF, et al. Azole resistance in *Aspergillus fumigatus*: a consequence of antifungal use in agriculture? Front Microbiol. 2017;8:1024.
3. Blum G, Perkhofer S, Haas H, et al. Potential basis for amphotericin B resistance in *Aspergillus terreus*. Antimicrob Agents Chemother. 2008;52:1553-5.
4. European Centre for Disease Prevention and Control. Risk assessment on the impact of environmental usage of triazoles on the development and spread of resistance to medical triazoles in *Aspergillus* species. Stockholm, Sweden: European Centre for Disease Prevention and Control; 2013.
5. Garcia-Rubio R, Cuenca-Estrella M, Mellado E. Triazole resistance in aspergillus species: an emerging problem. Drugs. 2017;77:599-613.
6. Jensen RH, Astvad KM, Silva LV, et al. Stepwise emergence of azole, echinocandin and amphotericin B multidrug resistance in vivo in *Candida albicans* orchestrated by multiple genetic alterations. J Antimicrob Chemother. 2015;70:2551-5.
7. Jensen RH. Resistance in human pathogenic yeasts and filamentous fungi: prevalence, underlying molecular mechanisms and link to the use of antifungals in humans and the environment. Dan Med J. 2016;63(10).
8. Kordalewska M, Lee A, Park S, et al. Understanding echinocandin resistance in the emerging pathogen *Candida auris*. Antimicrob Agents Chemother. 2018;62(6).
9. Mesa-Arango AC, Rueda C, Román E, et al. Cell wall changes in amphotericin B-resistant strains from *Candida tropicalis* and relationship with the immune responses elicited by the host. Antimicrob Agents Chemother. 2016;60:2326-35.
10. Rueda C, Cuenca-Estrella M, Zaragoza O. Paradoxical growth of *Candida albicans* in the presence of caspofungin is associated with multiple cell wall rearrangements and decreased virulence. Antimicrob Agents Chemother. 2014;58:1071-83.
11. Vanden Bossche H, Dromer F, Improvisi I, et al. Antifungal drug resistance in pathogenic fungi. Med Mycol. 1998;36(Suppl 1):119.
12. Vermeulen E, Lagrou K, Verweij PE. Azole resistance in *Aspergillus fumigatus*: a growing public health concern. Curr Opin Infect Dis. 2013;26:493-500.
13. Vermeulen E, Maertens J, De Bel A, et al. Nationwide surveillance of azole resistance in *Aspergillus* diseases. Antimicrob Agents Chemother. 2015;59:4569-76.
14. Verweij PE, Chowdhary A, Melchers WJ, et al. Azole resistance in *Aspergillus fumigatus*: Can we retain the clinical use of mold-active antifungal azoles? Clin Infect Dis. 2016;62:362-8.

SPECIFIC FUNGAL INFECTIONS

15

Candidiasis

Monica Mahajan, Rajeev Upreti

■ INTRODUCTION

Candidiasis is a fungal infection caused by yeasts of the genus *Candida*. *Candida* is the dominant genus responsible for fungal diseases in humans. Although over 20 species of *Candida* infect humans, the most common opportunistic fungal pathogen is *Candida albicans*. *Candida* is a normal commensal of skin, mucous membranes, and gastrointestinal (GI) tract in 70% of the population; however, overgrowth of the yeast causes infection. The three major forms of the disease are oropharyngeal candidiasis, vulvovaginal candidiasis (VVC), and invasive candidiasis. *Candida* can exist as a yeast, mycelial/pseudohyphal and chlamydospore phase. The normal desquamation and regeneration of the intact healthy skin is an important defense mechanism. A breakdown in the immune processes results in opportunistic infection by the yeast. Symptoms of candidiasis depend on the area of the body that is infected.

■ MORPHOLOGY

Candida belongs to the phylum Ascomycota and class Saccharomycetes. About 95% cases of candidiasis are due to these species: *C. albicans*, *C. tropicalis*, *C. glabrata*, *C. dubliniensis*, and *C. parapsilosis*. *Candida* is a polymorphic fungus. It has several different morphological forms ranging from unicellular budding yeast to pseudohyphae and hyphae. The pathogenic form is an ovoid-shaped budding yeast with parallel-walled true hyphae. The yeast form is important for dissemination and hyphal form for adhesion, invasion, and proteolytic activity. The pseudohyphal form is intermediate between yeast and hyphae. The factors impacting the morphology include temperature, pH, carbon dioxide levels, starvation, and quorum-sensing molecules, such as tyrosol. In 5–10% cases, multiple *Candida* species can be isolated from a single specimen (Table 15.1).

■ TRANSMISSION

Candida albicans is transmitted from mother to infant during childbirth and becomes part of the normal microflora. *Candida* colonizes in oropharyngeal cavity of 31–60% healthy adults and is found in 40–65% of normal stool samples. Overgrowth of this reservoir of microflora

Table 15.1: Characteristics of *Candida* species.

Species	Teleomorph	Natural habitat	Culture characteristics	Antifungal resistance	Industrial use
Candida albicans (*Candida stellatoidea*)	None	Normal flora of mucous membrane and GI tract	Colonies cream, glistening (Fig. 15.4) or sometimes waxy, soft and smooth; some strains—wrinkled. Forms hyphae in liquid culture in the presence of sera—"germ tube test"	Fully susceptible, azole resistance in wild-type isolates. Resistance to flucytosine after exposure. Echinocandin and AmB resistance rare	■ Removal of textile dyes before discharge of industrial effluents. ■ To degrade phenol compounds and formaldehyde
Candida glabrata	None	Human saprophyte, found in baker's yeast, birch wood, orange and passion fruit juice	■ Colonies cream colored, soft, smooth, glossy. ■ Does not produce hyphae/pseudohyphae. ■ Reproduces by budding	■ Develops secondary resistance to fluconazole—avoid using in infections by this species. ■ Exception Candida glabrata UTI	Biosurfactant agent
Candida krusei	*Issatchenkia orientalis*	Atmosphere, soil, sewage, fruits, and foodstuffs	■ Rough, white to yellow, matt appearance ■ Only species that can grow in vitamin-free media	■ Inherently resistant to fluconazole ■ Reduced susceptibility to AmB. Acquired resistance to itraconazole and voriconazole	Wine and chocolate production
Candida parapsilosis	Three groups: *Candida parapsilosis*; *Candida orthopsilosis*; *Candida metapsilosis*	■ Human commensal mucosa, skin, nails. Insects, domestic and marine animals. ■ Physical surfaces in hospitals	Pin-like colonies on CHROMagar. White, cream, and smooth on SAB and Columbia horse blood agar	■ Less susceptible to echinocandins. ■ Occasional acquired resistance to azoles	Stereospecific synthesis of chiral alcohols
Candida tropicalis	None	Seawater, marine fish, algae, fruits, feces, soil	Colonies cream-colored or off-white to gray, dull, smooth, soft and creamy, or wrinkled or rough. Absent terminal chlamydospores	Generally susceptible to all	Production of long-chain dicarboxylic acids and xylitol

AmB, amphotericin B; GI, gastrointestinal; UTI, urinary tract infection.

causes symptoms. There is no animal vector. Invasive candidiasis occurs when the pathogen from the commensal population enters the blood stream. Hospital outbreaks occur in immunocompromised individuals when they acquire infection from healthcare workers. It is the fourth leading cause of nosocomial bloodstream infections. *Candida* infection rarely spreads through the sexual route. Imbalances in the environment promote fungal growth. Antibiotic use eliminates the bacterial competition and is one of the most important mechanisms for increasing *Candida* population. It decreases the amount of lactobacillus bacteria which in turn decreases the pH of the vagina. About 75% women will experience at least one episode of VVC in their lifetime with almost 50% recurrence rate. Pregnancy, uncontrolled diabetes, and impaired immunity promote *Candida* infection. The incidence is very high in HIV, transplant recipients, chemotherapy, and low-birth-weight (LBW) babies.

VIRULENCE FACTOR FOR *CANDIDA*

Adhesins and Invasins

Apart from polymorphism, other virulence factors include "adhesins" and "invasins." Adhesins are glycosylphosphatidylinositol-linked cell surface glycoproteins that help in adhesion via hydrophobic interactions and biofilm formation. Invasins help *Candida* in invasion of the host epithelial and endothelial cells. Invasin genes also encode for heat-shock proteins mediating binding to host ligands. This induces host cells to engulf fungal pathogen.

Biofilm Formation

Surface-associated *Candida* can grow embedded in extracellular matrix that is composed of carbohydrates and proteins and is referred to as a biofilm. *Candida* forms biofilms by adhering to the surface of catheters, intrauterine devices, and mucous membranes. This protects the yeast from neutrophil attack and deters the formation of reactive oxygen species. Hyphae develop on the upper part of the biofilm forming a more resistant and mature biofilm. This increases the virulence of the fungus. The biofilm among individual *Candida* strains can differ greatly, and urinary isolates can be differentiated into low and high biofilm formers.

Hydrolases

The main classes of hydrolases secreted by *Candida* are proteases, lipases, and phospholipases. These assist in the penetration of the yeast into the host cell and uptake of nutrients from the environment.

Metabolic Adaptation

Candida is part of the normal gut microbiome due to easy access to nutrients. When the yeast encounters a hostile gut environment, it undergoes metabolic adaptation by glycolysis, gluconeogenesis, and starvation response. In the case of candidemia, the fungus relies on the high glucose levels in the bloodstream for its nutrition. Starvation response comes into play to resist phagocytosis by macrophages and damage by reactive oxygen species (ROS).

Host Immune Responses

Candida albicans manages to exist as a commensal on the mucosal surfaces by evading the host's immunological surveillance. The innate and adaptive immune systems play a role in the clearing of the yeast. Th-1 cells produce cytokines that activate phagocytosis. On the contrary, Th-2 cells appear to be producing cytokines that turn off the fungicidal capabilities of Th-1 cells. Neutrophils have an essential immunoregulatory role by releasing important cytokines, such as interleukin (IL)-10 and IL-12. Neutropenic patients have high risks for fungal infection. *C. albicans* elicits two different responses by dendritic cells when phagocytozed in yeast or hyphal form, respectively. Whenever yeast cells are phagocytozed, dendritic cells produce a typical antifungal immune response, whereas hyphal cells are able to break out of the phagosome of dendritic cells. Interferon-γ can inhibit the transformation of *Candida* blastoconidia to the more invasive hyphal phase. Since the CD4+ T-cell response is the normal GI defense mechanism against *Candida*, patients with low CD4+ cell count have a higher incidence of oropharyngeal and esophageal candidiasis.

▉ PREDISPOSING FACTORS FOR CANDIDAL INFECTIONS IN CRITICAL CARE PATIENTS

- Number and duration of antibiotics
- Parenteral feeding
- Use of multiple invasive devices
- The length of intensive care unit (ICU) stay
- Acute Physiology and Chronic Health Evaluation II Score (APACHE II-Score)
- Mechanical ventilation

Candida auris

Candida auris is a budding yeast that almost never forms pseudohyphae or germ tubes. It grows well at 40–42°C on CHROMagar to form white, pink, or red colonies. *C. auris* is emerging as a global threat because of the following reasons:

- It is often multidrug resistant.
- It is difficult to identify by standard laboratory techniques and is often misidentified.
- It has been responsible for hospital outbreaks and needs to be quickly curtailed once identified.

The infection was first described in Japan in 2009 but retrospectively detected in South Korea in 1996. Countries where *C. auris* transmission has been identified include United States, Canada, Israel, India, Pakistan, South Africa, Kenya, Kuwait, United Kingdom, and Venezuela. Approximately 54% of *C. auris* have been isolated from bloodstream, while the remaining cases were identified but not limited to urine, sputum, bile, and wounds. *C. auris* should not only be identified as a species from sterile sites, including blood and cerebrospinal fluid (CSF) but also from nonsterile sites. Even if *C. auris* can be causing colonization in nonsterile sites, infection control measures need to be implemented. Colonization can persist for even longer than a year. When a case of *C. auris* has been isolated from a healthcare facility, species identification must be performed on isolates from nonsterile sites for at least the next 1 month to determine further transmission. The traditional phenotypic yeast identification systems, including VITEK 2 YST, API 20C, BD Phoenix, and Microscan, misidentify *C. auris* as *Candida haemulonii, Candida duobushaemulonii, Candida sake, Candida famata, Candida guilliermondii, Candida lusitaniae, C. parapsilosis*, etc.

The last three species make pseudohyphae on cornmeal agar, and absence of pseudohyphae on cornmeal agar should raise suspicion of *C. auris*. Matrix assisted laser-desorption / ionisation time-of flight (MALDI-TOF) can distinguish *C. auris* from other species. Antifungal susceptibility testing helps in identifying resistance. Susceptibility breakpoints have not been determined for *C. auris*. There has been 90% fluconazole, 30% amphotericin B (AmB), and 5% echinocandin resistance noted with *C. auris*.

▮ CLINICAL MANIFESTATIONS OF CANDIDIASIS (TABLE 15.2)

Mucocutaneous Candidiasis

Mucocutaneous candidiasis can be divided into nongenital disease and genitourinary disease. Oropharyngeal candidiasis is the most common form of nongenital involvement, while VVC is the most frequent form of genitourinary candidiasis.

Intertrigo

Intertrigo is the superficial infection of the moist skin folds in the groin, armpits, and under the breasts caused by *Candida*. The predisposing factors for intertrigo include the following:
- Hot and damp environment of skin folds
- Increased friction in skin folds
- Immunocompromised state

Table 15.2: Clinical manifestations of candidiasis.	
Local mucocutaneous infections	*Chronic disseminated/hepatosplenic candidiasis*
• Intertrigo • Paronychia and onychomycosis • Oral • esophageal • Chronic mucocutaneous • Respiratory—laryngitis, tracheobronchitis, and pneumonia • Genitourinary—vulvovaginal, balanitis, candiduria, and UTI	*Candidemia* • *Candida* endocarditis • Suppurative thrombophlebitis *Disseminated candidiasis* • Endophthalmitis • Meningitis • Renal • Musculoskeletal • Peritonitis and intra-abdominal • Pericarditis and myocarditis • Mediastinitis • Intrauterine
UTI, urinary tract infection.	

- Occlusive clothing and footwear
- Hyperhidrosis
- Obesity
- Diabetes mellitus
- HIV
- Corticosteroid and chemotherapy use.

The patient presents with a pruritic rash. It begins with vesiculopustules that ultimately lead to macerated erythematous, fissured base surrounded by a scaly white rim of necrotic epidermis. Satellite papules or pustules are hallmark of *Candida* infection. Infants may develop diaper dermatitis. *Candida* can involve the toe webs similar to dermatophytes, resulting in "athlete's foot." Interdigital candidiasis may involve the hands.

Differential diagnosis includes *Tinea cruris*, seborrheic or atopic dermatitis, flexural psoriasis, impetigo, and herpes simplex infection.

Management includes maintaining cool and moisture-free skin, using drying agents, such as talcum powder, diabetes control, avoiding tight clothing, and weight loss. Topical antifungals such as clotrimazole cream are first line of treatment. More severe cases may require fluconazole or itraconazole.

Paronychia and Onychomycosis (Figs. 15.1 and 15.2)

It is a multifactorial inflammatory reaction of the proximal nail fold to allergens and irritants. It is commonly seen when hands are immersed in water for long period, especially while cooking and washing. There is damage to the cuticle which exposes the nail fold and the nail groove. *Candida* is often isolated in chronic cases of paronychia. There is a painful,

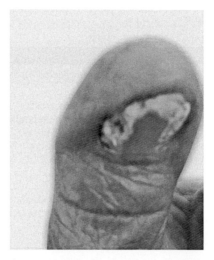

Fig. 15.1: *Distal and lateral onychomycosis:* White discoloration and hyperkeratosis of toe nail.

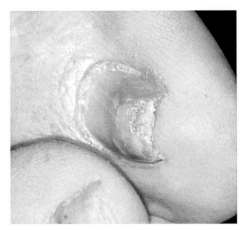

Fig. 15.2: *Distal onychomycosis:* Yellow discoloration and onycholysis of toenail.

erythematous swelling of the nail fold along with extension beneath the nail. Nail plate may show thickening and longitudinal grooving. Pitting and hypertrophy can be present due to involvement of the nail matrix. There can be pus discharge, discoloration, and loss of nail. Although antifungals have been the mainstay of treatment, topical steroids have been found to be more effective. Surgical treatment includes en bloc excision of the proximal nail fold or an eponychial marsupialization. A new surgical technique called Swiss roll technique has the advantage of retaining the nail plate and allows rapid healing without creating a defect in the skin.

Oral Candidiasis (Table 15.3)

Oral candidiasis has been described since the time of Hippocrates. It is also known as moniliasis, oral thrush, or candidosis and is the most common opportunistic infection of oral mucosa. It is caused by *C. albicans* but other species including *C. tropicalis, C. glabrata,* or *Candida krusei* may also be responsible for the disease. Predisposing factors include the use of broad-spectrum antibiotics, aerosolized inhaled and systemic corticosteroids, chemotherapeutic agents, radiotherapy, dentures, orthodontic appliances, diabetes, leukemia, lymphoma, HIV, malnutrition, extremes of age-groups, xerostomia, poor oral hygiene, endocrinopathies, pregnancy, and smoking. Over 90% of patients with AIDS will develop oropharyngeal candidiasis at some time during their illness.

Pseudomembranous candidiasis is the prototype of oral mucosal involvement characterized by desquamation of the epithelial cells and formation of pseudomembrane composed of necrotic debris, desquamated cells, and fungal hyphae. These appear as patchy white curd-like plaques or flecks on the mucosal surface. Once the white plaques are cleared off by gentle rubbing or scraping, there is erythema or mild ulceration of the underlying surface of tongue or oral mucosa. There is altered taste and burning sensation in the mouth.

Table 15.3: Classification of oral candidiasis
Acute: Pseudomembranous, erythematous/atrophic
Chronic hyperplastic Candida lesions: Candidal leukoplakia, papillary hyperplasia of palate, nodular variety of median rhomboid glossitis
Chronic atrophic Candida lesions: Denture stomatitis, angular stomatitis, median rhomboid glossitis
Keratinized lesions with secondary Candida infection: Lichen planus, leukoplakia
Candidiasis-associated syndromes: CMC, thymic aplasia, DiGeorge syndrome, HIV
CMC, Chronic mucocutaneous candidiasis; HIV, Human immunodeficiency virus

Acute atrophic candidiasis presents as erythematous, raw, painful mucosal lesions with depapillation of tongue, and minimal evidence of pseudomembrane formation. Patient has oral burning and sore throat after a course of antibiotics. Patients with iron-deficiency anemia may also develop acute atrophic candidiasis.

Chronic atrophic candidiasis includes denture stomatitis, angular cheilitis, and median rhomboid glossitis. There are numerous palatal petechiae, diffuse erythema involving denture covered mucosa and development of tissue granulation, involving the central areas of the hard palate and alveolar ridges. It involves the maxillary denture more than the mandibular denture.

Angular cheilitis or infection of the lip commissures generally coexists with denture stomatitis.

Median rhomboid glossitis is characterized by erythematous patches of atrophic papillae on the central area of dorsum of the tongue. When these lesions become nodular, it is called hyperplastic median rhomboid glossitis.

Candidal leukoplakia is a form of chronic hyperplastic candidiasis where firm leathery white hyperplastic plaques can be present on the cheeks, lips, palate, or tongue.

Chronic multifocal candidiasis presents with multiple areas of atrophic candidiasis.

Differential diagnosis includes hairy leukoplakia and lichen planus.

Microscopic examination of the lesion reveals inflammation, ulceration, and a fibrinoid exudate containing hyphae and pseudohyphae.

Severe oral candidiasis may result in impaired quality of life with poor food and liquid intake. If left untreated, it extends to the esophagus.

Esophageal Candidiasis

Candida is the most common cause of infectious esophagitis. The incidence of *Candida* esophagitis has increased mainly due to its association with HIV. However, the frequent use of screening endoscopy has led to more frequent diagnosis of esophageal candidiasis in healthy individuals. The organism identified from the esophageal surface is the same as the organism identified in oral secretions. Esophageal candidiasis develops as a two-step process consisting of colonization of the esophagus and subsequent invasion of the epithelial layer. *Candida* is known to colonize the esophagus of 20% of healthy adults. HIV infection, hematological or solid organ malignancy, impaired immunity, proton pump inhibitors, H_2-receptor antagonists, antibiotic use, corticosteroids, functional or mechanical obstruction of esophagus, and prior vagotomy increase the risk.

The patient presents with dysphagia, odynophagia, and retrosternal pain. Occasionally, the patient can be asymptomatic. The distal two-thirds of the esophagus are involved more frequently than the upper one-third. Diagnosis is made on the basis of direct visualization of the esophagus by endoscopy and histological evidence of tissue invasion by the fungus. The differential diagnosis includes viral esophagitis due to cytomegalovirus or herpes simplex virus, idiopathic HIV ulcers, and gastroesophageal reflux disease (GERD).

Chronic Mucocutaneous Candidiasis

Chronic mucocutaneous candidiasis (CMC) is a rare genetic syndrome that manifests in childhood. There is chronic and persistent involvement of the skin, nails, and mucosal sites due to widespread *Candida* infection. CMC occurs due to an impairment of cell-mediated immune response against *Candida*. It is associated with a heterogeneous group of autoimmune, genetic, and endocrine disorders.

- The disorder may have an autosomal dominant or autosomal recessive inheritance. Autosomal dominant CMC is associated with gain-of-function signal transducer and activator of transcription 1 mutations resulting in IL-17 deficiency.
- Chronic mucocutaneous candidiasis is associated with autoimmune polyendocrinopathy-candidosis–ectodermal dystrophy; in which, there is mutation of the *AIRE* (autoimmune regulator gene on 21q22.3) gene which encodes a protein to maintain tolerance in the thymus. This is more prevalent in the Jewish population.
- Endocrinopathies associated with CMC include hypothyroidism, hypoparathyroidism, diabetes mellitus, Addison disease, thymomas, dental dysplasia, and antibodies to melanin-producing cells.
- There can be defects in T-cell functioning as is seen in DiGeorge syndrome.
- Rarely, CMC may develop in adults in association with a thymoma, myasthenia gravis, aplastic anemia, alopecia areata, vitiligo, biliary cirrhosis, idiopathic thrombocytopenic purpura, pernicious anemia, neutropenia, or hypogammaglobulinemia.
- HIV and hyperimmunoglobulin E syndrome may present with CMC.

The clinical features include recurrent or persistent superficial candidiasis presenting as chronic white adherent plaques of oral thrush, angular cheilitis, diaper dermatitis, paronychia and onychomycosis, crusted hyperkeratotic plaques on the scalp or hands or feet, granulomas in the mouth/skin/nails, scarring alopecia, esophageal or laryngeal or vaginal stenosis, tympanic membrane calcification, dental enamel hypoplasia, and iron deficiency. Nails are discolored, thickened, and fragmented with erythematous periungual skin.

Despite having a protracted course, there is very little tendency to disseminate. Life expectancy is normal in most patients. Complications include secondary bacterial sepsis, pneumonia, mycotic aneurysms, and premature death. Infection with *Staphylococcus aureus* is common in CMC. Certain malignancies including ear, nose, throat and esophageal cancers and skin cancers may have a higher incidence in patients with CMC. Patients can be more prone to human papilloma virus (HPV), warts and *Pneumocystis jirovecii* pneumonia.

Diagnosis is made on the basis of clinical features, microscopy, and culture of skin scrapings. Additional tests conducted in patients with CMC include thyroid function tests, glycosylated hemoglobin, liver function test, corticotrophin testing and serum cortisol levels, short synacthen test, parathormone levels, follicle-stimulating hormone, luteinising hormone, complete blood count, and enzyme-linked immunosorbent assay for HIV. The differential diagnosis includes cutaneous candidiasis, DiGeorge syndrome, mucosal candidiasis, and pediatric severe combined immunodeficiency (SCID).

Respiratory Tract Candidiasis

Candida Laryngitis

Laryngeal fungal infection is a rare clinical entity. *Candida* species are the most common cause. Other fungi which may cause laryngitis include *Histoplasma, Blastomyces, Aspergillus,* etc. Candidal infection of the larynx may occur after pulmonary, pharyngeal and esophageal candidiasis, or as part of disseminated disease. The three typical patterns of fungal laryngitis are follows:

- Focal thick, whitish lesions involving one or both vocal folds with hoarseness of voice as the primary symptom.
- Diffuse mucosal involvement of the larynx and occasionally hypopharynx with hoarseness, pain, and dysphagia.
- Acute epiglottitis with airway embarrassment and respiratory distress.

The symptoms are gradual in onset. Endoscopy of the larynx shows white patchy lesions of *Candida* which may form a pseudomembrane in the glottis. At times, the supraglottic larynx, pyriform fossa, and the posterior pharyngeal wall are involved. The vocal folds can be involved in isolation. The lesions may mimic premalignant or malignant lesions of the larynx and sometimes may result in unnecessary surgical interventions. Fungal stains and culture of swabs from plaques can be performed. Treatment involves oral antifungal therapy and the removal of predisposing factors. Asthmatic patients should be instructed to lower the frequency of inhaled steroids, use spacers, and rinse the mouth after inhaler use.

Candida Tracheobronchitis

It is an uncommon form of invasive candidiasis where *Candida* invades the bronchial mucosa and causes fever, cough with expectoration, and dyspnea. There can be patchy exudates in the tracheobronchial tree, and histopathology confirms the presence of *Candida*.

Fungal bronchitis should be considered in patients with chronic sputum production or mucous plugging, especially in patients whose symptoms and findings do not resolve with antibiotic therapy and have fungi on sputum smear or culture.

Candida Pneumonia

It is a rare infection of the lungs and is most commonly seen as part of disseminated candidiasis. There is airspace opacification due to infection by *Candida*. Since the pathogen is normally present as part of the oropharyngeal flora, the diagnosis is challenging and requires endobronchial or transthoracic biopsy. A positive culture can be consistent with a pathogen or can be a contaminant. Three histologic patterns of pulmonary candidiasis include embolic/arterial invasive pulmonary candidiasis, disseminated/capillary invasive pulmonary candidiasis, and bronchopulmonary/airspace invasive pulmonary candidiasis.

Candida pneumonia radiologically resembles other forms of pneumonia. There is no specific clinical or radiological presentation. There can be multifocal patchy airspace opacification without a zonal predilection. Focal cavitation may develop. Computed tomography (CT) scan can vary depending on the pathological pattern. Apart from the findings similar to those on plain film, CT scan may also reveal small pulmonary abscesses or a miliary nodular pattern. The nodules range from 3 mm to 30 mm in diameter and tend to be multiple. These can be in association with tree-in-bud changes, ground-glass opacities, and air-space consolidation. Sometimes there can be a halo sign around the nodules. *Candida* pneumonia has a high morbidity and is often fatal. The incidence of *Candida* isolation from pulmonary biopsies in critically ill, mechanically ventilated, non-neutropenic patients who die is high. However, definite *Candida* pneumonia established by histopathology is much less. In one series, the incidence of *Candida* isolation from pulmonary biopsies was 40%, whereas the incidence of definite *Candida* pneumonia was 8%. Therefore, the presence of *Candida* in lung cultures is a frequent event in critically ill patients who die in the ICU but does not represent *Candida* pneumonia.

Genitourinary Tract Candidiasis

Vulvovaginal Candidiasis (VVC)

- "Colonization" of the vagina is defined as the presence of *Candida* in the vagina in the absence of immunosuppression, damaged mucosa, or signs of disease.
- "VVC" is defined as signs and symptoms of inflammation in the presence of *Candida* species and in the absence of other infectious etiology.
- "Uncomplicated VVC" is the sporadic or infrequent occurrence of mild-to-moderate VVC in immunocompetent females.
- "Complicated VVC" includes severe VVC, non-*albicans Candida* VVC, infection during pregnancy, uncontrolled diabetes or immunosuppression with VVC, or recurrent VVC (RVVC).
- "RVVC" is defined as at least four episodes of VVC during 1 year. These patients may have up to 50% recurrence after the discontinuation of suppressive therapy.

Risk factors for VVC include frequent sexual intercourse, receptive oral sex, high-estrogen oral contraceptives, spermicides, antibiotic use, uncontrolled diabetes, and genetic predisposition. Antibiotic use alters the microflora of the GI tract and vagina and allows for the overgrowth of *Candida*. Reduction in lactobacilli in the vaginal tract predisposes women to VVC. Lactobacilli play a vital role in protection against pathogenic invasion by producing hydrogen peroxide, bacteriocins, and lactic acid. Most episodes of VVC occur in the reproductive age-group and are rare in the premenstrual or postmenopausal age-groups. VVC is associated with increased vaginal shedding of HIV virus.

VVC presents as pruritus and burning in the vagina associated with soreness and irritation leading to dysuria and dyspareunia. On physical examination, findings include vulval and vaginal edema, erythema, fissures, and thick curdy white discharge. The differential diagnoses include bacterial vaginosis, trichomoniasis, gonorrhea, and *Chlamydia* infection. Symptoms cause distress and altered self-esteem. Yeast cells and hyphae are seen on a wet mount vaginal culture which helps in species identification. CHROMagar *Candida* is a selective fungal medium that includes chromogenic substances allowing for quick identification of different *Candida* species based on their color.

Candidal Balanitis

Candidal balanitis is defined as the inflammation of the glans penis due to *Candida* species in the absence of other infectious etiology. When the prepuce is also involved, it is called balanoposthitis. The glans penis can be asymptomatically colonized with *Candida* species. The predisposing factors include diabetes, immunosuppression, and being uncircumcised. Poor hygiene and accumulation of smegma make uncircumcised men more prone to candidal balanitis. Candidal balanitis is sexually acquired. Patients complain of penile pruritus and local burning. Diagnosis is based on clinical examination. Vesicles on the penis develop into patches of whitish exudate. There is erythema with papules and pustules. The adhesive tape method is better than swab for microscopy and culture.

Candiduria

The definition of candiduria is not precise and mostly relies on the microscopic visualization of *Candida* in urine and culture of urine. Colony forming unit (CFU) criteria to diagnose candiduria range from 1,000 CFU/mL to 100,000 CFU/mL urine. Standard bacterial culture techniques are less sensitive in recovering *Candida* species. Variable cutoff definitions and unreliable culture techniques create confusion in the analysis of candiduria. Hospitalized patients have a high incidence of candiduria linked to antibiotic usage. The incidence is higher in ICUs and burns units. *C. albicans* is the most common nosocomial pathogen associated with urinary tract infection (UTI). Fungal UTI is more frequent in catheterized patients. *C. albicans* accounts for 50–70% of all *Candida*-related urinary isolates, followed by *C. glabrata* and *C. tropicalis*. In neonates, *C. parapsilosis* is dominantly responsible for candiduria.

Predisposing factors include extremes of age, female gender, antibiotic usage, diabetes, neutropenia, indwelling urinary catheter, obstructive uropathy, anatomic urinary tract abnormalities, abdominal surgery, ICU admission, and renal transplant. Fluconazole use is associated with *C. glabrata*-mediated candiduria.

Urinary Tract Infection

Fungal UTI is mostly asymptomatic. Most patients do not develop fever or dysuria. Some patients with pyelonephritis may have fever, chills, renal angle tenderness, and hematuria. Leukocyturia is absent in candiduria. Candiduria can result in uncomplicated cystitis and/ or pyelonephritis due to ascending infection. A very small percentage of patients develop candidemia with incidence being higher in the ICU setting. Concomitant fungal septicemia develops only in a minority of patients. Prostatitis and epididymitis can also result in candiduria. Some patients may develop an abscess in the tissue. A rare manifestation of candiduria is pneumaturia consequent to emphysematous tissue invasion or perinephric abscess formation. Fungal ball or bezoars may form due to the accumulation of fungal hyphae in the renal pelvis and lead to intermittent urinary tract obstruction.

CHRONIC DISSEMINATED CANDIDIASIS/HEPATOSPLENIC CANDIDIASIS

Hepatosplenic candidiasis is a very rare disease and yet is the most frequent form of chronic disseminated candidiasis. Most cases have been documented in patients with hematologic malignancy, who are recovering from neutropenia. It has been reported in acute leukemia, lymphoma, aplastic anemia, and sarcoma. It is characteristically seen in patients with long-lasting neutropenia defined by more than 10 days of absolute neutrophil counts (ANC) below 500/mL. This causes a breach in mucosal integrity resulting in spread of *Candida* species from the GI tract into the bloodstream. Intravascular catheters and administration of broad-spectrum antibiotics predispose to the infection. Since the portal system receives the highest load of the fungus, the liver and spleen are predominantly involved. Rare cases have been reported in non-neutropenic patients as well. Acute and chronic disseminated candidiasis is differentiated by the presence or absence of sepsis syndrome, respectively. The incidence of hepatosplenic candidiasis has reduced due to the early initiation of empiric antifungal therapy in neutropenic patients. Therefore, patients who do not receive antifungal prophylaxis or are on extended courses of corticosteroids are more likely candidates for the disease. The fungi most commonly isolated are *C. albicans, C. tropicalis, C. parapsilosis, C. glabrata,* and *C. krusei.*

Most patients with long-lasting neutropenia will experience at least one febrile episode which resolves after the neutropenia recovers. A persisting, high-spiking fever just beginning after the recovery of ANC in a previously afebrile patient should raise suspicion for hepatosplenic candidiasis. Other accompanying symptoms include right upper abdominal pain, diarrhea, anorexia, nausea, vomiting, and occasionally jaundice. The clinical symptoms are a result of fungal abscesses and immune reconstitution inflammatory syndrome (IRIS).

Laboratory findings may show a pattern of more than threefold increased serum alkaline phosphatase with deranged liver function tests. These abnormalities may persist for many months. In hepatosplenic candidiasis, blood cultures can be sterile. A potential explanation for the low blood culture yield can be that hematogenous invasion is limited to the portal vasculature without dissemination into the venous blood elsewhere. *Candida* can be positive in biopsies but blood cultures are often negative. Biopsy reveals multiple granulomas with yeast and hyphal forms.

If chronic disseminated candidiasis cannot be proven by biopsy, imaging is important to define "probable" hepatosplenic candidiasis. Ultrasound, CT, or magnetic resonance imaging (MRI) scans detect multiple microabscesses in the liver, spleen, and occasionally the kidney. MRI is more sensitive, whereas CT scan is a less expensive modality to diagnose the infection. Lesion enhancement pattern differs for acute, subacute, and chronic stage of disease. The most sensitive CT phase for liver involvement in the acute stage is the arterial phase, i.e. 25-35 seconds after injection of contrast. It shows a hyperattenuating rim surrounding a hypoattenuating center giving a "bull's eye" appearance. In the portal venous phase, i.e. 60–80 s after the injection of contrast, microabscesses appear as hypoattenuating lesions of approximately 1-cm diameter. Initially hypodense lesions in the acute phase on nonenhanced CT can become hyperdense secondary to hemorrhage or calcification in the subacute or chronic stage of the disease. Differential diagnoses include lymphoma, leukemic infiltrates, and metastases. A typical ultrasound phenotype of hepatic candidiasis is the bull's eye or target pattern with a peripheral hypoechoic halo encircling a central hyperechoic core. Contrast-enhanced ultrasound (CEUS) with sulfur hexafluoride contrast shows a late-phase washout, i.e. 90–240 s after injection. In the arterial phase, i.e. 5–25 s after injection, lesions often have a hyperechoic rim enhancement with a growing central washout in the portal venous and late phase. Sometimes, the lesions exhibit an isoechoic rim enhancement; others may be hypoechoic in all contrast phases without any peripheral rim enhancement. Advantages of CEUS are a bedside examination and absence of nephrotoxicity and radiation exposure.

Systemic Candidiasis

Systemic candidiasis comprises two distinct syndromes:
1. Candidemia
2. Disseminated candidiasis.
Invasive candidiasis can be divided into three subgroups:
1. Candidemia without deep-seated or visceral involvement
2. Candidemia with deep-seated or visceral *Candida* infection
3. Deep-seated or visceral candidiasis without candidemia.

Risk Factors for Systemic Candidiasis

- *Neutropenia and bone marrow transplant recipients:* Neutrophils are a major defense mechanism against candidiasis. Neutropenia, functional impairment of bone marrow, loss of mucosal integrity while on chemotherapy, and the use of broad-spectrum antibiotics make these patients more prone to systemic candidiasis. Use of antifungal prophylaxis in the past few decades has resulted in increased incidence of non-*albicans* candidiasis.
- *Solid organ transplant recipients:* Impairment of T-cell immunity leads to increased mucosal and cutaneous candidiasis in these patients. Breakthrough *Candida* infection can be due to fluconazole-resistant strains.
- *Nonsurgical critically ill patients:* Patients with multiorgan failure are not only on broad-spectrum antibiotics but also have indwelling intravascular catheters, endotracheal tubes, Foley's catheters, and nasogastric tubes which are colonized by *Candida* species. *Candida* has a tendency to form biofilms on these surfaces. This results in catheter-associated *Candida* infections even in the absence of severe immune compromise.
- *Critically ill abdominal surgery patients:* Any perforation of abdominal viscera will contaminate the peritoneal cavity with bowel flora. Recurrent peritonitis, anastomotic leakage, or nonfunctional bowel results in the progression of *Candida* colonization to invasive candidiasis. Prolonged antibiotic use, septic shock, and multiorgan failure

precipitates the infection. Peritonitis or intra-abdominal abscess secondary to invasive candidiasis is defined by one of the culture criteria from specimens obtained at surgery:

◆ Monomicrobial growth of *Candida* species.
◆ Any amount of *Candida* species growth in a mixed-flora abscess.
◆ Moderate-to-heavy growth of *Candida* species in a mixed-flora peritonitis which has been treated with appropriate antibiotics as per culture sensitivity.

Some studies do suggest the role of antifungal prophylaxis in patients of anastomotic leakage to prevent the development of invasive candidiasis.

Fungal infection develops in 10% of patients with necrotizing pancreatitis not treated with antibiotics. This is due to progressive colonization of the bowel and translocation of the fungus into necrotic tissue.

■ *Critically ill with respiratory colonization:* Mechanically ventilated patients have colonization with *Candida,* and true *Candida* pneumonia is rare. *Candida* has low affinity for alveolar pneumocytes. Most of the patients with lung involvement are secondary to hematogenous spread of *Candida* leading to fungal abscesses. Isolation of *Candida* from respiratory tract is considered colonization and does not warrant treatment unless histology shows fungal pneumonia.

Candida Colonization Index

Candida colonization index (CI) is defined as the ratio of the number of distinct nonblood body sites colonized by *Candida* species to the total number of body sites cultured. Blood culture is not considered. The *Candida* species isolated from each site should be genetically identical.

Both exogenous nosocomial and endogenous colonization of *Candida* can coexist in the same individual but most invasive candidiasis infections are due to endogenous colonization. Contaminated solutions and hands of health-care workers are exogenous sources.

Colonization index = Number of sites colonized/number of sites cultured

Use of the CI: In patients perceived to be at a higher risk of developing invasive candidiasis, twice-weekly surveillance culture of the following sites is done:

■ Oropharynx swab or tracheal secretions
■ Urine sample
■ Perineal swab or stool sample
■ Gastric fluid
■ Surgical wound swab or abdominal drain fluid
■ Catheter insertion sites

The corrected CI takes into account the amount of *Candida* species measured by semiquantitative cultures. Patients with a CI >0.5 can be empirically treated with antifungals. The limitation of CI is the limited bedside practicality and expenditure involved.

GI tract is normally colonized by *Candida,* and isolation of yeast from stool does not require treatment.

Candidemia

Candidemia is defined as the presence of *Candida* species in blood. *Candida* species are responsible for most Invasive fungal infection (IFI) in humans and the fourth most common pathogen isolated from the blood stream. The prevalence worldwide has been reported at 6.9 per 1,000 ICU patients. This nosocomial blood stream infection is not restricted to patients with hematological malignancy but is also being reported in ICUs, organ transplant recipients, internal medicine wards, LBW babies, patients on parenteral nutrition, indwelling catheters and devices, and abdominal surgery patients.

The three major routes by which *Candida* species enter the bloodstream are as follows:
1. Through the GI mucosal barrier
2. Via an intravascular catheter, especially central venous catheter (CVC). *Candida* colonization can be at either the insertion site or the hub leading to candidemia.
3. From a localized focus of *Candida* infection, e.g. *Candida* UTI with obstructive uropathy.

Non-*albicans Candida* species, such as *C. glabrata, C. parapsilosis, C. tropicalis,* and *C. krusei,* are more frequently being implicated. Other species responsible for candidemia are *C. lusitaniae, C. guilliermondii,* and *Candida rugosa.* Widespread use of fluconazole is responsible for the emergence of these non-*albicans* strains which are intrinsically resistant to the drug. Bulk consumption of fluconazole has changed the ecology of the fungus. On the other hand, use of fluconazole prophylaxis in appropriate setting like stem cell transplant patients has reduced probability of candidemia in these patients. Early empirical treatment for severe candidiasis has improved survival but is majorly responsible for overuse of antifungals.

The clinical signs and symptoms are nonspecific and may vary from the absence of symptoms to septic shock with hypotension, tachycardia, and tachypnea. Fever is unresponsive to broad-spectrum antibiotics.

The diagnosis is confounded by poor yield on blood cultures (<50%) and more frequent exposure of patients to fluconazole. Patients on fluconazole may develop acquired resistance to the drug and experience drug toxicity. Serological markers such as β-D-glucan aid diagnosis. Echinocandins are the preferred antifungals and will also show efficacy in fluconazole-resistant candidemia. Species identification and susceptibility testing are important in guiding the clinician.

Suppurative thrombophlebitis: This is a form of candidemia associated with prolonged central venous catheterization. It causes fever with sepsis and septic shock despite the removal of catheter, incision and drainage or the resection of the vein and appropriate antifungal therapy. Resection is not possible when central veins are involved.

Candida endocarditis: *Candida* endocarditis (CE) is one of the most serious manifestations of candidiasis. *Candida* is the most common cause of fungal endocarditis, followed by *Aspergillus* species and *Histoplasma capsulatum.* It is seen in patients with candidemia. The major species of *Candida* causing CE include *C. albicans, C. tropicalis,* and *C. glabrata.*

The risk factors predisposing to CE include valvular heart disease, indwelling CVCs, prosthetic heart valves, bacterial endocarditis, intravenous (IV) drug use, chemotherapy, and LBW. Infection of the prosthetic valve can occur at the time of surgery or later.

The patient presents with breathlessness, chest pain, new or changing murmur or features of congestive heart failure. Systemic complaints include fever, malaise, weight loss, and night sweats. Embolic phenomena involve the vessels of the brain, GI tract, and extremities. Fungal vegetations are larger in size and cause arterial embolization more frequently than bacterial vegetations. Other complications include meningitis, osteomyelitis, and endophthalmitis. Classical signs of endocarditis including Osler nodes, Janeway lesions, and Roth spots, may be absent.

Diagnosis of CE is based on blood culture showing candidemia. Echocardiography reveals large valvular vegetations. Transesophageal echocardiography is more sensitive than transthoracic echocardiography in detecting the vegetations.

Disseminated Candidiasis

Disseminated candidiasis involves one or more organs due to dissemination of the infection to the deeper viscera by hematogenous spread. Single or multiple organs may be simultaneously involved. Majority of the patients will have a negative blood culture. It presents as pyrexia of unknown origin with a negative blood culture and unresponsiveness to broad-spectrum antibiotics. Clinical manifestations may include chorioretinitis, skin lesions, or muscle abscesses.

Skin lesions can be clusters of painless pustules or large necrotic nodules. Punch biopsy from these lesions may aid in diagnosis.

Candida endophthalmitis: Almost all the cases of yeast endophthalmitis are due to *Candida* species. Other yeasts including *Cryptococcus* are less frequently implicated. The most common species of *Candida* causing endophthalmitis is *C. albicans*, followed by *C. tropicalis*. Postsurgical outbreaks have been described with *C. parapsilosis* due to its high propensity to survive in irrigation fluid. *Candida* endophthalmitis can be:

- Exogenous—Accidental penetrating trauma or iatrogenic injury to the eye causing fungal inoculation from the environment.
- Endogenous—Hematogenous spread of *Candida* to the eye; it is a marker of disseminated candidiasis.

It may involve the chorioretinal structures or extend to involve the vitreous (vitritis). It is an ophthalmological emergency. The patient may present with progressively diminishing vision, ocular pain, photophobia, scotomas, and floaters. Systemic symptoms may include fever and chills. Fundus examination reveals early pinhead-sized whitish lesions in the posterior vitreous. Vitreous haze may be present. Subsequent larger lesions appear as fluffy white "cotton balls" or "snow balls" or a "string of pearls" and can be multiple, extending from the chorioretinal surface into the vitreous. The degree of vitreous inflammation is graded from 0 to 4. White blood cells may settle at the bottom of aqueous to form a hypopyon or may form an inflammatory membrane in the anterior chamber.

Intraocular samples should be sent for both bacterial and fungal stains and cultures. A fungal stain, such as calcofluor-white, will show fluorescence of the cell wall of yeasts and molds.

Central Nervous System Candidiasis

Exogenous central nervous system (CNS) infections due to *Candida* result from trauma, surgery, craniotomy, ventricular shunt placement, or lumbar puncture. The endogenous CNS involvement is due to hematogenous spread to the brain parenchyma. The infection is most often caused by *C. albicans* but other species, including *C. parapsilosis* and *C. tropicalis*, may also be responsible. *C. glabrata* is rarely isolated. The clinical spectrum of the disease may include meningitis, diffuse cerebritis, microabscesses, mycotic aneurysms, and granulomatous vasculitis.

Patients present with fever, headache, neck stiffness, confusion, obtundation, and altered sensorium. *Candida* meningitis occurs most frequently in premature neonates. Device and shunt infections occur within several months of the surgical procedure and indicate intraoperative contamination rather than hematogenous spread. Shunt malfunction results in increased intracranial pressure. Bacterial meningitis and antibiotic use promotes *Candida* meningitis. Other signs of dissemination may be present, including endophthalmitis, endo-carditis, and pyelonephritis. Chronic *Candida* meningitis is rare and resembles tuberculosis and cryptococcosis. It may cause cranial nerve palsies.

CNS candidiasis is suspected if *Candida* is isolated from the CSF or if CSF shows pleocytosis and *Candida* is isolated from another normally sterile site. Candidemia on blood culture should also raise suspicion of *Candida* meningitis in the appropriate clinical scenario. CSF culture can be positive in approximately 80% cases. There can be a neutrophilic or a lymphocytic pleocytosis. The serum and CSF β-D-glucan can be a useful adjunctive test. CT scan can be normal or may detect hydrocephalus. MRI can detect microabscesses as multiple, small ring-enhancing lesions. These may occasionally have a hemorrhagic component.

Renal Candidiasis

Invasive renal involvement is a consequence of candidemia or disseminated candidiasis. *Candida* species are responsible for most cases of fungal infection of kidney. Other fungi which can involve the kidney as a result of hematogenous dissemination include *Aspergillus*, *Fusarium, Rhizopus, Mucor, Cryptococcus, Trichosporon*, and dimorphic fungi.

Candida infection involving the kidneys can be due to lower UTI ascending to the upper urinary tract or via hematogenous dissemination. The fungus attaches to the endothelial surfaces and penetrates into tissues.

Candiduria is very frequent in ICU patients and may represent colonization, ascending infection, or dissemination of *Candida* to renal tract. The main complications of asymptomatic candiduria are ascending infection and candidemia. Ascending infection occurs in association with obstructive uropathy due to the formation of fungus balls. Perinephric abscess can form. Papillary necrosis and emphysematous pyelonephritis are rare. Involvement is mostly unilateral, involves the renal pelvis and medulla but spares the cortex. The course is subacute or chronic, and fever may be absent. Candidemia secondary to candiduria occurs in patients who have undergone urological procedures or have urinary tract abnormalities/obstruction, prostatic hypertrophy, chronic bladder catheterization, or neurogenic bladder.

In contrast, kidneys are the organ most frequently involved in disseminated candidiasis. There can be other signs and symptoms in addition to candiduria. The renal involvement is bilateral and is characterized by microabscesses in the cortex and medulla of the kidney. The patient may be asymptomatic or may have flank pain and renal angle tenderness. Papillary necrosis provides the required nidus for fungal bezoar formation. CE may cause embolization, vascular involvement, and renal infarction. Neonates may have more severe manifestations, frequent formation of fungal balls, and renal impairment. Identification of fungal casts in urine by periodic acid–Schiff (PAS) or silver stains indicates renal involvement.

Musculoskeletal Candidiasis

The incidence of musculoskeletal involvement due to *Candida* is on the rise due to increased frequency of candidemia and invasive candidiasis. The male:female ratio is >2:1. The patients may not necessarily be neutropenic or immunocompromised. Risk factors in neonates and infants include LBW, necrotizing enterocolitis, and umbilical vein catheterization. *Candida* osteomyelitis may be the first manifestation of invasive candidiasis or may appear in patients who already have candidemia or disseminated candidiasis. It may be diagnosed before the initiation of antifungal therapy or may occur as a breakthrough infection while on antifungal drugs. Bone involvement can be due to hematogenous dissemination (endogenous), direct inoculation (exogenous), and contiguous infection. Direct inoculation can be due to:

- External trauma with open wound or ulcer.
- Intraarticular injection.
- Surgical manipulation or prosthesis implantation.
- Median sternotomy for coronary artery bypass grafting.
- IV drug users may develop septic arthritis along with endophthalmitis and folliculitis.

Coinciding with hematogenous infection, most patients have ≥2 infected bones. Once a single focus is identified, search should be made for other osseous sites of infection. The bones most frequently involved are vertebrae, ribs, sternum, femur, and humerus. Vertebrae are the most common site in adults versus femur in children. The synovial joints most commonly infected are knee, hip, and sacroiliac joint. Patients may have costochondral, costosternal, or costoclavicular joint involvement.

Proven osteomyelitis: Compatible clinical characteristics, consistent radiographic features, and isolation of *Candida* on culture and/or from histology samples of bone or samples from metal hardware obtained by percutaneous biopsy or surgery.

Probable osteomyelitis: Compatible clinical and radiological features along with evidence of positive culture of *Candida* and/or histology from other than bone tissue or metal hardware specimens, including disk, cartilage, adjacent abscess, blood, or synovial fluid.

Most patients present with local pain, tenderness, erythema, and edema. Fever may be absent. The symptoms are insidious and may be present for many weeks or months before the diagnosis is established. This may result in limitation in range of movement, draining pus, sinus tracts, or fracture as a sequel of osteomyelitis. Infection in children begins in the cartilaginous portion of long bones causing destruction and growth retardation.

There can be a concomitant bacterial and fungal infection highlighting the need for biopsy and cultures. Even a scanty growth of *Candida* on biopsy or synovial fluid is pathological. *S. aureus* and other bacteria can be identified on mixed cultures. Biopsy can be percutaneous, closed, guided, or open biopsy at the time of surgery. Non-*albicans Candida* including *C. glabrata*, *C. tropicalis*, and *C. parapsilosis* are being frequently isolated as a cause of fungal osteomyelitis. *Candida* arthritis can concomitantly occur. Markers of inflammation, such as erythrocyte sedimentation rate, C-reactive protein, and leukocyte count, may show a mild-to-moderate rise.

The radiological findings include bone erosion or destruction and involvement of surrounding tissue. There can be reduction in articular space, bone abscess, or sequestrum. Spine involvement on MRI reveals decrease in intervertebral space, epidural abscess, paraspinal or psoas abscess, or spinal cord compression. Compared to bacterial osteomyelitis, *Candida* involvement tends to be multifocal and spares the intervertebral disks. MRI shows decreased signal intensity on T1-weighted image and increased signal intensity on T2-weighted image. There is increased uptake on radionuclide scan.

Differential diagnoses include tuberculosis, bacterial osteomyelitis, and metastasis to bones.

Candida Peritonitis and Intra-abdominal Infections

Candida peritonitis develops as a consequence of abdominal surgery, viscus perforation, fecal peritonitis, anastomotic leak after bowel surgery, necrotizing pancreatitis or continuous peritoneal dialysis in patients with End-stage renal disease (ESRD). Multiple antibiotics and diabetes increase the risk. It can be a component of a polymicrobial infection.

Other intra-abdominal infections caused by *Candida* include gangrenous cholecystitis, common bile duct obstruction by a fungal bezoar, or a pancreatic abscess.

The clinical signs and symptoms resemble those of a bacterial peritonitis, including fever, chills, abdominal pain and distension, rebound tenderness, absent bowel sounds, localized mass, continued purulent discharge from a peritoneal drain, or cloudy bags in the case of peritoneal dialysis. About 15% cases may result in candidemia or dissemination. Diagnosis is confirmed by culture of peritoneal fluid obtained by ultrasound or CT-guided aspiration or during surgery. Isolation of *Candida* from a drain site may indicate colonization or contamination. *Candida* polymerase chain reaction (PCR) on blood or peritoneal fluid and/or serum β-D-glucan detection is likely to be diagnostic.

Candida Pericarditis and Myocarditis

Candida spreads to the pericardium and myocardium by hematogenous route or from contiguous structures, including sternum or esophagus. It can be a complication of cardio-thoracic surgery. Apart from *C. albicans*, the other species responsible for the infection are *C. tropicalis* and *C. glabrata*. Diffuse abscesses are scattered throughout the myocardium. Purulent pericarditis is a rare but life-threatening manifestation of disseminated candidiasis. The clinical signs and symptoms are nonspecific, including fever, hypotension, new or changing murmur, tachycardia, and shock. Chest radiograph shows cardiomegaly. Echocardiography reveals pericardial effusion and/or cardiac tamponade. The fungus can be cultured from the pericardial fluid or pericardial biopsy.

Candida Mediastinitis

Candida mediastinitis occurs following cardiothoracic surgery causing fever, chest wall erythema, and instability of sternum. It resembles bacterial mediastinitis. Treatment includes mediastinal drainage with debridement of sternum along with antifungal therapy. Treatment is same as that of candidemia. Therapy is continued till clinical response, and resolution of CT scan findings is achieved.

Intrauterine Candidiasis

Intrauterine candidiasis results from ascending infection of the maternal genital tract. It presents as multiple yellow-white lesions on the surface of the umbilical cord. Once the amniotic fluid is infected, the infection spreads to the fetus and can cause spontaneous abortion or congenital cutaneous candidiasis.

Congenital cutaneous candidiasis results from infection in utero or at the time of delivery. The risk factors include premature rupture of membranes, intrauterine device, or vaginal candidiasis. The infant is born with erythematous macules or papules which turn vesicular or bullous. Unlike miliaria, palms and soles are frequently involved. Oral thrush may be present. Examination of umbilical cord lesions may offer a clue. The lesions respond to topical antifungals and resolve by desquamation. Occasionally, it may progress to candidemia (Table 15.2).

DIAGNOSES OF CANDIDIASIS

Differential Diagnosis

- Cutaneous candidiasis—Contact dermatitis, folliculitis
- Esophageal candidiasis–Herpes simplex esophagitis, GERD, radiation esophagitis
- Pulmonary candidiasis—Bacterial or viral pneumonia, *Aspergillus* pneumonia
- Genitourinary candidiasis—Bacterial cystitis and pyelonephritis
- CMC—Chronic granulomatous disease
- Hepatosplenic candidiasis—Hepatic abscesses, ascending cholangitis, granulomatous hepatitis, graft-versus-host disease, malignancy
- Candidemia—Bacterial sepsis
- *Candida* endocarditis—Bacterial endocarditis
- Disseminated candidiasis—Bacterial meningitis, bacterial osteomyelitis, bacterial endo-carditis, tuberculosis

Laboratory Diagnosis

- Wet mounts from scrapings and smears obtained from skin, nails, oral or vaginal mucosa are examined for the presence of the yeast. A potassium hydroxide smear (Fig. 15.3), culture on SDA (Fig 15.4) and Gram stain (Fig 15.5) demonstrate the presence of the fungus.

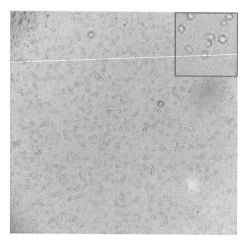

Fig. 15.3: Budding yeast cells on potassium hydroxide mount.

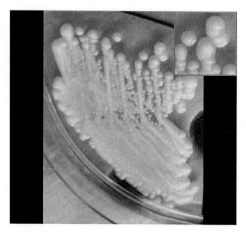

Fig. 15.4: Colony of *Candida albicans* on Sabouraud dextrose agar.

- ◆ CHROMagar *Candida* uses color reactions in specialized media to differentiate different colored colonies of the various *Candida* species.
- ▪ Fluorescence *in situ* hybridization (FISH) allows identification of *C. albicans* and *C. glabrata* from blood culture bottles by hybridization.
- ▪ Blood culture is the gold standard for the diagnosis of invasive candidiasis. The overall blood culture positivity for invasive candidiasis is approximately 50%. The limit of detection of blood culture is ≤1 CFU/mL. The turn around time for blood cultures is 2–3 days and can be up to 7 days. Certain species, such as *C. glabrata* take a longer time to grow, whereas *C. tropicalis* takes a shorter time. The reasons for negative blood cultures may include extremely low level candidemia, intermittent candidemia, deep-seated

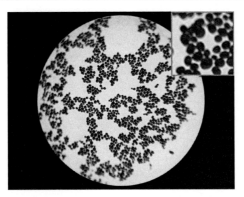

Fig. 15.5: Budding yeast cells on Gram stain

candidiasis in the absence of candidemia. Cultures from nonsterile sites including the GI, urinary, or respiratory tract may indicate colonization and may not always be indicative of true invasive candidiasis.

- *Antigen and antibody detection*: A combined mannan/antimannan antibody assay (*Platelia Candida* Ag and Ab) becomes positive much before the blood culture and before radiographic features of *Candida* develop.
- β-D-*Glucan*: It is useful as an adjunct to culture for the diagnosis of invasive fungal infections including *Candida, Aspergillus, P. jirovecii,* and other fungi. It shortens the time for the initiation of antifungal therapy. The causes of false positivity include bacteremia, IV amoxicillin-clavulanate, hemodialysis using gluten containing membranes, fungal colonization, albumin or immunoglobulin infusion, use of surgical gauze containing glucans, mucositis, and disruption of GI tract. The role of β-D-glucan testing in samples other than serum is not well established.
- *Germ-tube test*: *C. albicans, Candida stellatoidea,* and *C. dubliniensis* are identified by the germ-tube formation since these yeast cells form hyphae after 2–3 hours of incubation.
- *Polymerase chain reaction*: These assays give rapid results compared to cultures but lack standardization and validation. It is a labor-intensive technique. Its advantages include species identification, detection of molecular markers of drug resistance and multiplex formatting.
- *T2 Candida*: It is a US Food and Drug Administration–approved *Candida* detection panel that detects the five main *Candida* species: *C. albicans, C. tropicalis, C. glabrata, C. parapsilosis,* and *C. krusei*. It detects the pathogens in 3–5 hours with 91.1% sensitivity and 99.4% specificity. It runs on a fully automated T2Dx instrument. The limits of detection are as low as 1 CFU/mL. It works by measuring how water molecules react in the presence of magnetic fields. It is the same principle on which conventional MRI machines work but this is on a miniaturized scale. T2 magnetic resonance uses super paramagnetic particles coated with one or more binding agents specific to particular fungal species. The patient's blood sample contains the target pathogen. The particles bind, and cluster around the pathogen. This disrupts the microscopic fields experienced by the surrounding water molecules. This alteration in signals confirms the presence of the pathogenic species.

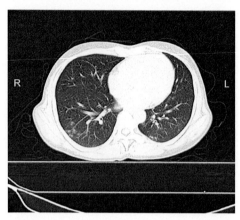

Fig. 15.6: Chest computed tomography scan, axial section shows multiple ill-defined nodular opacities in right lower lobe, posterior segment, with ground-glass haze. Few nodular opacities are also noted in left posterobasal segment.

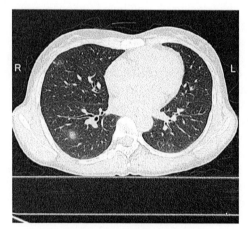

Fig. 15.7: Chest computed tomography scan, axial section shows nodular opacity in right lower lobe with surrounding halo.

Imaging Studies

- Chest radiographs—Nonspecific findings of multilobar pneumonia indistinguishable from a bacterial pneumonia.
- Ultrasonography—Helps in the detection of hepatosplenic and abdominal abscesses, renal abscesses, and fungal balls in urinary tract.
- Computerized tomography confirms the findings of radiographs and ultrasonography (Figs. 15.6 and 15.7).
- Echocardiography detects fungal vegetations in the case of CE.

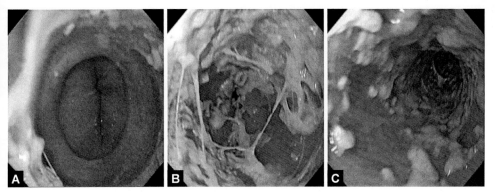

Figs. 15.8A to C: Upper gastrointestinal endoscopy of a patient with esophageal candidiasis showing multiple scattered lesions of candidal infection throughout the esophagus.

■ TREATMENT AND MANAGEMENT

Invasive Procedures

Bronchoscopy, bronchoalveolar lavage (BAL), and lung biopsy confirm *Candida* pneumonia differentiating it from colonization.

Endoscopy is required to diagnose esophageal candidiasis (Figs. 15.8A to C).

Histology of biopsy specimens and stains, including PAS, Grocott silver-methenamine, and methylene blue, identifies *Candida* as yeast cells, pseudohyphae or hyphae (*See* Table 15.3).

All major categories of antifungal drugs are used for the treatment of candidiasis (Table 15.4).

Ketoconazole is no longer prescribed orally due to associated toxicities, including severe hepatotoxicity, adrenal insufficiency, and adverse drug reactions.

Echinocandins are preferred agents for candidemia and invasive candidiasis (with the exception of CNS, eye, and UTIs) due the following reasons:

- Early fungicidal activity
- Better outcomes.
- Good safety profile
- Convenience of dosing
- Usefulness in azole-resistant *Candida.*

Each *Candida* species has unique virulence and susceptibility patterns. It is important to collect epidemiological data regarding prevalent species in a hospital setup and also monitor for antifungal resistance.

Candidiasis during Pregnancy

Amphotericin B is the treatment of choice in pregnancy. Azoles and flucytosine may cause birth defects when used in the first trimester. There is insufficient data regarding the use of echinocandins in pregnancy.

Table 15.4: Antifungal therapy for candidiasis.

Drug	Dose	Salient features
AmBd	0.5–1 mg/kg IV daily	• May be used for less susceptible *Candida* spp. including *C. glabrata* and *C. krusei* • Nephrotoxicity and AKI, renal tubular acidosis
LAmB	3–5 mg/kg IV daily	• Same efficacy as AmBd but less nephrotoxic • Not preferred in UTI due to reduced renal excretion
Fluconazole	Loading dose 800 mg (12 mg/kg), average daily dose 400 mg (6 mg/kg) Dose reduction if CrCl <50 mL/min For *C. glabrata*, use higher dose—800 mg/day	• Less active against *C. glabrata* and *C. krusei* • Standard treatment for oropharyngeal, oesophageal, vaginal candidiasis, and UTI • Oral bioavailability >90% • Achieves good penetration in CSF, vitreous, and urine
Itraconazole	200 mg thrice daily for 3 days followed by twice daily	• Used for mucosal candidiasis if treatment failure with fluconazole • Capsule absorbed better with food, oral suspension better if empty stomach
Voriconazole	Loading dose 400 mg (6 mg/kg) twice daily for two doses, maintenance dose 200–300 mg (3–4 mg/kg) twice daily Same dose for both oral and IV formulation	• Works in both mucosal and invasive candidiasis • As step-down oral therapy for *C. krusei* and fluconazole-resistant, voriconazole-sensitive *C. glabrata* • CSF and vitreous concentrations >50% serum concentration • Does not accumulate in active form in urine, avoid in UTI • Cyclodextrin in IV nephrotoxic • Oral voriconazole dose adjusted in moderate hepatic impairment; not for renal impairment • Gene polymorphism effects drug levels • Causes hepatic injury, visual side effects, photosensitivity, CNS side effects
Posaconazole	Loading dose 300 mg twice daily for two doses, maintenance dose 300 mg once daily, same dose for oral and IV	• Inadequate data regarding efficacy in primary candidiasis
Echinocandins	*Caspofungin:* Loading 70 mg IV stat, maintenance 50 mg IV daily *Anidulafungin:* Loading 200 mg IV stat, maintenance 100 mg IV daily *Micafungin:* No loading dose, maintenance 100 mg IV daily	• Low MICs for most *Candida* species • Some *C. glabrata* strains resistant to echinocandins • *C. parapsilosis* has innately higher MICs and may be less responsive • Achieve lower therapeutic concentrations in eye, CNS, urine • No dosage adjustment in renal insufficiency or dialysis • Caspofungin dose reduced in moderate-to-severe hepatic insufficiency
Flucytosine	25 mg/kg orally four times daily	• Efficacy against most *Candida* species except *C. krusei* • Bioabsorption 80–90% most drug excreted unchanged and dose adjustment needed in renal dysfunction, has high penetration in CNS and eye • Early resistance if used as monotherapy • Causes bone marrow and hepatic toxicity, used in refractory endocarditis, meningitis, endophthalmitis and UTI

AKI, acute kidney injury; AmBd, amphotericin B deoxycholate; CrCl, creatinine clearance; CSF, cerebrospinal fluid; IV, intravenous; LAmB, liposomal amphotericin B;

Therapeutic Drug Monitoring

Therapeutic drug monitoring is recommended for itraconazole, voriconazole, posaconazole, and flucytosine to optimize efficacy and reduce toxicity.

Candidemia in Non-neutropenic Patients

No clinical trial has demonstrated the clear superiority of one antifungal over the other agents in management of candidemia. Some *Candida* strains can be multidrug resistant.

The choice of the antifungal agent will depend on the following:
- Recent azole exposure
- Recent echinocandin exposure
- Dominant *Candida* species and its susceptibility in a particular center
- Severity of illness/invasive candidiasis
- CNS ocular, or cardiac involvement
- Comorbidities
- History of intolerance to an antifungal in the past.

Echinocandins are used as initial drugs for candidemia for previously mentioned reasons. They demonstrate similar efficacy and may be used interchangeably. They provide a survival benefit. Once the patient is clinically stable and blood cultures have become negative, step-down therapy involves the use of azoles. Fluconazole can be used for sensitive strains of *C. albicans, C. parapsilosis*, and *C. tropicalis*. Voriconazole is used for *C. krusei*. This transition generally occurs within a week of start of therapy.

Fluconazole is used as first-line therapy in patients who *do not* have hemodynamic compromise, prior azole exposure, high risk of *C. glabrata*, uncontrolled diabetes, or malignancy.

Recent data indicate no difference in patients with *C. parapsilosis* infection treated with echinocandins or fluconazole as initial therapy.

Voriconazole is active against most *Candida* species, including *C. krusei, C. guilliermondii*, and *C. glabrata* which are voriconazole sensitive. Disadvantages of using this drug include unpredictable pharmacokinetics and more drug interactions.

Itraconazole has limited role in the management of candidemia.

Posaconazole and isavuconazole demonstrate excellent in vitro activity against *Candida* and could be useful once more clinical efficacy data is available.

Amphotericin B is active against most *Candida* species except *C. lusitaniae*. Liposomal AmB (LAmB) is preferred over AmB deoxycholate (AmBd). AmB is preferred in the following scenarios:
- Intolerance to echinocandins and/or azoles.
- Infection is refractory to other therapies.
- The pathogen is resistant to other agents.
- There is suspicion of infection with non-*Candida* fungi, including *Cryptococcus neoformans* and *H. capsulatum*.

Echinocandin and/or azole-resistant *Candida* isolates, especially *C. glabrata*, are preferably treated with LAmB.

Ocular involvement can be a sight-threatening complication of candidemia and dilated fundus examination by an ophthalmologist is a must in the first week of therapy.

Appropriate duration of antifungal therapy is determined by blood cultures drawn every day or every other day till they become sterile. If there is no dissemination, systemic antifungal therapy is continued for at least 14 days following the documented clearance of *Candida* on cultures and the resolution of signs and symptoms.

Central venous catheters and intravascular devices are a source of development and persistence of candidemia. The fungus forms biofilms on these surfaces. *C. parapsilosis* candidemia is especially associated with CVCs. CVCs should be removed as early as possible if the CVC is the presumed source of infection, and it is safe and feasible to remove the catheter. It offers a survival benefit.

Candidemia in Neutropenic Patients

Candidemia in neutropenic patients is associated with complications, including dissemination, multiorgan failure, sepsis, and death. Hepatosplenic candidiasis or chronic disseminated candidiasis can be a consequence of GI mucositis in a neutropenic patient not on antifungal prophylaxis.

Echinocandins are the drug of choice for the initiation of therapy with LAmB as an alternative. Since fluconazole is used as prophylaxis for the prevention of candidiasis in neutropenic patients, it is not advisable to use this as initial treatment in patients who have had prior azole exposure. It is used for step-down or maintenance therapy in clinically stable patients with infection from *Candida* strains which are fluconazole sensitive. In *C. krusei* infection, the use of voriconazole as step-down therapy is recommended. The recommended duration of therapy is for at least 2 weeks after blood cultures become negative and neutropenia as well as symptoms resolve. When neutropenia is protracted, antifungal therapy should be continued till engraftment.

The fundus examination by an ophthalmologist is to be performed within the first week after recovery from neutropenia as the vitreoretinal findings are more apparent at this stage.

Since the GI tract is the more likely source of candidemia in neutropenic patients, the decision regarding the removal of CVCs needs to be individualized because of difficult IV access in these patients.

Granulocyte colony-stimulating factor mobilized granulocyte transfusions can be beneficial in patients with persistent candidemia and prolonged neutropenia.

Chronic Disseminated/Hepatosplenic Candidiasis

Suspected diagnosis on the basis of clinical picture, laboratory parameters, and imaging results should prompt early initiation of treatment. LAmB and echinocandins are used as primary therapy with step-down therapy with fluconazole. In patients who have had a previous episode of fluconazole-resistant candidemia, voriconazole or posaconazole is preferred. Treatment duration is based on the resolution or calcification of lesions on imaging or periods of immunosuppression. Most patients show resolution of lesions in approximately 6 months. Premature discontinuation of therapy leads to relapse. Fluconazole dose is adjusted in the cases of renal insufficiency and caspofungin dose adjustment in moderate-to-severe hepatic insufficiency.

Based on the hypothesis that chronic disseminated candidiasis is driven by IRIS, concomitant glucocorticosteroids and nonsteroidal anti-inflammatory drugs are prescribed in a few cases with persistent fever but there are no consensus recommendations regarding the same. The dosage of corticosteroids is 0.5–1 mg/kg daily of oral prednisone but the duration of therapy is not well defined. Splenectomy is performed if microabscesses are mainly restricted to the spleen. In the cases where chemotherapy or hematopoietic stem cell transplantation is required, it should not be delayed because of hepatosplenic candidiasis, and the antifungals should be continued throughout the period of immunosuppression.

Empiric Treatment of Suspected Invasive Candidiasis in Non-neutropenic Patients in the Intensive Care Unit

Empiric antifungal therapy is based on the following:
- Critically ill patient with risk factors for invasive candidiasis including *Candida* colonization, severe illness, recent major surgery, exposure to broad-spectrum antibiotics, necrotizing pancreatitis, CVCs, dialysis, parenteral nutrition, corticosteroid use.
- No other known cause of fever.
- Surrogate markers for invasive candidiasis including β-D-glucan, mannan–antimannan antibodies, and PCR and T2 *Candida*, and/or culture data from nonsterile sites.
- Clinical signs of septic shock.

The empiric therapy has to be initiated as early as possible to improve survival. Echinocandins are the preferred drugs. Fluconazole is an alternative for patients who have not had a recent azole exposure. LAmB is an alternative for patients intolerant to echinocandins and azoles. The duration of therapy is for 2 weeks in patients who show improvement with empiric therapy.

Justifications for stopping empiric therapy are as follows:
- Lack of signs of improvement after 4–5 days of starting therapy
- Negative nonculture-based diagnostic assays for *Candida*
- No subsequent evidence of invasive candidiasis after the start of therapy.

Prophylaxis for Preventing Invasive Candidiasis in Intensive Care Unit

Prophylaxis is offered to high-risk patients in ICUs with a rate of invasive candidiasis in excess of the expected rate of <5%. Fluconazole prophylaxis may reduce incidence of invasive candidiasis in these patients but may not necessarily translate into lesser candidemia or better survival chances. The disadvantages of fluconazole prophylaxis include adverse reactions, emergence of fluconazole resistance, and ecological shifts in *Candida* species.

Daily bathing of ICU patients with chlorhexidine decreases the incidence of catheter-associated and noncatheter-associated bloodstream infections, including *Candida*.

Neonatal Candidiasis and Candidemia

Amphotericin B deoxycholate 1 mg/kg daily is recommended for the treatment of invasive candidiasis and candidemia in neonates. Fluconazole 12 mg/kg IV or oral daily may be used as an alternative in patients who have not been on fluconazole prophylaxis. LAmB is not a good option in the presence of UTI. Echinocandins are reserved for use as salvage therapy. Imaging is mandatory to evaluate liver, spleen, and renal involvement in culture-positive neonates. Lumbar puncture and dilated retinal examination are recommended for the evaluation of meningoencephalitis and ocular involvement. CVC removal is strongly recommended to reduce prolonged candidemia and mortality. The duration of therapy is for 2 weeks after documented negative cultures and resolution of signs of candidemia.

Candiduria in extremely LBW infants should be evaluated further by blood culture, ultrasound, and lumbar puncture. If untreated, it is associated with dissemination, neurodevelopmental impairment, and death.

Central Nervous System Candidiasis in Neonates

Amphotericin B deoxycholate 1 mg/kg daily may be used as initial therapy. LAmB 5 mg/kg daily is an alternative regimen as it achieves good CSF levels albeit poor urine levels. Fluconazole 12 mg/kg is used as step-down therapy for susceptible strains. Flucytosine is considered salvage therapy. Infected devices including ventriculoperitoneal shunts should be removed if possible. Therapy is continued till complete clinical and radiological resolution of signs of disease. Data on use of echinocandins in neonates is still emerging.

Prophylaxis in Neonatal Intensive Care Unit

In nurseries with invasive candidiasis rates >10%, fluconazole prophylaxis 3–6 mg/kg twice weekly for 6 weeks is recommended in babies with birth weight <1,000 g. Oral nystatin and oral bovine lactoferrin may be considered alternatives. Lactoferrin is a mammalian milk glycoprotein involved in innate immunity and may reduce incidence of invasive candidiasis.

Intra-abdominal Candidiasis

Candida abscesses require surgical or percutaneous drainage. Echinocandins are the drugs of choice. In susceptible strains, fluconazole may be used. In continuous ambulatory peritoneal dialysis *Candida* peritonitis, remove the peritoneal dialysis catheter and shift the patient to hemodialysis. Concomitant bacterial peritonitis should also be treated.

For fluconazole-sensitive species, fluconazole 800 mg loading dose followed by fluconazole 400 mg orally daily can be used. It achieves excellent concentrations in bile and peritoneal fluid. For *C. glabrata*, echinocandins are the choice for initial therapy followed by voriconazole. Therapy should be continued for at least 2 weeks or till the resolution of peritonitis.

Candida Pneumonia

Unlike *Candida* bronchitis, colonization of the airways is the presence of *Candida* in the absence of symptoms and signs of infection. Patients with diabetes, cystic fibrosis, long-term antibiotics, and corticosteroid use have increased colonization and do not need treatment.

Candida pneumonia is rare and is limited to severely immunocompromised patients with hematogenous spread of infection into the lungs. The diagnosis is supported by isolation of the yeast from BAL specimen but the diagnostic test is histopathology for evidence of invasive infection. Treatment is initiated for pneumonia and not for colonization.

Candida Endocarditis

Management of CE requires a combined medical and surgical approach. Valve replacement is recommended for the treatment of both native and prosthetic valve endocarditis.

- *Initial antifungal therapy for native or prosthetic valve endocarditis:*
  - ◆ Liposomal amphotericin B (3–5 mg/kg) IV daily with or without flucytosine (25 mg/kg) orally four times daily in patients with normal renal function.
    Or
    An echinocandin at a high dose, which includes caspofungin 150 mg IV daily, micafungin 150 mg IV daily, or anidulafungin 200 mg IV daily.
  - ◆ Amphotericin B deoxycholate is associated with nephrotoxicity. Flucytosine is associated with bone marrow toxicity. Serum flucytosine levels need to be monitored. Echinocandins have the advantage of being active against biofilm-embedded *Candida*.
  - ◆ Resection of the valve is essential. Antifungal therapy should be continued for at least 6 weeks post-surgery.
- *Step-down therapy:*
  - ◆ Once the patient stabilizes and the blood culture becomes negative, the therapy may be changed to oral fluconazole 400–800 mg daily. Patients with perivalvular abscess may be treated for months or lifelong instead of the conventional 6 weeks of therapy. Fluconazole should not be used as initial monotherapy for CE.
  - ◆ All patients who cannot undergo surgical resection of the affected valve and patients with prosthetic valve endocarditis should receive lifelong antifungal therapy with oral fluconazole (6–12 mg/kg) (400–800 mg daily) if the isolate is fluconazole susceptible. For strains resistant to fluconazole, oral voriconazole 200–300 mg twice daily (3–4 mg/kg) or delayed release posaconazole (300 mg daily) should be used as chronic suppressive therapy.
  - ◆ In neonates with CE, antifungal therapy alone can be effective. Flucytosine toxicity is more common in neonates than in adults.
  - ◆ Relapse is common even after surgical resection and treatment with AmB.
  - ◆ For pacemakers and implantable cardiac defibrillator infections, the entire device should be removed. For infections limited to generator pockets, 4 weeks of antifungal therapy after removal of the device is recommended. For infection involving the wires, the duration of therapy is at least 6 weeks after wire removal. For ventricular assist devices that cannot be removed, treatment recommendations are the same as for native valve endocarditis with lifelong immunosuppression.

Candida Pericarditis and Myocarditis

Treatment involves pericardiocentesis, decompression of tamponade, pericardiectomy, and antifungal therapy. Echinocandins are preferred as initial therapy. In the case of fluconazole-sensitive strains, the patient is switched to oral fluconazole after stabilization. LAmB may be used as an alternative therapy. For *C. glabrata,* use echinocandins followed by voriconazole. The treatment is continued till complete resolution of pericardial inflammation.

Candida Suppurative Thrombophlebitis

The initial therapy for *Candida* thrombophlebitis is either LAmB (3–5 mg/kg IV daily) or fluconazole (6–12 mg/kg IV or orally) or an echinocandin at a higher dose (caspofungin 150 mg IV daily, micafungin 150 mg IV daily, and anidulafungin 200 mg IV daily). Step-down therapy is with fluconazole. Antifungal therapy is discontinued once the thrombus has resolved. There is insufficient evidence to support use of systemic anticoagulants or thrombolytic therapy.

Candida Osteoarticular Infections

Combined surgery and antifungal therapy are used in majority of the patients. Surgical procedures may involve debridement, drainage, decompression, stabilization, intervertebral fusion, or bone grafting.

Prosthetic joint infection requires removal of infected prosthesis and implantation of new prosthesis 3–6 months later. If the prosthetic device cannot be removed, chronic suppression with fluconazole 400 mg orally daily should be given if the isolate is fluconazole sensitive.

Septic arthritis caused by fluconazole-sensitive strains is treated with oral fluconazole 400 mg/day for at least 6 weeks or an IV echinocandin daily for 2 weeks with oral fluconazole for 4 weeks. LAmB may be used alternatively in the first 2 weeks at 3–5 mg/day IV. Intraarticular instillation of AmB is not recommended as it causes synovial irritation. The antifungal therapy for osteomyelitis can be continued for 6–12 months. For *C. glabrata,* initial therapy is with echinocandins, followed by step-down therapy with voriconazole. *C. krusei* is resistant to fluconazole and needs treatment with voriconazole, echinocandins, or AmB. *C. parapsilosis* can be less susceptible to echinocandins, and fluconazole can be preferred.

Relapsed infection after complete or partial response can be due to inadequate duration of therapy or acquired drug resistance in the strains responsible for osteomyelitis.

Candida Endophthalmitis

The penetration of systemically administered antifungals is highly variable and achieving adequate concentrations of the drugs in the infected tissues is crucial. The choroid and retina are highly vascular compared to the vitreous. The intraocular structures are separated from the vascular compartments by the blood–ocular barrier. Chorioretinal lesions sparing the macula and the vitreous are treated solely with systemic antifungal agents. Drugs that achieve adequate concentrations in the vitreous are fluconazole, voriconazole, and flucytosine. All formulations of AmB and echinocandins do not achieve sufficient concentrations in vitreous when administered systemically. Fluconazole is most widely used. Flucytosine should not be used as a sole therapy.

For sight-threatening macular involvement and vitritis, intravitreal injection of AmB (5–10 μg AmBd/0.1 mL sterile water) or voriconazole (100 μg/0.1 mL sterile water or normal saline) is helpful in achieving high local antifungal concentrations. Repeated intravitreal injections may be required.

Vitrectomy is recommended for sight-threatening endophthalmitis with vitritis. Vitrectomy permits removal of loculated areas of infection not amenable to systemic antifungals reducing the burden of the disease. Cultures sent at the time of vitrectomy guide therapy.

Treatment with antifungals is continued for at least 4-6 weeks with the final duration of therapy being determined by the repeated ophthalmologic examination. It is important to detect macular or vitreal involvement early to preserve visual acuity.

The Infectious Diseases Society of America (IDSA) recommends a dilated retinal examination in all patients with candidemia within the first week of diagnosis. Neutropenic patients should additionally have a second retinal examination after the recovery of neutropenia.

Central Nervous System Candidiasis

For *Candida* meningitis, LAmB (5 mg/kg IV daily) with or without flucytosine (25 mg/kg four times daily) is preferred. Flucytosine is added due to good anti-*Candida* efficacy and excellent penetration into the CSF. Amphotericin deoxycholate is preferred in neonates as they tolerate it better than adults, and there is limited experience with LAmB. Flucytosine is avoided in neonates.

Lumbar puncture is repeated every week till the pleocytosis decreases and the culture becomes sterile. Step-down therapy after several weeks of LAmB is with oral fluconazole at 400-800 mg daily. Oral formulation of fluconazole has good oral bioavailability. Voriconazole may be preferred in the case of infection with *C. krusei* or voriconazole-sensitive *C. glabrata*. Posaconazole and isavuconazole do not achieve adequate CSF levels. Echinocandins do not achieve adequate CSF concentrations and are not used for *Candida* meningitis. Treatment is continued till the following targets are achieved:

- Patient's signs and symptoms resolve.
- Cerebrospinal fluid examination becomes normal.
- All microabscesses resolve on MRI.

Infected ventricular devices and other implanted devices, such as deep brain stimulators, should be removed. If removal of the device is not possible, AmBd (0.01-0.5 mg in 2 mL 5% dextrose in water) should be administered through the device.

Genitourinary Candidiasis

Vulvovaginal Candidiasis

Treatment of uncomplicated VVC involves use of intravaginal agents including 2% butoconazole, 1% or 2% clotrimazole cream, 100-mg clotrimazole vaginal tablet, 2% miconazole cream, 100-mg or 200-mg miconazole vaginal suppository, 100,000 unit nystatin vaginal tablet, 0.8% terconazole cream, or 80-mg terconazole vaginal suppository. The duration of therapy varies from 1 day to 14 days depending on the agent and formulation used. As an oral antifungal therapy, a single dose of fluconazole at 150 mg is recommended.

Treatment of complicated VVC and RVVC with azole-susceptible strains requires intravaginal topical therapy for 7 days in combination with multiple doses of fluconazole. Oral fluconazole is used at 150 mg every 72 hours for three doses. RVVC is treated with long-term weekly dose of fluconazole. Non-*albicans Candida* species are likely to be azole resistant. Vaginal boric acid capsules are efficacious in management of *C. glabrata*. Treatment with amphotericin B pessaries is another option. Most probiotics contain lactobacilli which are likely to inhibit or reduce the growth of *Candida* in the vaginal tract.

Candiduria and Urinary Tract Infection

Fluconazole is the mainstay of treatment as high concentrations are attained in the urine. Echinocandins are poorly renally excreted, and there is insufficient data to support their role in management of funguria. AmBd is used at a dose of 0.3–0.6 mg/kg IV daily. Flucytosine (25 mg/kg) orally four times daily may be used to treat cystitis or added to AmBd in the cases with pyelonephritis. Bladder irrigation with AmB is rarely recommended. LAmB achieves low drug levels in renal tissue and is not the drug of choice in pyelonephritis. Voriconazole, posaconazole, and isavuconazole do not achieve adequate drug levels in urine to treat UTI.

Asymptomatic candiduria: When yeast is isolated in urine, clinical evaluation is warranted to determine its relevance and to make an appropriate decision regarding the initiation of treatment. The debate is unresolved due to the following facts:

- Asymptomatic candiduria can resolve spontaneously or by catheter removal alone.
- Fluconazole clears candiduria in only half of the patients and does not improve survival.
- There is decreased survival in candiduria patients compared to matched controls thereby favoring treatment.
- Excessive treatment and prophylaxis may affect the overall microbiome adversely.

The IDSA guidelines recommend observation of asymptomatic patients and elimination of predisposing factors if possible. Removal of the indwelling catheter, urologic stents, or discontinuation of antibiotics can be sufficient treatment intervention. Asymptomatic patients who are immunocompromised, including LBW infants (<1,500 g), neutropenic patients, or are to undergo urinary tract manipulation should receive IV antifungals for a prolonged period. Neutropenic patients and LBW babies should be treated on the lines of candidemia. Other asymptomatic candiduria patients do not need antifungal treatment. If any urologic procedure is being conducted, fluconazole should be administered preoperatively as well as postoperatively at a dose of 6 mg/kg daily. In the case of fluconazole-resistant non-*albicans Candida* species, conventional AmB is used at a dose of 0.3–0.6 mg/kg daily. Renal transplant is no longer considered an absolute indication for the treatment of asymptomatic candiduria. Candiduria is treated early in the course of transplant when the ureteric stent is still in situ or there is a risk of graft involvement. Imaging of urinary tract is recommended in persistent candiduria to rule out fungal ball formation, hydronephrosis, or perinephric abscess.

Symptomatic candiduria: Symptomatic *Candida* cystitis is treated with oral fluconazole 200 mg/day for 14 days. Pyelonephritis is treated with fluconazole 200–400 mg/day for 14 days. Dosing of fluconazole is reduced in patients with renal insufficiency. Azole-resistant *Candida* strains are treated with conventional AmBd with or without flucytosine. Bladder irrigation with AmB will clear funguria albeit transiently. For *C. glabrata* infection or management of pyelonephritis, flucytosine is continued for 7–14 days. It should not be used as monotherapy due to the risk of development of resistance. Patients should be monitored for bone marrow and hepatic toxicity. *C. krusei* is inherently resistant to flucytosine. Emphysematous pyelonephritis can be life-threatening and requires surgical intervention. A perinephric abscess may require surgical or percutaneous drainage. *Candida* prostatitis and epididymo-orchitis require both antifungal therapy and surgical intervention.

Renal Candidiasis

Complications of renal candidiasis include perinephric abscess, emphysematous pyelonephritis, fungal bezoar, renal artery invasion, or aneurysm formation. Management of perinephric abscess and emphysematous pyelonephritis involves drainage and irrigation with a wide bore catheter. Open drainage may be required in the case of fistulae or multiple loculations. Percutaneous nephrostomy or retrograde catheterization is required to access fungal balls. Systemic antifungals are started to prevent dissemination secondary to manipulation. Fungal ball is extracted through the catheter, and lavage is attempted. Irrigation of the upper tract with AmB (25–50 mg in 500 mL sterile water) is performed. Balloon dilatation of ureteric stricture may be required. Oral fluconazole is used at a dose of 200–400 mg/day. Alternatively, AmBd with or without flucytosine may be used.

Oropharyngeal Candidiasis

Treatment includes withdrawal of antibiotics, topical treatment including use of clotrimazole oral troches, nystatin oral pastille or suspension, AmB oral solution, mycostatin or iodoquinol cream, or rinses.

For mild disease, clotrimazole troches 10 mg five times per day or a mucoadhesive buccal tablet of miconazole 50 mg applied on the mucosal surface over the canine fossa once daily is recommended for 1–2 weeks.

Alternative therapy for mild disease includes nystatin suspension 100,000 U/mL used as 4–6 mL four times daily or 1–2 nystatin pastilles (200,000 U each) four times daily for 1–2 weeks.

Systemic treatment for moderately severe disease includes fluconazole 100–200 mg orally once daily for 1–2 weeks.

For fluconazole refractory patients, itraconazole solution 200 mg once daily or posaconazole suspension 400 mg twice daily for 3 days followed by 400 mg daily for up to 4 weeks is recommended. Voriconazole 200 mg twice daily or AmBd suspension 100 mg/mL four times daily are alternatives for fluconazole-refractory disease.

For HIV-positive patients, initiate highly active antiretroviral therapy (HAART).

For denture-related candidiasis, dentures need to be disinfected.

Esophageal Candidiasis

Topical antifungals have minimal value in esophageal candidiasis. Minimize all possible predisposing factors including steroids, antimicrobials, and chemotherapeutic drugs. Oral fluconazole is preferred 200–400 mg (3–6 mg/kg) daily for 14–21 days because of its efficacy and safety profile. Itraconazole oral solution may be used as an alternative. Voriconazole used at a dose of 200 mg twice daily has broader spectrum of activity compared to fluconazole in esophageal candidiasis but more drug–drug interactions due to its effect on cytochrome P450 enzyme. More potent azoles will offer only modest advantage but with the disadvantage of added cost and more drug interactions. Posaconazole use has been associated with less common relapse compared to fluconazole and is used as suspension 400 mg twice daily or extended release tablets 300 mg once daily. Concerns have been raised about increased frequency of *C. glabrata* isolation in HIV patients on prolonged fluconazole.

For patients who cannot tolerate oral fluconazole, IV fluconazole or an echinocandin is recommended. AmBd is a less preferred alternative.

For patients who have recurrent esophagitis, chronic suppressive therapy with fluconazole 100–200 mg three times weekly is strongly recommended.

For HIV-positive patients, initiate HAART.

Chronic Mucocutaneous Candidiasis

Patients should follow a healthy lifestyle and maintain good oral and general hygiene. Systemic antifungals including azoles, LAmB, and IV echinocandins are used. Relapse is common on discontinuing therapy. Drug toxicity and resistance pose a challenge. Clotrimazole troches or oral nystatin solution are used for oral lesions.

Annual screening for associated endocrinopathies may be performed. Routine MR angiography to screen for aneurysms is not a universal recommendation. Immune status may be improved by using transfer factor, Janus kinase 1/2 tyrosine kinase inhibitors, such as ruxolitinib, IV immunoglobulin G, granulocyte-macrophage colony-stimulating factor infusions, and interferon-α. Transfer factor is a cell-free protein extracted from the T-lymphocytes of *Candida*-immune donors. Treating underlying endocrinopathy does not reduce severity of *Candida* infection. Oral or parenteral iron may be needed to correct iron-deficiency anemia.

MORTALITY

Candidemia is associated with up to 47% attributable mortality when it is complicated by septicemic shock. Early initiation of appropriate antifungals, source control, removal of contaminated catheters, and drainage of infected material is cardinal to reducing morbidity and mortality associated with the disease. Risk of death is higher with increasing age, higher Acute Physiology and Chronic Health Evaluation II score, immunosuppressed state, renal dysfunction, and CVC retention.

CLINICAL PEARLS

- *Candida* is the fourth most common nosocomial bloodstream infection.
- Echinocandins are the drugs of choice for both neutropenic and non-neutropenic patients.

- Fluconazole may be used as step-down therapy for fluconazole-sensitive strains.
- Ophthalmology examination is a must to identify endophthalmitis.
- Central venous catheters should be removed from most patients with candidemia.
- *Candida auris* is a challenge since it is multidrug resistant.

■ SUGGESTED READING

1. Bassetti M, Merelli M, Righi E, et al. Epidemiology, species distribution, antifungal susceptibility, and outcome of candidemia across five sites in Italy and Spain. J Clin Microbiol. 2013;51:4167-72.
2. Centers for Disease Control and Prevention. Clinical alert to U.S. healthcare facilities—global emergence of invasive infections caused by the multidrug-resistant yeast *Candida auris*. [online] Available from <https://www.cdc.gov/fungal/diseases/candidiasis/candida-auris-alert.html>.
3. Cornely OA, Bassetti M, Calandra T, et al. ESCMID* guideline for the diagnosis and management of *Candida* diseases 2012: non-neutropenic adult patients. Clin Microbiol Infect. 2012;18(Suppl. S7):19-37.
4. Cuenca-Estrella M, Verweij PE, Arendrup MC, et al. ESCMID* guideline for the diagnosis and management of *Candida* diseases 2012: diagnostic procedures. Clin Microbiol Infect. 2012;18(Supp7):9-18.
5. European Conference on Infections in Leukaemia (ECIL): Guidelines for the treatment of invasive candidiasis, aspergillosis and mucormycosis in leukemia and hematopoietic stem cell transplant patients.
6. Fisher JF, Kavanagh K, Sobel JD, et al. *Candida* urinary tract infection: pathogenesis. Clin Infect Dis. 2011;52(Suppl 6):S437.
7. Kauffman CA. Diagnosis and management of fungal urinary tract infection. Infect Dis Clin North Am. 2014;28:61.
8. Leon C, Ruiz-Santana S, Saavedra P, et al. A bedside scoring system ("*Candida* score") for early antifungal treatment in nonneutropenic critically ill patients with *Candida* colonization. Crit Care Med. 2006;34:730-7.
9. Pappas PG, Kauffman CA, Andes DR, et al. Clinical practice guideline for the management of candidiasis: 2016 update by the Infectious Diseases Society of America. Clin Infect Dis. 2016;62:e1.
10. Pappas PG, Rotstein CM, Betts RF, et al. Micafungin versus caspofungin for treatment of candidemia and other forms of invasive candidiasis. Clin Infect Dis. 2007;45:883.
11. Pfaller MA, Jones RN, Doern GV, et al. International surveillance of blood stream infections due to *Candida* species in the European SENTRY Program: species distribution and antifungal susceptibility including the investigational triazole and echinocandin agents. SENTRY Participant Group (Europe). Diagn Microbiol Infect Dis. 1999;35:19-25.
12. Shorr AF, Wu C, Kothari S. Outcomes with micafungin in patients with candidaemia or invasive candidiasis due to *Candida glabrata* and *Candida krusei*. J Antimicrob Chemother. 2011;66:375.
13. Tan BH, Chakrabarti A, Li RY, et al. Incidence and species distribution of candidemia in Asia: a laboratory-based surveillance study. Clin Microbiol Infect. 2015;21:946-53.
14. Tortorano AM, Prigitano A, Lazzarini C, et al. A 1-year prospective survey of candidemia in Italy and changing epidemiology over one decade. Infection. 2013;41:655-62.
15. Vallabhaneni S, Kallen A, Tsay S, et al. Investigation of the first seven reported cases of *Candida auris*, a globally emerging invasive, multidrug-resistant fungus—United States, May 2013-August 2016. MMWR Morb Mortal Wkly Rep. 2016;65:1234.
16. Weiss E, Timsit JF. Management of invasive candidiasis in nonneutropenic ICU patient. Ther Adv Infect Dis. 2014;2:105-15.

16

Cryptococcosis

Monica Mahajan

INTRODUCTION

Cryptococcosis is an invasive fungal infection caused by the encapsulated yeast *Cryptococcus*. It was isolated in 1894 when Otto Busse and Abraham Buschke isolated *Cryptococcus* species from a chronic granuloma in the infected tibia of a 31-year-old female patient. This leads to the eponym *Busse–Buschke* disease. Most of the cases of cryptococcosis occur in immunocompromised hosts with defects in their cell-mediated immune responses. The magnitude of problem caused by this environmental saprophyte became apparent with the AIDS pandemic in the 1980s when it was included as an AIDS-defining illness. Human-to-human transmission has never been documented. Although cryptococcosis predominantly affects immunocompromised patients, outbreaks have been noted in healthy individuals; the recent one being popularly known as the Pacific Northwest outbreak in Canada and North America. The cases of cryptococcosis are distributed worldwide.

Based on the host response, *Cryptococcus* can result in colonization, meningoencephalitis, or disseminated disease with pulmonary, cutaneous, or blood-stream infection.

TAXONOMY

Cryptococcus is an encapsulated saprophytic yeast. The genus *Cryptococcus* encompasses more than 50 species. Based on whole-genome sequencing and specific antigenic character of the capsular polysaccharide, *Cryptococcus neoformans* and *Cryptococcus gattii* are the main human pathogens. On the basis of the capsular agglutination reactions, the serotypes are designated A, B, C, and D.

C. neoformans is subclassified into two varieties—var. *grubii* and var. *neoformans*. Serotype A is *C. grubii* and is divided into three molecular subtypes: VNI, VNII, and VNB. Serotype D is classified under the variety *C. neoformans*.

Serotype B and C are called *C. gattii* species. It is useful to identify and track a strain during an outbreak. On the basis of genotyping studies, four genotypes of *C. gattii* are labeled VGI to VGIV.

For all practical purposes, the terminology used is "*C. neoformans* species complex" and "*C. gattii* species complex." *C. neoformans* var. *grubii* (capsular serotype A) is responsible for approximately 82% of cryptococcal infection globally.

MORPHOLOGY

Cryptococcus is an encapsulated, unicellular anaerobic yeast-like fungus with a thick polysaccharide capsule. The organism is round or oval shaped and roughly 6–8 μm in diameter. Unlike *Candida*, the pseudohyphae of *Cryptococcus* are absent or rudimentary. The colonies are fast growing and appear within 48 hours as soft, mucoid, or slimy, glistening to dull, cream, or yellowish brown in color. The backbone of the capsule is a mannose substituted with xylose and glucuronic acid. This is known as glucuronoxylomannan. Serological differences in serotypes A, B, C, and D are due to variation in the number of xylose side chains and extent of *O*-acetylation. India ink stain is the best staining technique for *Cryptococcus* since pigment particles are not able to cross the polysaccharide capsule, and a resultant halo is seen around the stained fungal cells. All *Cryptococcus* species produce urease and are nonfermentative. Nitrate may be assimilated or not but inositol is assimilated. *C. neoformans* can be differentiated from *C. gattii* by growth on L-canavanine-glycine-bromothymol blue (CBG) agar.

LIFE CYCLE

Cryptococcus is a "basidiomycete" yeast, since it produces spores which occur in a club-shaped structure called a "basidium." Asexual reproduction is by budding where a daughter cell buds off a parent cell. These are haploid and the only form of *Cryptococcus* isolated from humans.

Sexual reproduction begins with two cells each containing genetic material in a haploid state. These two different mating types "a" and "α" fuse with each other; mitotic cell divisions results in thread-like extensions called hyphae. A basidium is formed at the tip of the hypha and bears the basidiospores. The spores are unencapsulated to begin with but rapidly develop a capsule when released. The haploid spores are released to develop into fungal cells. Basidiospores form yeast cells at 37°C or transform into dikaryotic hyphae at 24°C. Inhalation of spores causes cryptococcosis.

EPIDEMIOLOGY

Cryptococcosis has a worldwide distribution. Both subtypes are present in avian guano, soil, and decomposing organic matter. *C. neoformans* is globally distributed, whereas *C. gattii* is a tropical or subtropical fungus found in Australia, Northern USA, Canada, Northern Europe, and Southeast Asia.

Avian excreta is rich in *C. neoformans*, and feral pigeons/city pigeons are responsible for the outbreaks of infection in crowded urban societies. When pigeons feed on contaminated vegetation, *Cryptococcus* survives in the gastrointestinal tract of these pigeons. The higher body temperature of >40°C protects the pigeons from developing the disease. However, a majority of patients will deny history of exposure to pigeons, and outbreaks have occurred where there has been no association with pigeon roosting areas and pigeon guano. There is no direct transmission from pigeons to humans. Contaminated vegetation may also cause exposure to humans.

In Australia, India, and other Asian countries the environmental reservoir for *C. gattii* is eucalyptus trees. There has been a higher prevalence of cryptococcosis amongst rural aborigines in areas abundant in eucalyptus, and there is epidemiological and molecular data to support the same. It has also been isolated from non-eucalyptus trees including fir, oak, cedar, and pine species. The fungus could have spread to other continents from trees native to Australia. *C. gattii* has been isolated from soil samples, fresh water, and sea water.

Whilst VGI is the main subtype in Australasia, VGII has been responsible for the outbreak in healthy individuals from British Columbia, Canada between 1999 and 2010. Vancouver Island recorded 218 cases of cryptococcosis in this duration. *C. gattii* has become endemic in the Pacific Northwest. The extent of cryptococcosis caused by *C. gattii* is underestimated since smaller laboratories do not identify *Cryptococci* at a species level. VGIV is mostly restricted to Africa.

Most cases in Australia are residing in rural areas while those in British Columbia are urban residents with no apparent exposure to endemic areas.

Discovery of the organism from heterogeneous biogeoclimatic zones suggests that climate change can be responsible for the expanding area of distribution of the disease.

PREDISPOSING FACTORS

- *Human immunodeficiency virus (HIV) and AIDS:* HIV-infected patients have the highest predisposition for cryptococcosis with the worsening in degree of immunosuppression and especially cluster of differentiation (CD)4 count <100 cells/μL. Globally, cryptococcosis accounts for more than 1 million cases annually in HIV-positive patients. With the development of effective highly active antiretroviral therapy (HAART), the upsurge of cases of cryptococcal disease has reversed and declined in the developed nations. The same is not true for low-income nations with resource crunch where there is delayed or incomplete access to HAART
- *Immunosuppression:* Other risk factors for cryptococcosis include patients on immu-nosuppressive medication including corticosteroids, calcineurin inhibitors, cytotoxic agents, monoclonal antibodies, such as alemtuzumab and infliximab, for cancer treatment, transplant conditioning, or rheumatological disorders.
- *Organ transplant and hematopoietic stem cell transplant:* Cryptococcosis ranks third after *Candida* and *Aspergillus* as a cause for invasive fungal infection in solid organ transplants (SOT) recipients. It occurs most frequently in kidney transplant recipients, followed by liver, heart, lung, and pancreas recipients. The median time of diagnosis is 20 months and is as a consequence of reactivation of latent disease in the recipient. The overall incidence does not vary between use of various primary immunosuppressants including tacrolimus, cyclosporine, or azathioprine. Rare instances have been recorded where infections have resulted from infected donor tissue. The diagnosis should be made if multiple recipients from a single donor develop the disease, surgical graft site infection, or in case the infection develops within 1 month of transplant. Donor screening is not mandatory unless the donor has pyrexia of unknown origin, unexplained central nervous system (CNS) or pulmonary involvement. *Cryptococcus* infection may rarely occur after corneal transplant. For unrecognized reasons the risk of acquiring cryptococcosis is higher in autologous transplant than in allogeneic stem cell transplant.

CRYPTOCOCCAL VIRULENCE

- *Cryptococcal capsule*:
  - ◆ Cryptococcal polysaccharide capsule mediates immune evasion through various mechanisms. It helps the yeast to go unrecognized by the phagocytic cells.

Glucuronoxylomannan is present in the patient's blood circulation and prevents the transmigration of leukocytes through the endothelium into the site of tissue injury. The leukocyte adhesion cascade involves steps including capture, rolling, adhesion, and transmigration.

- Cytokines IL-1 and tumor necrosis factor-α activate the endothelium at the site of infection and makes the leukocytes adhere to the activated endothelial surface.
- In the initial phase the selectins cause leukocyte adhesion and a slow rolling downstream over the activated endothelium based on the interaction of selectins and their complementary counterligands. Selectins are transmembrane molecules expressed on the surface of leukocytes and activated endothelium. L-selectins are expressed on leukocytes.
- The integrins are glycoproteins that bind the leukocyte to the ligands intercellular adhesion molecule and vascular cell adhesion molecule-1 present on endothelium, leading to final transmigration of the leukocytes.
- Glucuronoxylomannan in the cryptococcal capsule reaches the bloodstream during infection and disallows these binding processes leading to a reduced efflux of leukocytes toward the site of inflammation.
- Stimulation with the encapsulated *Cryptococcus* also downregulates the activity of macrophages, neutrophils, and dendritic cells.
- The fungal capsule stops the antibody from binding effectively to the epitope thereby interfering with the humoral immune response and the subsequent complement activation by classical pathway.
- The capsule accelerates the degradation of complement component C3b.
- *Melanin*: Melanin is a dark pigment produced by the polymerization of polyphenols by enzyme phenol oxidase in *C. neoformans*. High levels of dopamine in the CNS may serve as a phenolic substrate. It is a polyanionic molecule and differs structurally from human melanin. It is an antioxidant and protects *Cryptococcus* from oxidative injury and phagocytosis. Macrophages kill the engulfed foreign particles by the production of free radicals that damage the DNA and cellular proteins. Melanin protects against free radicals by neutralizing them. The presence of pigments in cells reduces susceptibility to oxidative killing.
- *Modulation of the adaptive immune response*: The reason for long-term persistence of cryptococcal infection is the capability of the fungus to alter the adaptive immune response. This is mediated through the following ways:
  - T-cell inhibition and apoptosis
  - Promotion of a nonprotective type 2 T helper (Th2) response
  - Interference with development of dendritic cells
  - Induction of immune tolerance
  - Interference with antibody production
  - Induction of IL-10 which inhibits type 1 T helper (Th1) responses.
- *Cell enlargement*: The cryptococcal cells may enlarge in vivo to up to 100 μm in diameter and resist phagocytosis. Enlargement of the cell is promoted by coinfection with strains belonging to the opposite mating type. DNA analysis of these cells shows polyploid, uninucleate cells capable of producing daughter cells in vivo.

Host Immune Responses

Immunocompetent individuals are able to contain the disease due to natural barriers, such as skin and nasal mucosa. Human saliva and serum have anticryptococcal activity. The main host responses are complement system and phagocytes.

- Activation of complement cascade produces inflammation and recruitment of macrophages and neutrophils. The triggers for phagocytosis can be two different mechanisms— the phagocytic cells may come into contact with the cryptococcal capsule or indirectly recognize the cells that have been opsonized by antibodies.
- Dendritic cells function as professional antigen presenting cells, process antigens, and then present them to the T cells to initiate cell-mediated immunity (CMI). They generate a more robust T-cell activation in comparison to alveolar or peritoneal macrophages.
- Rapid release of reactive oxygen species "respiratory burst" by human neutrophils acts to eliminate the fungus but paradoxically may damage the host cells.
- Defects in CMI in immunocompromised patients with HIV, myeloproliferative disorders, or prolonged steroid use may result in higher incidence of cryptococcosis. CMI involves the killing of the fungus through direct killing/cytotoxic effects or indirect killing by natural killer cells and T lymphocytes. The CD4 and CD8 cells counter the infection by the secretion of perforin and granzymes which cause cryptococcal lysis. HIV infection results in a low CD4$^+$ count and inhibits secretion of these serine proteases or granzymes.

PATHOGENESIS

Cryptococcal spores are inhaled and reach the lungs. From there, the organism disseminates hematogenously. There are several reasons for CNS tropism. Unlike serum, the cerebrospinal fluid (CSF) lacks anticryptococcal activity and favors fungal growth. Moreover, CSF exhibits very little complement activation. Dopamine levels in the brain provide a substrate for melanin production by *Cryptococcus*. Brain involvement generally diffuses but localized *cryptococcomas* also occur. Unlike polymorphonuclear infiltrates in bacterial meningitis, the mononuclear cells generate the inflammatory response.

CLINICAL FEATURES

Cryptococcosis is a chronic, subacute, or acute disease. Incubation period is uncertain and may vary from few weeks to few months. Cryptococcal infection involves the lungs or the CNS although other systems including skin, bones, urinary tract, eyes, myocardium, and other viscera may also get involved. Immunocompetent individuals may be asymptomatic.

Pulmonary Involvement

Most infections with *Cryptococcus* involve the lungs. The fungus may result in the following ways:

- Asymptomatic airway colonization, especially in chronic obstructive pulmonary disease and bronchiectasis.
- Pneumonia with fever, cough with scanty phlegm, malaise, weight loss, pleuritic chest pain, dyspnea, and night sweats if disseminated disease.

- A mass causing compression on mediastinal structures.
- Acute respiratory distress syndrome (ARDS).

Rare manifestations may include hemoptysis, pleural effusion, mediastinal lymphadenopathy, and cavitation. Fibrosis and calcification are absent. The lung involvement can be unilateral, bilateral, lobar, or multilobar. Immunocompetent patients may have a spontaneous resolution of disease. Immunocompromised patients may develop ARDS or chronic infection. Pulmonary disease manifests in the absence of extrapulmonary disease and vice versa.

Central Nervous System Involvement

When the infection crosses the blood–brain barrier, it results in cryptococcal meningoen-cephalitis. It is the most frequent presentation of CNS cryptococcosis. The disease is mostly subacute or chronic in nature. Neurological symptoms may develop gradually and include fever, headache, photophobia, diplopia, emesis, memory impairment, lethargy, personality changes, focal neurological signs, hallucinations, hearing defects, seizures, ataxia, aphasia, obtundation, and coma. Cryptococcomas cause focal neurological deficit. *C. gattii* is more likely to cause papilledema, seizures, focal neurological deficits, and severe neurological sequelae compared to *C. neoformans*. Symptoms are nonspecific, and HIV-positive patients may have no fever or only a mild increase in body temperature. In the absence of appropriate antifungal therapy, the disease may prove fatal any time from a fortnight to many years after disease onset. Complications include hydrocephalus and dementia.

Cryptococcal Skin and Bone Involvement

Cutaneous manifestations include umbilicated papules, pustules, ulcers, nodules, vasculitic lesions, or draining sinuses. Immunocompromised patients may develop cellulitis and necrotizing fasciitis. Bony lesions are osteolytic, and osteomyelitis may be mistaken for cold abscesses or malignancy.

Other forms of cryptococcosis include chorioretinitis, optic neuritis, endophthalmitis, renal abscesses, prostatitis, myocarditis, peritonitis, lymphadenitis, bone marrow involvement, and myositis.

Eye involvement leading to blindness may be due to choroiditis, optic nerve invasion, raised intracranial pressure (ICP), or local arachnoiditis.

C. gattii is more likely to cause large cryptococcomas in lungs and brain compared to *C. neoformans*. This can mimic pyogenic abscesses or neoplasms. *C. gattii* is more likely to affect immunocompetent patients in comparison to *C. neoformans* which predominantly involves immunocompromised individuals.

DIAGNOSIS

Cerebrospinal Fluid Examination

Lumbar puncture (LP) and CSF examination are necessary for the diagnosis of cryptococcal meningoencephalitis. Fundus examination for papilledema and imaging should be performed prior to carrying out the procedure to exclude mass lesions which could result in herniation. Patients with advanced HIV infection may generate inadequate immune response and may have a normal CSF examination except being positive on India ink or cryptococcal antigen testing (Table 16.1).

India Ink Preparation

India ink is a negative contrast. On India ink staining the capsule appears as a clear area amidst the surrounding ink particles in both the species when specimen is examined under the microscope (Fig. 16.1).

Fungal Culture

Cryptococcus produces brown-color effect when grown in niger seed/bird seed agar. The brown colonies effect is due to conversion of substrate to melanin by phenol oxidase enzyme present in *Cryptococcus*. On Sabouraud dextrose agar, the growth of *Cryptococcus* is yeast-like mucoid, cream to buff-colored (Fig. 16.2). Mucoid colonies, because of production of polysaccharides, the capsular material.

Histopathology

Cutaneous or mass lesions are biopsied and stained. Methenamine silver stain identifies the yeast form of the fungus in histopathology specimens. Mucicarmine stain is utilized to stain

Table 16.1: CSF findings in cryptococcal meningoencephalitis.	
Opening pressure	≥25-cm CSF
Cell count	Lymphocyte predominance, 0–50 cells/mm^3 in HIV-infected, 20–200 cells/mm^3 in non-HIV patients
Glucose levels	Low or normal
Protein level	Elevated or normal
India ink	Encapsulated yeast in 50–75% patients
Culture	Positive in 90%, grows over 3–5 days, use 5–15-mL CSF for better yield
Cryptococcal antigen	93–100% sensitive, rapid results

CSF, cerebrospinal fluid.

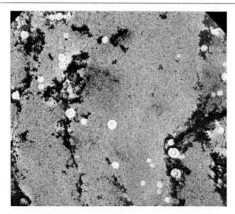

Fig. 16.1: *Cryptococcus* spp. on India ink mount.

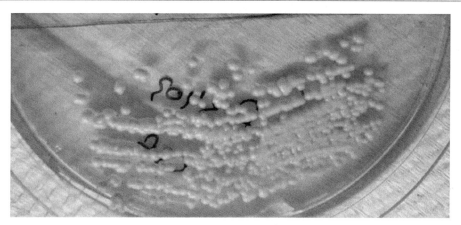

Fig. 16.2: Colony of *Cryptococcus* spp. on Sabouraud dextrose agar (SDA).

both the yeast form and the capsule specifically for *Cryptococcus* since the stain is taken up by mucopolysaccharides. Melanin pigment in *C. neoformans* is best observed with Fontana-Masson stain.

Serum Cryptococcal Antigen

This antigen is more likely to be positive in disseminated disease, CNS involvement, and transplant patients. It cannot entirely rule out cryptococcal meningitis in non-HIV patients as its sensitivity is lower in these patients vis-à-vis HIV-infected patients. Antigen titers in serum or CSF correlate with the fungal load but may not be reliable in assessing response to treatment. Lateral flow assays or enzyme immunoassay testing provide rapid results.

The causes of false-positive serum cryptococcal antigen include infections due to *Trichosporon asahii*, *Stomatococcus*, or soap/disinfectants. False-negative test is due to prozone phenomenon (when the amount of antibody in the sample is higher than the amount of antigen in the assay). Titers can remain elevated from months to years.

Blood and Cerebrospinal Fluid Culture

Positivity is higher in HIV-associated meningoencephalitis. Always confirm positive smears by appropriate cultures. Bronchoalveolar lavage (BAL) culture is better than culture from transbronchial lung biopsy. Lysis centrifugation method for blood culture gives faster and better results. *Cryptococcus* assimilates inositol and produces urease. *C. neoformans* produces melanin. Use of CBG agar distinguishes *C. gattii* from *C. neoformans*. *C. gattii* colonies turn CBG agar blue, whereas *C. neoformans* does not change the original yellow-green color of CBG agar.

- HIV antibody testing
- Cluster of differentiation 4 count (idiopathic CD4 lymphopenia)

- Immunoglobulin levels
- *Fundus examination*—For papilledema
- Bronchoscopy and BAL for culture.

Matrix-assisted Laser Desorption/Ionization Time-of-flight Mass Spectrometry

Matrix-assisted laser desorption/ionization time-of-flight mass spectrometry can provide reliable species identification but the accuracy of results relies on the quality of database.

Radiography

Magnetic resonance imaging (MRI) or computed tomography (CT) of brain can be normal or reveal diffuse cerebral atrophy, cerebral edema, or focal/diffuse areas of contrast enhancement. Cryptococcomas appear as mass lesions and may be single or multiple. The most common CT finding is small, ring-enhancing lesions. Nonenhancing "pseudocysts" are more frequently noted in immunocompromised hosts. A single large cryptococcoma >3 cm may be indistinguishable from a pyogenic abscess. MRI identifies masses or dilated perivascular spaces. These findings on the scan are nonspecific. MRI with gadolinium shows basilar meningeal enhancement and smaller mass lesions better than CT scans.

Pulmonary involvement on X-rays and CT scans appears as alveolar or interstitial infiltrates, patchy pneumonitis, granulomas, circumscribed cryptococcomas/nodules, or miliary shadows. Cavitation, mediastinal lymphadenopathy, and pleural effusion are rare (Figs. 16.3 and 16.4).

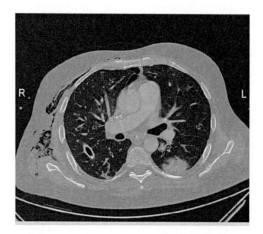

Fig. 16.3: Chest CT scan, axial section shows nodular area of consolidation with surrounding ground-glass halo in left lower lobe apical segment. Moreover, note the ICD with pneumothorax with subcutaneous emphysema. CT, computed tomography; ICD, intercostal chest drains.

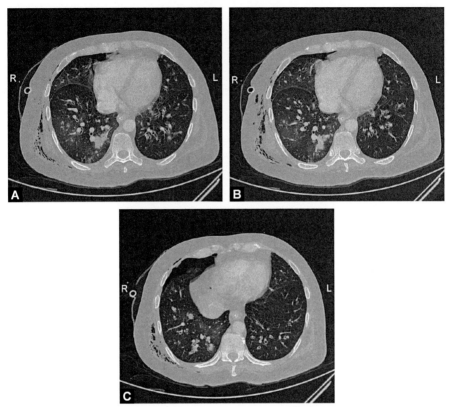

Figs. 16.4A to C: Chest CT scan. Axial section shows patchy ill-defined opacities in bilateral lower lobes with surrounding ground-glass haze. Moreover, note the ICD with pneumothorax with subcutaneous emphysema. CT, computed tomography; ICD, intercostal chest drains.

DIFFERENTIAL DIAGNOSES

- Differential diagnoses of pulmonary cryptococcosis include the following:
    - *Mycobacterium tuberculosis* infection
    - *Pneumocystis jirovecii* pneumonia
    - *Histoplasma capsulatum* infection
    - Acute respiratory distress syndrome
    - Wegener's syndrome
    - *Nocardia* infection
    - Septic emboli
    - Malignancy.
- *Differential diagnoses of CNS cryptococcosis*:
    - Tuberculosis
    - Chronic benign lymphocytic meningitis
    - Other mycoses

- ◆ Syphilis
- ◆ Meningeal metastases
- ◆ Sarcoidosis
- ◆ *Herpes simplex* infection
- ◆ Arbovirus infections
- ◆ *Aspergillus, Nocardia,* or pyogenic abscess
- ◆ Toxoplasmosis
- ◆ Brain tumors
- ◆ Lymphoma.
- ■ *Differential diagnoses of cutaneous cryptococcosis:*
  - ◆ *Molluscum contagiosum*
  - ◆ Basal cell carcinoma
  - ◆ Acne
  - ◆ Lipoma
  - ◆ Syphilis.
- ■ *Differential diagnoses of bone cryptococcosis:*
  - ◆ Tubercular cold abscess
  - ◆ Neoplasm.

■ MANAGEMENT

Cryptococcal disease in HIV always warrants therapy (Table 16.2).

Alternative Therapy for Induction

- ■ In patients intolerant to amphotericin B, fluconazole 800–1,200 mg/day is used along with flucytosine 100 mg/kg/day for at least 6 weeks and has been found to be moderately effective.
- ■ Amphotericin B deoxycholate (AmBd) (0.7–1 mg/kg/day) or liposomal amphotericin B (LAmB) (3–4 mg/kg/day) intravenous (IV) for 4–6 weeks. Doses of 6 mg/kg/day of LAmB used in the case of treatment failure or high fungal burden of disease.

Table 16.2: Cryptococcal meningoencephalitis in human immunodeficiency virus.

Drug	Dose	Duration
Induction: Amphotericin B deoxycholate or liposomal amphotericin B	0.7–1 mg/kg/day or 3–4 mg/kg/day, respectively	Initial 2 weeks
Induction: Flucytosine	100 mg/kg/day in four divided doses in addition to amphotericin B	Initial 2 weeks
Consolidation: Fluconazole	400 mg/day	After initial 2 weeks of induction therapy and is continued for minimum 8 weeks
Maintenance: Fluconazole	200 mg/day	≥1 year

- Amphotericin B deoxycholate (0.7–1 mg/kg/day) plus fluconazole (800 mg/day orally) for 2 weeks followed by fluconazole (800 mg/day orally) for 8 weeks.
- Fluconazole 800–2,000 mg/day orally for 10–12 weeks with a dosage of ≥1,200 mg/day being preferred, if fluconazole alone is used.

Indications for Continuing Induction Therapy beyond 2 Weeks

- Patient remains comatose.
- Clinical deterioration
- Symptomatic patient with a persistent elevation in ICP
- Cerebrospinal fluid culture is expected to remain positive despite 2 weeks of induction therapy.

In these patients the induction phase may be prolonged by an additional 1–6 weeks.

Response to Therapy

The positive consequences of therapy are elimination of *Cryptococcus* from host, and negative consequences are immune reconstitution inflammatory syndrome (IRIS). Initial therapy is considered adequate only after CSF culture is negative for *Cryptococci*, and the patient shows improvement in clinical signs. Induction phase is successful if a CSF culture at 2 weeks is negative and indicates a good outcome. High load of *C. neoformans* per mL of CSF and cerebral dysfunction are associated with early death. Flucytosine use is associated with cytopenias, and complete blood count should be frequently monitored. Therapeutic drug levels for flucytosine are determined in 3–5 days to target 2-hour postdose level of 30–80 µg/mL; levels >100 µg/mL are associated with toxicities.

Maintenance Suppressive and Prophylactic Therapy

- Fluconazole 200 mg/day orally is preferred.
- In azole intolerant patients, AmBd 1 mg/kg/week IV can be used although there is poor evidence to support this.
- Itraconazole 200 mg twice daily orally is also a weak recommendation.
- Highly active antiretroviral therapy is to be initiated 2–10 weeks after the commencement of antifungal therapy. The exact timing for the initiation of HAART to avoid IRIS is not well determined. Long delays in initiating HAART increases risk of mortality. At the same time, consider drug interaction with antifungals and HAART.
- Suppressive therapy is discontinued once CD4$^+$ counts exceed 100 cells/µL, and HIV viral load is undetectable/very low for more than 3 months (continue antifungal therapy for minimum of 12 months).
- Reinstitute therapy if CD4+ count subsequently falls to less than 100 cells/µL.
- For asymptomatic antigenemia, perform LP and blood culture. If cultures are positive, treat as per recommendations for symptomatic meningoencephalitis. If there is no evidence of meningoencephalitis, use fluconazole 400 mg/day orally.
- Primary antifungal prophylaxis for cryptococcosis is not routinely recommended in HIV-positive individuals.

Cryptococcal Meningoencephalitis in Organ Transplant Recipients

Cryptococcosis has been documented in an average of 2.8% of SOT patients.

Induction Therapy

- Liposomal amphotericin B (3–4 mg/kg/day IV) or amphotericin B lipid complex [ABLC (5 mg/kg/day IV)] + flucytosine (100 mg/kg/day in four divided doses) for at least 2 weeks.
- Alternatively, LAmB 6 mg/kg/day IV or ABLC 5 mg/kg/day for 4–6 weeks.

Consolidation Therapy

Fluconazole (400–800 mg/day orally) for 8 weeks.

Maintenance Therapy

Fluconazole (200–400 mg/day orally) for 6–12 months.

- Concurrent use of AmBd and calcineurin inhibitors increases the risk of nephrotoxicity; LAmB is preferred for use as induction agent.
- Higher doses of LAmB (6 mg/kg/day) might be considered in the cases of relapse or high burden of disease.
- A positive serum cryptococcal antigen test in a transplant recipient warrants investigations for meningoencephalitis or disseminated disease.
- Isolation of *C. neoformans* in sputum of an SOT patient warrants further investigation for invasive pulmonary disease.

Non-Human Immunodeficiency Virus, Nontransplant Host with Meningoencephalitis

Induction Phase

- Amphotericin B deoxycholate (0.7–1 mg/kg/day IV) + flucytosine (100 mg/kg/day in four divided doses) for at least 4 weeks for induction therapy. This 4-week induction is applicable for patients where there are no severe neurological complications, and CSF culture becomes negative in 2 weeks after the initiation of the therapy. For AmBd toxicity issues, LAmB may be substituted in the second week at 3–4 mg/kg/day.
- In the case of patients with severe neurological complications, extend induction therapy for a total of 6 weeks.
- In case flucytosine is not given, lengthen induction with AmBd or LAmB for at least 2 weeks.
- In the cases of mild disease, immunocompetent patient with good clinical response and low chances of treatment failure, induction with AmBd and flucytosine can be cut short to 2 weeks with consolidation phase with fluconazole 800 mg/day for 8 weeks.

Consolidation Phase

Consolidation phase is with fluconazole 400 mg/day for 8 weeks (800 mg/day or 12 mg/kg/day if induction phase is 2 weeks).

Maintenance Phase

After induction and consolidation therapy, maintenance therapy is with fluconazole 200 mg/day (3 mg/kg) for 6–12 months.

Control of Cerebrospinal Fluid Pressure

Higher CSF pressure corresponds to higher burden of yeast in the CSF. Target opening pressure around 20 cm CSF. The ICP must be lowered gently to avoid the risk of cerebral herniation. Perform a CT scan or MRI in patients with focal neurological deficits, papilledema, or impaired mentation before performing LP. In case, pressure is 25 cm CSF or higher, manage with the following steps:

- Regular spinal taps daily until the CSF pressure and symptoms have been stabilized for >2 days.
- Spinal fluid drain or ventriculostomy for patients who need repeated LP on a daily basis.
- Ventriculoperitoneal (VP) shunt, if more conservative measures fail. VP shunt procedure can be performed even during active infection as long as antifungal treatment has been started before the shunt placement.
- Mannitol has no proven benefit.
- Acetazolamide or steroids are beneficial in the cases of raised pressure and IRIS.
- If there is obstructive hydrocephalus that needs decompression, ventriculostomy or VP shunt are required for drainage.
- Control of CSF pressure reduces headache.

Management of Immune Reconstitution Inflammatory Syndrome

Immune reconstitution inflammatory syndrome (IRIS) may develop if antiretroviral therapy is started early in cryptococcal meningitis in HIV. It has also been known to occur in immunocompetent patients during treatment for *C. gattii* and in SOT patients. IRIS is a clinical rather than a laboratory diagnosis. IRIS in cryptococcosis can manifest in two forms:

1. "Unmasking" IRIS wherein starting HAART unmasks the symptoms of cryptococcosis and these become apparent for the first time.
2. "Paradoxical" IRIS in which a patient is already a diagnosed case of cryptococcosis on treatment and later on IRIS appears on administration of HAART.

It can occur early or as late as 12 months after initiating therapy. It causes rapid deterioration in the patient's condition due to sudden enhanced host immune response. It is thought to be caused due to a shift from a predominantly anti-inflammatory Th2 immune response to a proinflammatory Th1 response on starting antifungal therapy. There are new neurological deficits, visual impairment, hydrocephalus, fever, mediastinal or abdominal lymphadenitis during the course of an otherwise successful antifungal treatment. It needs to be distinguished from microbiological progression of disease, drug-related side effects, and other opportunistic infections to tumors. It can prove fatal or cause graft rejection in SOT patients.

Risk factors for IRIS include:
- Very low CD4 cell count
- Fungemia
- Lack of previous use of antiretroviral therapy
- Introduction of HAART too early in the induction phase
- Rapid fall in viral load on starting HAART
- Lack of CSF sterilization at 2 weeks of induction therapy.

Manage severe IRIS with prednisone 0.5–1 mg/kg/day or high-dose dexamethasone. The duration of empirical steroid therapy may be 2–6 weeks. The manifestations may even resolve spontaneously in a few days to weeks. There is no need to alter antifungal therapy or add new antifungal agents. There is little evidence supporting the use of nonsteroidal anti-inflammatory drugs or thalidomide.

Management of Cerebral Cryptococcomas

Cerebral cryptococcomas require prolonged antifungal drugs, reduction in increased ICP, corticosteroids for mass effect, and surrounding edema. Induction phase is extended to 6 weeks. Consolidation and maintenance fluconazole should be continued for 6–18 months. Surgery may be stereotactic-guided debulkment and/or removal or performing open surgery. It is considered for lesions >3 cm which are producing a mass effect and are in an accessible location. Brain biopsy may be required when a differential diagnosis of a tumor or a second pathogen is being considered or if the mass is enlarging. Cryptococcomas are more often associated with *C. gattii* infection. Brain lesions can persist for long duration and may develop edema during effective antifungal therapy due to immunological response. Shunting is indicated for symptomatic hydrocephalus with dilated cerebral ventricles. Adjunctive recombinant interferon gamma (IFN-γ) is of unproven benefit although it has been tried as salvage therapy.

Cerebrospinal Fluid Examination during the Therapy

Perform weekly CSF examination till culture conversion is documented, and cultures remain negative for 4 weeks. CSF protein levels may be misguiding as these can remain elevated for years despite successful therapy.

Persistent Infection

Definition: Persistently positive results of cultures of CSF after 4 weeks of proven antifungal therapy at an established effective dose. Measures to counter persistence include the following:
- Decrease immunosuppression.
- Introduce HAART.
- Reinstitute induction phase of primary therapy for longer duration (4–10 weeks)

- Increase dose of AmBd or LAmB.
- Use of intraventricular or intrathecal AmBd is discouraged.
- Recheck isolates for changes in the minimal inhibitory concentration from the original isolate. A ≥3-dilution difference suggests the development of direct drug resistance.
- In azole-exposed patients, increasing dosage of azole alone is unlikely to be successful.
- Adjunctive recombinant IFN-γ can be considered for refractory infection but a positive impact on outcome is not definitive.

Relapse of Infection

Relapse of infection is defined as recovery of viable cryptococcosis from a previously checked sterile body site and recrudescence of signs and symptoms at the previous site of disease. In a relapsed infection, both of these features have normalized and then recurred. Most cases of relapse occur if duration or dosage of primary therapy is inadequate, or there is noncompliance during consolidation/maintenance phase. Restart induction and determine susceptibility. Salvage consolidation therapy may be instituted with the following:

- Fluconazole—800–1,200 mg/day
- Voriconazole—200–400 mg twice daily
- Posaconazole—200 mg orally four times per day or 400 mg twice per day orally

Pulmonary Cryptococcosis

- Some immunocompetent, asymptomatic patients with positive cultures, serology, or histopathology may have spontaneous recovery in the absence of antifungal therapy.
- In immunocompromised patients with pulmonary cryptococcosis, meningitis should be ruled out by LP. Blood and CSF cultures should be performed.
- Antifungal treatment is recommended in immunocompromised host, coexisting CNS or extrapulmonary cryptococcosis.
- Pneumonia associated with CNS disease, disseminated disease, or ARDS is treated like CNS disease.
- Corticosteroid treatment may be considered if ARDS is present in the context of IRIS.
- Patient may be kept under observation with no antifungal treatment if immunocompetent, small or stable, or shrinking pulmonary lesion and no evidence of dissemination.
- Antifungal treatment for mild-to-moderate disease (in the absence of diffuse infiltrates or severe immunosuppression) is fluconazole 400 mg/day orally for 6–12 months.
- In cases with severe disease, treat like CNS disease.
- In HIV-infected patients who are receiving HAART with a CD4 cell count >100 cells/µL and a cryptococcal antigen titer that is ≤1:512 and/or not increasing, fluconazole may be stopped after 1 year of treatment.
- For mild-to-moderate symptoms in immunocompetent patients, use fluconazole 400 mg/day for 6–12 months. For severe disease, treat like CNS infection (Table 16.3).
- Alternatives to fluconazole include itraconazole (200 mg twice daily), voriconazole (200 mg twice daily), or posaconazole (400 mg twice daily).
- Perform LP to rule out CNS involvement.

Table 16.3: Treatment of pulmonary cryptococcosis.		
Patient group	*Antifungal drug*	*Duration (months)*
Mild-to-moderate disease in immunocompetent/ immunocompromised	Fluconazole 400 mg/day	6–12
Severe disease in immunocompetent/ immunocompromised	Same as Central nervous system (CNS) disease	12

Nonmeningeal Nonpulmonary Cryptococcosis

Disseminated disease with involvement of at least two noncontiguous sites or evidence of high fungal burden with antigen titers of ≥1:512 should be treated similar to CNS disease. A single site infection can be treated with fluconazole 400 mg/day for 6–12 months.

Cryptococcosis in Pregnancy

- Immunological alteration in pregnancy may increase severity of cryptococcosis with mortality rates of up to 25%.
- Treat disseminated or CNS disease with AmBd or LAmB. It is category B rating in pregnancy. Use for a duration to ensure antifungal treatment throughout pregnancy.
- Flucytosine is category C, use only if benefits outweigh risks. It has been used in second and third trimesters without any increased risk to neonates in some studies.
- Avoid fluconazole in first trimester. In the last two trimesters, use after considering benefit versus risks. Fluconazole use in pregnancy has been associated with craniofacial ossification defects and renal pelvis defects.
- Patients with limited/stable pulmonary cryptococcosis can be observed during pregnancy and administered fluconazole postpartum.
- Fluconazole concentration in breast milk is similar to that of plasma concentration of the drug.
- Cryptococcosis symptoms may worsen in the third trimester and postpartum due to IRIS.

Cryptococcus gattii Infection

- Treat same as *C. neoformans* infection.
- Cryptococcomas are more frequent with *C. gattii* and managed as above.
- Certain genotypes of *C. gattii* are associated with reduced azole sensitivity.

Mortality

Without appropriate antifungal therapy, cryptococcocal meningoencephalitis in HIV may have 100% mortality within 2 weeks after the onset of clinical disease. Despite advanced medical care and access to HAART, the 3-month mortality during management of acute meningoencephalitis is approximately 20%.

■ CLINICAL PEARLS

- Test patients with cryptococcal meningoencephalitis or disseminated disease for HIV.
- Induction treatment is with amphotericin B and flucytosine. Monitor for nephrotoxicity and flucytosine cytotoxicity. After 2 weeks of induction therapy for meningoencephalitis, confirm sterilization of the CSF.
- Lower raised ICP ≥ 25 cm H_2O by repeated LPs, lumbar drain, ventriculostomy, or VP shunt.
- Monitor for IRIS.
- Cryptococcomas may need surgical management.
- Serum cryptococcal antigen does not correlate with disease progression or response to treatment.

■ SUGGESTED READING

1. Baddley JW, Schain DC, Gupte AA, et al. Transmission of *Cryptococcus neoformans* by organ transplantation. Clin Infect Dis. 2011;52:e94.
2. Bamba S, Lortholary O, Sawadogo A, et al. Decreasing incidence of cryptococcal meningitis in West Africa in the era of highly active antiretroviral therapy. AIDS. 2012;26:1039.
3. Chang LW, Phipps WT, Kennedy GE, et al. Antifungal interventions for the primary prevention of cryptococcal disease in adults with HIV. Cochrane Database Syst Rev. 2005;(3):CD004773.
4. Chaturvedi V, Chaturvedi S. *Cryptococcus gattii*: a resurgent fungal pathogen. Trends Microbiol. 2011;19:564.
5. Chen SC, Meyer W, Sorrell TC. *Cryptococcus gattii* infections. Clin Microbiol Rev. 2014;27:980.
6. Firacative C, Trilles L, Meyer W. MALDI-TOF MS enables the rapid identification of the major molecular types within the *Cryptococcus neoformans/C. gattii* species complex. PLoS One. 2012;7:e37566.
7. Hagen F, Khayhan K, Theelen B, et al. Recognition of seven species in the *Cryptococcus gattii/Cryptococcus neoformans* species complex. Fungal Genet Biol. 2015;78:16.
8. Harris J, Lockhart S, Chiller T. *Cryptococcus gattii*: Where do we go from here? Med Mycol. 2012;50:113.
9. Jarvis JN, Meintjes G, Rebe K, et al. Adjunctive interferon-γ immunotherapy for the treatment of HIV-associated cryptococcal meningitis: a randomized controlled trial. AIDS. 2012;26:1105.
10. Kwon-Chung KJ, Bennett JE. Epidemiologic differences between the two varieties of *Cryptococcus neoformans*. Am J Epidemiol. 1984;120:123.
11. Panel on Opportunistic Infections in HIV-infected Adults and Adolescents. Guidelines for the prevention and treatment of opportunistic infections in HIV-infected adults and adolescents: recommendations from the Centers for Disease Control and Prevention, the National Institutes of Health, and the HIV Medicine Association of the Infectious Diseases Society of America. [online] Available at http://aidsinfo.nih.gov/contentfiles/lvguidelines/adult_oi.pdf.
12. Pappas PG. Managing cryptococcal meningitis is about handling the pressure. Clin Infect Dis. 2005;40:480.
13. Perfect JR, Dismukes WE, Dromer F, et al. Clinical practice guidelines for the management of cryptococcal disease: 2010 Update by the Infectious Diseases Society of America. Clin Infect Dis. 2010;50:291.

14. Qu J, Zhou T, Zhong C, et al. Comparison of clinical features and prognostic factors in HIV-negative adults with cryptococcal meningitis and tuberculous meningitis: a retrospective study. BMC Infect Dis. 2017;17:51.

15. Thompson GR 3rd, Rendon A, Ribeiro Dos Santos R, et al. Isavuconazole treatment of cryptococcosis and dimorphic mycoses. Clin Infect Dis. 2016;63:356.

16. Vilchez RA, Fung J, Kusne S. Cryptococcosis in organ transplant recipients: an overview. Am J Transplant. 2002;2:575.

17

Aspergillosis

Monica Mahajan

INTRODUCTION

Aspergillosis is defined as an infection caused by one or more molds of the genus *Aspergillus*. It is a ubiquitous fungus, and exposure to its spores/conidia is frequent. The aerosolized conidia reach the tissues and germinate to form invasive fungal hyphae. The disease may be localized to lungs, sinuses, or other tissues. The invasive form of the disease is seen in immunocompromised individuals where invasive infection of lungs or sinuses disseminates to other organs and is potentially life-threatening. *Aspergillus* species may cause allergic manifestations in both atopic and nonatopic individuals.

TAXONOMY

Aspergillus species have a worldwide distribution. Although more than 100 species have been identified, fewer than 40 cause diseases in humans and animals. The most common species causing human illness are *Aspergillus fumigatus*, *Aspergillus niger*, and *Aspergillus clavatus*. Recent reports indicate increased incidence of invasive disease by *Aspergillus terreus*, a mold resistant to amphotericin B (AmB). *A. fumigatus* is an important human allergen. *A. fumigatus* and *A. clavatus* have been associated with extrinsic allergic bronchoalveolitis.

Aspergillus species is found on decaying matter and can withstand temperatures as high as 50°C. Inside the houses, *Aspergillus* can be isolated from basements, ventilation ducts, humidifiers, potted plants, and condiments, such as pepper.

Nosocomial aspergillosis occurs due to the presence of *Aspergillus* spores in the hospital environment. The outbreaks have occurred during new construction or building renovation. The contaminated ventilators, unfiltered air, or hospital water supply have been responsible for the nosocomial infections. However, most aspergillosis cases are sporadic, and it is difficult to determine whether an immunocompromised host acquired the infection inside or outside the hospital setting. The cases of invasive mold disease with the onset of symptoms ≥7 days after hospital admission are more likely to be nosocomial.

Aspergillus flavus produces a very potent carcinogen called Aflatoxin that causes hepatic necrosis and hepatocellular carcinoma. *A. flavus* grows on stored food grains and spices.

Aspergillus hyphae are dichotomously branched, Y-shaped with frequent septae, and branching at acute angle. This distinguishes them from the Mucorales that are pauci-septate and branch at right angle.

Inhalation of the *Aspergillus* spores is the most frequent route of infection. It may also occur from direct inoculation from contaminated dressings, corneal trauma/infection, or taking shower with contaminated water. Mold exposure can also occur following the consumption of contaminated food products.

PATHOGENESIS

Host Defenses

On inhalation of the conidia, the human host defenses get activated with the mucous layer and ciliary action of the airway epithelium. The macrophages and neutrophils engulf the fungus and eradicate it. They secrete inflammatory mediators after recognition of key cell wall components, such as β-D-glucan. The mediators cause recruitment of neutrophils. This results in killing of the invasive hyphae producing secondary inflammation. Corticosteroids and immunosuppressive therapy impair macrophages and neutrophil function.

Microbial Factors

Aspergillus produces mycotoxins and proteases which affect the host defense mechanisms adversely by inhibiting macrophage phagocytosis and killing by inhibiting nicotinamide adenine dinucleotide phosphate (NADPH) oxidase activation. They also interfere with the functional T-cell responses.

The fungal hyphae bind to the vascular wall and damage the basement membrane, extracellular matrix, and cellular constituents. This causes angioinvasion, infarction, and tissue necrosis.

RISK FACTORS FOR INVASIVE ASPERGILLOSIS

Invasive aspergillosis (IA) is seen in immunocompromised hosts, including patients with hematological malignancy, hematopoietic stem cell transplant, solid-organ transplant (SOT), corticosteroid use, AIDS, chronic obstructive pulmonary disease (COPD), intensive care unit (ICU), tumor necrosis factor (TNF) blockers, etc. The duration and degree of neutropenia during chemotherapy regimens for remission induction, consolidation, or relapse is predictive of occurrence of IA.

- *Hematopoietic stem cell transplant*: The risk of IA is higher in allogeneic hematopoietic stem cell transplantation (HSCT) compared with autologous HSCT. In human leukocyte antigen (HLA)-mismatched donor recipients, there is delayed engraftment and higher chances of graft-versus-host disease (GVHD). These patients are most vulnerable to IA during the following conditions:
  - Neutropenia following the conditioning regimen
  - Acute GVHD requiring exogenous immunosuppression.

- ◆ Chronic GVHD (>100 days after transplant) requiring exogenous immunosuppression
- ◆ Concomitant cytomegalovirus (CMV) infection is an additional risk factor for IA. T cell-depleted or CD34 selected stem cell products increase the risk.
- *Solid-organ transplant*: Lung transplant patients have the higher risk of IA. The predisposing factors include pretransplant *Aspergillus* airway colonization, especially among cystic fibrosis patients, CMV infection, obliterative bronchiolitis, graft rejection, and increased immunosuppression. Heart, lung and liver transplant patients are at higher risk of IA compared with renal transplant recipients. The risk increases with poor allograft function and impaired renal function requiring hemodialysis. Donor CMV seropositivity is a risk factor for late-onset IA in renal transplant recipients.
- *Inherited immunodeficiencies*: Chronic granulomatous disease (CGD) is characterized by recurrent bacterial and fungal infections. Patients with CGD have an inherited disorder of the phagocyte NADPH oxidase. Mannose-binding lactic deficiency has also been associated with IA.
- *Human immunodeficiency virus (HIV) infection*: With the introduction of highly active antiretroviral therapy, the incidence of AIDS-associated aspergillosis is reducing. Risk factors include neutropenia, steroid use, and concurrent opportunistic infections.
- *Immunosuppressants*: Newer agents target the immune cell populations and signaling pathways. Tumor necrosis factor (TNF)-α antagonists have a greater risk of IA associated with their use compared with nonbiological antirheumatic drugs. Use of infliximab in severe GVHD is associated with higher risk of IA. Alemtuzumab (anti-CD52) makes patients more prone to IA and CMV reactivation.
- *Chronic obstructive pulmonary disease*: Use of glucocorticoid therapy in patients with COPD is associated with IA.
- *Critical illnesses*: Admission in ICUs, prolonged ventilation and multiorgan failure, and comorbidities are heterogeneous risk factors that increase the risk of IA.
- *Gene polymorphism*: Various gene polymorphisms involved in innate immune response, e.g. interleukin (IL)-1-beta and toll-like receptor 4 gene have been associated with increased risk of IA. Genetic deficiency of the soluble pattern-recognition receptor called PTX3 (long pentraxin 3) in the *PTX3* gene of donor cells leads to impaired neutrophil antifungal capacity and increased IA in recipients of HSCT.

CLINICAL MANIFESTATIONS

Aspergillosis can have a wide range of clinical manifestations from acute invasive to chronic and allergic. These are distinguished from each other on the basis of clinical progression, radiological features, and histopathology.

Acute Invasive Pulmonary Aspergillosis

Acute invasive pulmonary aspergillosis (IPA) occurs most frequently due to inhalation of conidia and less often due to direct inoculation into the skin or spread from the gastrointestinal tract. It most commonly involves the lungs but hematogenous dissemination to distant organs including the central nervous system (CNS) can occur.

Angioinvasion by the fungus causes hemorrhagic infarction. This process leads to the formation of a necrotic center surrounded by a ring of hemorrhage and edema. This produces the "halo sign" surrounding the nodular density on imaging studies.

The classic triad of aspergillosis in neutropenic patients is fever, pleuritic chest pain, and hemoptysis. However, there can be neutropenic patients where the only manifestation of the disease is fever which is unresponsive to broad-spectrum antibiotics. Patients may have nonproductive cough and dyspnea.

Lung imaging may reveal focal pulmonary infiltrates, nodules, and wedge-shaped infarcts. The focal infiltrates may lead to the formation of a cavity during the recovery phase of neutropenia.

Empyema

Aspergillus empyema may manifest as pleural effusion.

Tracheobronchitis

Tracheobronchial aspergillosis (TBA) is seen most frequently in lung transplant recipients. The typical presentation of the patient is with dyspnea, cough, and wheeze. The cough may be associated with expectoration of intraluminal mucus plugs. The various patterns of *Aspergillus* tracheobronchitis are the following:

- *Pseudomembranous tracheobronchitis*: The pseudomembrane is composed of fungal hyphae admixed with necrotic debris and forming an inflammatory layer over the mucosa.
- *Ulcerative tracheobronchitis*: There is focal invasion of the tracheobronchial mucosa and cartilage by fungal hyphae leading to ulceration.
- *Obstructive bronchial aspergillosis*: The airways are filled with mucus plugs formed by fungal hyphae. These plugs lead to segmental or lobar atelectasis.

  Aspergillosis of the bronchial stump can develop from infection of the silk sutures. The incidence can be reduced by using nylon monofilaments instead of silk. In lung transplant patients, tracheobronchitis develops in the first month after transplantation and may be associated with complications, including:

  a. Anastomotic dehiscence
  b. Bronchial stenosis
  c. Bronchial necrosis
  d. Bronchoarterial fistula formation.

Bronchoscopic examination is diagnostic.

Acute Invasive Rhinosinusitis

Invasive *Aspergillus* rhinosinusitis resembles rhinocerebral mucormycosis in its clinical manifestations. However, the major predisposing factor for aspergillosis and mucormycosis are neutropenia and uncontrolled diabetes, respectively.

Aspergillus flavus and *A. fumigatus* have higher propensity for rhinosinusitis. The patient presents with fever, unilateral sinusitis, facial pain, and nasal congestion. Nasal endoscopy may reveal an eschar over the nasal septum or turbinates. Orbital involvement causes proptosis,

ptosis, and ophthalmoplegia. Aspergillosis of the ethmoid or sphenoid sinuses can cause cavernous sinus thrombosis with III, IV, V, and VI nerve involvement. Spread of infection to the CNS can prove fatal. Some patients may have a milder form of the disease with focal rhinitis.

Central Nervous System Aspergillosis

Central nervous system involvement in aspergillosis may occur as hematogenous spread as part of disseminated disease or as contiguous spread from rhinosinusitis. The patients may present with focal neurological deficits, paresis, seizures, or cranial nerve involvement. The characteristic features of CNS aspergillosis are abscesses and cortical or subcortical infarcts. A SOT patient developing a cerebral abscess early post-transplant should be investigated for aspergillosis. Focal meningitis and solid intracerebral lesions/cerebral granuloma can be other manifestations of CNS aspergillosis. Cerebrospinal fluid (CSF) culture may be negative but *Aspergillus* galactomannan (GM) may be detected in the CSF. Vascular occlusion by fungal hyphae may reduce antifungal penetration.

Aspergillus Endophthalmitis

Aspergillus endophthalmitis can be a consequence of hematogenous spread of disseminated infection to the eye. Rarely, it may result from an ocular trauma or a corneal infection. *A. fumigatus* is most frequently implicated. The presenting symptoms include eye pain and impaired vision. Physical signs include iridocyclitis, vitritis, or retinitis. Other features may include hypopyon formation, yellow-white retinal lesions, and retinal hemorrhage. Progressive involvement of the various structures of the eye carries a poor visual prognosis and may require enucleation.

Aspergillus Osteomyelitis

Aspergillus osteomyelitis may mimic tubercular osteomyelitis or caries spine. Although it is an uncommon condition but is seen more in children with CGD. The most frequent sites of infection are the ribs and the spine. The infection can occur as a direct spread from the underlying lung in the cases of pulmonary aspergillosis, hematogenous spread, or from direct inoculation during a surgical procedure. The clinical features include fever, soft tissue tenderness over the involved bone, or a paraspinal abscess. *Aspergillus* osteomyelitis may spread to the adjacent joint leading to fungal arthritis.

Cardiac Aspergillosis

Cardiac involvement in aspergillosis may result most frequently in valvular or mural endocarditis. However, there may be myocardial or pericardial infection in some instances.

Aspergillus is the second most frequent etiological agent for fungal endocarditis, the most common being *Candida* spp. The infection occurs primarily in patients with prosthetic heart valves or in parenteral drug abusers. The onset may be early if the fungus contaminates the surgical site. Endocarditis may also develop in relation to central venous catheters. *Aspergillus* has been isolated in some cases of vascular prosthetic grafts of the aorta in immunocompetent individuals.

The clinical presentation of *Aspergillus* endocarditis is with fever and embolic complications. Patient may experience anorexia, fatigue, and weight loss. The valvular vegetations are large and friable with tendency to embolism to major arteries. Physical examination may reveal cardiac murmurs and splenomegaly. The microscopic examination of the embolus may reveal *Aspergillus* hyphae. Despite medical and surgical interventions, endocarditis may have 100% mortality. *Aspergillus* myocarditis is a postmortem diagnosis in patients with disseminated disease. *Aspergillus* pericarditis may arise from transmural infection from endocardial infection, contiguous pulmonary or mediastinal lesions or intraoperative contamination.

Gastrointestinal Aspergillosis

It is primarily seen in neutropenic patients with mucositis. Direct inoculation of the gastrointestinal tract can cause abdominal pain, gastrointestinal bleed, appendicitis, typhlitis, or ulceration of colonic mucosa.

Renal Aspergillosis

Aspergillosis limited to the urinary tract is rare. This can be a focus of disseminated disease in immunocompromised or intravenous (IV) drug abusers. *A. fumigatus* is the most common isolate. Three different patterns of renal involvement include: (1) disseminated aspergillosis with hematogenous renal involvement, (2) aspergillosis of the renal pelvis with bezoar formation, and (3) ascending panurothelial aspergillosis. Renal involvement is silent if disease is limited to cortex of kidney. Renal pelvis involvement may be unilateral or bilateral. *Aspergillus* bezoars/masses may cause hydronephrosis. Both bladder and prostate involvement have been reported. Outflow obstruction symptoms similar to benign prostatic hyperplasia are noted.

Cutaneous Aspergillosis

Cutaneous aspergillosis can be in two forms:
1. Primary cutaneous aspergillosis due to direct inoculation of fungal spores into the skin
2. Secondary cutaneous aspergillosis due to contiguous spread from underlying infected tissue or hematogenous spread, especially from the lungs.

Cutaneous aspergillosis is seen more frequently in burn victims, neonates, malignancies, HSCT, and SOT patients. Cutaneous ulcers in healthy individuals have been due to traumatic inoculation, use of contaminated adhesive tapes and armboards/splints.

The cutaneous lesion begins as an erythematous, indurated plaque which further progresses to a necrotic ulcers with a black eschar. Secondary cutaneous aspergillosis lesions may be multiple which may enlarge and coalesce. Similar cutaneous lesions are seen with other fungi, including mucormycosis and *Fusarium*. It is important to perform a deep skin biopsy to demonstrate the hyphae invading the blood vessels.

Disseminated Aspergillosis

Aspergillus can disseminate to multiple organs, including the brain, eye, kidneys, liver, skin, and bone. Disseminated disease has poor prognosis.

> **Box 17.1:** Predisposing factors for chronic pulmonary aspergillosis
>
> - Pulmonary tuberculosis especially with cavities ≥2 cm
> - Nontuberculous mycobacteria—*Mycobacterium avium* complex, *Mycobacterium xenopi*, *Mycobacterium malmoense*
> - Asthma requiring glucocorticoids
> - Chronic obstructive pulmonary disease
> - Fibrocavitary sarcoidosis stage II/III
> - Allergic bronchopulmonary aspergillosis
> - Bullae formation secondary to pneumothorax
> - Silicosis
> - Pneumoconiosis
> - Rheumatoid arthritis
> - Ankylosing spondylitis
> - Hyperimmunoglobulin E syndrome
> - Genetic defects in immune function, e.g. TLR4, TREM-1, VEGFA
>
> Treated lung cancer
>
> Radiotherapy chest
>
> Cannabis lung
>
> TLR, toll-like receptor; TREM, triggering receptor expressed on myeloid cells; VEGFA, vascular endothelial growth factor A.

Chronic Pulmonary Aspergillosis

Chronic pulmonary aspergillosis has a spectrum of manifestations ranging from aspergilloma to chronic necrotizing aspergillosis (also called subacute IPA), chronic cavitary pulmonary aspergillosis (CCPA), and *Aspergillus* nodules. The chronic and relapsing nature of the disease poses a challenge to effective treatment.

A patient suffering from aspergillosis for longer than 3-month duration is said to be suffering from chronic pulmonary aspergillosis. Chronic pulmonary aspergillosis occurs in immunocompetent patients who have either prior pulmonary damage or disease. The underlying diseases predispose to chronic aspergillosis (Box 17.1).

Aspergilloma

An aspergilloma is a dense fungus ball composed of a rounded conglomerate of *Aspergillus* hyphae matted together, fibrin, mucus, and cellular debris in a preexisting pulmonary cavity colonized by *Aspergillus* species. The risk of developing an aspergilloma within a cavity of 2 cm in diameter is 15–20%. Patients with pulmonary tuberculosis (TB), fibrocystic sarcoidosis, histoplasmosis, pneumoconiosis, bullae, lung cancer (primary or metastatic) treated with radiofrequency ablation, and bronchiectasis are more likely to develop aspergillomas. Patients recovering from neutropenia may develop aspergillomas in consolidated lesions in the lungs. HIV patients with prior *Pneumocystis jiroveci* pneumonia may develop aspergilloma in the cystic areas of the lung. In countries with a high burden of TB, a cavity resulting from TB is the most common cause of a simple aspergilloma.

The usual site of aspergilloma is the upper lobe, reflecting the predilection for cavities to form there but sometimes these may be located in the apical segments of the lower lobes. Mycelial growth arises from the cavity wall, subsequently spreading to the lumen of the cavity. Layers of mycelia accumulate over months to form a fungal ball. Since the fungal ball does not completely fill the cavity, it may be mobile and same can be documented on imaging. The air crescent between the aspergilloma and the cavity wall may not always be obvious, as there may be mycelial fronds in that space. Endobronchial aspergillomas have also been reported.

Aspergilloma may be noticed as a radiographic abnormality in an asymptomatic individual with a preexisting lung cavity. Other patients may present with fever, cough, weight loss, fatigue, chest pain, or hemoptysis. Hemoptysis occurs in 50–90% of the cases. However, 40–60% patients may have massive hemoptysis that can be life-threatening. Spontaneous lysis of the aspergilloma has been noted in 10% patients. Pleural aspergillosis may be a complication of aspergilloma resection or result from a bronchopleural fistula.

Chronic Necrotizing Pulmonary Aspergillosis or Subacute IPA

Chronic necrotizing pulmonary aspergillosis (CNPA) is a subacute form of IPA characterized by a slowly progressive inflammatory destruction of lung tissue superimposed on a chronic lung disease. It develops in patients with COPD, alcoholism, prolonged corticosteroid use, or HIV. The symptoms progress over 1–3 months including fever, cough, and weight loss. Patients are unresponsive to prolonged courses of antibiotic therapy, and the radiograph reveals areas of cavitating pneumonia or consolidation. Some patients may receive empiric antitubercular therapy without any response.

Chronic Cavitary Pulmonary Aspergillosis

Chronic cavitary pulmonary aspergillosis (CCPA) was previously termed "complex aspergilloma" since significant number of patients did not have a demonstrable aspergilloma inside the cavities. Immunocompetent patients develop one or more pulmonary cavities that expand and coalesce over months. This leads to loss of functional lung tissue. Symptoms include cough, fever, weight loss, breathlessness, and hemoptysis.

Chronic fibrosing pulmonary aspergillosis is a late stage of CCPA which is characterized by extensive fibrosis and destroyed lung.

Chronic cavitary pulmonary aspergillosis differs from aspergilloma as there is less pleural thickening, multiple enlarging cavities that may or may not have a fungus ball in them in CCPA compared with the latter.

Diagnostic criteria for CCPA include the following:
- A period of 3 months of chronic pulmonary symptoms or progressive radiographic abnormalities with cavitation, pleural thickening, pericavitary infiltrates, and sometimes a fungal ball
- Elevated *Aspergillus* immunoglobulin G (IgG) antibody or other microbiological data
- No or minimal immunocompromised, usually with one or more underlying pulmonary disorders.

The *Aspergillus* IgG antibody test is the most sensitive microbiological test. Sputum polymerase chain reaction (PCR) for aspergillosis has better sensitivity than sputum culture.

Table 17.1: Differences between Chronic invasive *Aspergillus* rhinosinusitis and Chronic granulomatous *Aspergillus* sinusitis.

Chronic invasive Aspergillus rhinosinusitis	Chronic granulomatous Aspergillus sinusitis
Aspergillus fumigatus is the most common cause	*Aspergillus flavus* is the most common cause
Worldwide distribution, largest number of cases reported in North America	Reported more from North Africa, the Middle East and Southeast Asia (India, Pakistan, Saudi Arabia)
The sinus mass is necrotic, friable, or purulent with dense accumulation of hyphae infiltrating mucosa, blood vessels and adjacent tissues, necrosis of tissue	The sinus mass is firm, adherent and difficult to remove with noncaseating granuloma with scanty fungal hyphae within Langerhans-type giant cells, vasculitis perivascular fibrosis
Infection commences in deeper sinuses— posterior ethmoid and sphenoid. The infection spreads to contiguous structures—orbit leading to orbital apex syndrome, cavernous sinus or anterior cranial fossa	Chiefly involves maxillary and ethmoid sinuses, nose, orbit, and cheek. The infection causes tissue destruction by pressure necrosis and expansion of the mass which is also called paranasal granuloma
Presenting symptoms include thick, purulent mucus discharge, anosmia, persistent headache, proptosis or cavernous sinus thrombosis	Presenting symptoms include nasal obstruction, facial discomfort or silent unilateral proptosis or an enlarging painless, irregular mass in the cheek, orbit, nose, or paranasal sinuses mimicking an orbital tumor
Occurs in patients with subtle immunosuppression as in diabetes, corticosteroid use and human immunodeficiency virus (HIV)	Develops in immunocompetent patients or well controlled diabetics

Aspergillus Nodules

Aspergillus nodules can be single or multiple, may or may not have cavitation within them, and occur in immmunocompetent individuals. The nodule is composed of a necrotic center containing fungal hyphae. This is surrounded by inflammatory granuloma formation containing multinucleate giant cells. Patient can be asymptomatic or may experience mild cough. It is important to rule out carcinoma of the lung which may have a similar appearance on radiography. These nodules are usually non-spiculated. Problem arises in differential diagnosis as *Aspergillus* nodules can be moderately or strongly fluoro deoxy glucose (FDG) avid in positron emission tomography (PET) scanning and mimic carcinoma lung. Histopathology and a positive *Aspergillus* IgG titer in blood are useful.

Aspergillus Otomycosis

This is a chronic manifestation of aspergillosis involving the external auditory canal in patients with diabetes mellitus, hypogammaglobulinemia, eczema, or HIV. The symptoms include pain, pruritus, and/or discharge. In the cases of tympanic membrane perforation the middle ear and mastoid sinus get involved.

Chronic Aspergillus Rhinosinusitis (Table 17.1)

Fungal organisms are the etiology for chronic rhinosinusitis in 6–12% of patients, *Aspergillus* species being the leading cause. A fungal etiology is suspected in patients with refractory or

> **Box 17.2:** Diagnostic criteria for ABPA: International Society for Human and Animal Mycology (ISHAM) Working Group.
>
> - *Predisposing conditions* (one must be present)
>   - Asthma
>   - Cystic fibrosis
> - *Obligatory criteria* (both must be present)
>   - *Aspergillus* skin test positivity or detectable IgE levels against *Aspergillus fumigatus*
>   - Elevated total serum IgE (typically >1,000 IU/mL), but if the patient meets the other criteria, an IgE level <1,000 IU/mL can be acceptable
> - *Other criteria* (at least two must be present)
>   - Precipitating serum antibodies to *A. fumigatus*
>   - Radiographic pulmonary opacities consistent with ABPA
>   - Total eosinophil count >500 cells/μL in glucocorticoid naive patients (can be historical)
>
> ABPA, allergic bronchopulmonary aspergillosis; IgE, immunoglobulin E.

recurrent sinusitis. Diagnosis is often delayed, especially in immunocompetent individuals. Chronic *Aspergillus* rhinosinusitis can present as follows:

- Chronic invasive *Aspergillus* rhinosinusitis
- Chronic granulomatous *Aspergillus* sinusitis
- *Allergic manifestations of aspergillosis.*

Allergic Manifestations of Aspergillosis

The allergic forms of aspergillosis include: (1) Allergic bronchopulmonary aspergillosis (ABPA), (2) Extrinsic allergic alveolitis, and (3) Allergic *Aspergillus* sinusitis (AAS).

Allergic Bronchopulmonary Aspergillosis (Box 17.2)

Allergic bronchopulmonary aspergillosis (ABPA) is a complex hypersensitivity reaction of the lungs due to inhalation and colonization of the airways with spores of *A. fumigatus*. It occurs in atopic individuals with asthma or in patients with cystic fibrosis. It causes episodic airway obstruction, mucus plug impaction, and eosinophilia secondary to a humoral immune response.

Allergic bronchopulmonary aspergillosis occurs in 1–2% of patients with persistent asthma and 2–9% patients with cystic fibrosis. Other predisposing conditions associated with ABPA include bronchiectasis, CGD, hyperimmunoglobulinemia E, and lung transplant.

As a response to *Aspergillus* antigens, T-cells generate cytokines including IL-4, IL-5, and IL-13. These ILs increase immunoglobulin E (IgE) levels and cause eosinophilia in ABPA patients. When *Aspergillus* colonizes in the airways, there is a significant IgE- and IgG-mediated immune response. Despite this vigorous immune response, the fungus is able to colonize, release mycotoxins, and cause airway damage. There is T-helper CD4+ cells-mediated eosinophilic inflammation and IL-8-mediated neutrophilic inflammation.

Mucus plugs impacting the bronchi contain the fungal hyphae but the fungus does not invade the mucosa. Eosinophilia is present in sputum, blood, and lung tissue. This complex hypersensitivity reaction leads to inflammation, bronchiectasis, fibrosis, and respiratory compromise. There is the development of apical fibrosis.

Genetic susceptibility has been reported in patients with ABPA. Certain HLA alleles, especially HLA-DR2, increase susceptibility to ABPA, whereas HLA-DQ2 is protective.

The clinical presentation is that of recurrent exacerbations of bronchial asthma with accompanying fever, malaise, cough, expectoration with brownish mucus plugs due to fungal hyphae, and weight loss. Occasionally, the patients may have hemoptysis. Wheezing may be noted on auscultation. Some patients may have asymptomatic consolidation lung with no obvious wheeze. ABPA may be associated with AAS. The patients have frequent relapses and remissions and progress from steroid-responsive to steroid-dependent asthma. Bronchiectasis and disabling fibrosis with end-stage lung disease are late complications of ABPA.

Extrinsic Allergic Alveolitis

This unusual allergic manifestation of *Aspergillus* is seen in malt workers. The causative organism is *Aspergillus clavatus*. It is a hypersensitivity pneumonitis that develops within few hours after exposure and manifests as fever, dyspnea, reticulonodular infiltrates, and a positive IgG precipitin test. Unlike ABPA, eosinophilia is not a feature of extrinsic allergic alveolitis.

Allergic Aspergillus Sinusitis (AAS)

This is a noninvasive allergic manifestation of aspergillosis seen in immunocompetent patients. They experience recurrent bouts of rhinosinusitis which do not resolve with antihistaminics, antibiotics, or nasal corticosteroids. Some patients may have coexisting asthma or ABPA.

Symptoms include thick, yellowish-green sinus discharge, nasal polyps, proptosis if the allergic mucin enters orbit or deviated nasal septum. It differs from invasive rhinosinusitis as there is no true tissue invasion despite mucosal thickening and bone erosion.

Sinus aspirate obtained at the time of surgery or nasal endoscopy yields mucinous material that contains eosinophils, Charcot–Leyden crystals, and hyphal elements.

■ DIFFERENTIAL DIAGNOSES

- Infections causing pulmonary involvement and similar radiological features as aspergillosis include the following:
  - *Mucorales*
  - *Fusarium* spp.
  - *Scedosporium apiospermum*
  - *Scedosporium prolificans*
  - Tuberculosis
  - *Pseudomonas aeruginosa*
  - Granulomatosis with polyangitis (Wegener's granulomatosis)
  - Acute respiratory distress syndrome
  - Bronchiectasis
  - Lung abscess
  - Sarcoidosis.

- Differential diagnosis of *Aspergillus* rhinosinusitis with CNS involvement:
  - Mucormycosis
- Differential diagnoses of *Aspergillus* brain abscess:
  - *Mucorales*
  - *Fusarium* spp.
  - *Scedosporium* spp.
  - Dematiaceous fungi
  - Pyogenic abscess
  - Tuberculomas
  - Central nervous system lymphoma.
- Differential diagnoses of ABPA:
  - Asthma with fungal sensitization with positive serum precipitins to *Aspergillus* but do not meet with full criteria for the diagnosis of ABPA. They may experience recurrent mucoid impaction, atelectasis, bronchiectasis, and elevated serum total IgE.
  - Pulmonary eosinophilia due to causes other than ABPA, including:
    - Acute or chronic eosinophilic pneumonia
    - Drug or toxin-induced eosinophilia, e.g. nonsteroidal anti-inflammatory drugs, nitrofurantoin, phenytoin
    - Tropical pulmonary eosinophilia (*Wuchereria bancrofti, Brugia malayi*)
    - Loeffler's pneumonia (*Ascaris, Ancylostoma*)
    - Hypereosinophilic syndromes
    - Eosinophilic granulomatosis and polyangiitis (Churg–Strauss).
  - Bronchiectasis secondary to cystic fibrosis, ciliary dysfunction, hypogammaglobulinemia.
  - *Mucoid impaction and bronchocentric granulomatosis:* Half the cases of broncho-centric granulomatosis are not associated with ABPA. Bronchocentric granulomatosis characterizes lung injury due to various etiologies, including ABPA, TB, Wegener's granulomatosis, rheumatoid arthritis, influenza A, red cell aplasia, glomerulonephritis, or bronchogenic carcinoma.

DIAGNOSIS

Tissue and fluid specimens are collected for histopathology and culture.

Laboratory Investigations

Blood eosinophil count is elevated in ABPA. Total serum IgE levels of >1,000 IU/mL, IgE and IgG antibodies specific to *Aspergillus* may be present in the serum. Sputum contains eosinophils and Charcot–Leyden crystals. Other causes of elevated IgE levels need to be excluded (Table 17.2).

Histopathology

It is vital to demonstrate histopathologic evidence of *Aspergillus* to determine the significance of a positive culture. Specimens can be obtained by bronchoscopy and bronchoalveolar lavage

Table 17.2: Causes of elevated IgE levels.

Atopy	ABPA, allergic rhinitis, allergic asthma, allergic dermatitis
Infections	Parasites, EBV, CMV, TB, HIV
Neoplasms	Hodgkins, IgE myeloma
Immunodeficiency syndromes	Hyperimmunoglobulin E, DiGeorge, Wiskott–Aldrich
Inflammatory disorders	Churg–Strauss
Miscellaneous	Bullous pemphigoid, nephrotic syndrome, cystic fibrosis, smoker, BMT

ABPA, allergic bronchopulmonary aspergillosis; BMT, bone marrow transplantation; CMV, cytomegalovirus; EBV, Epstein–Barr virus; HIV, human immunodeficiency virus; IgE, immunoglobulin E; TB: tuberculosis.

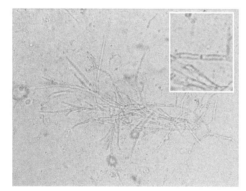

Fig. 17.1: Hyaline, septate fungal hyphae with branching at acute angle.

(BAL), video-assisted thoracoscopic biopsy, or percutaneous needle aspiration. The optical brighteners, Calcofluor or Blankophor, are used as special stains. Fixed tissues can be stained with Gomori methenamine silver (GMS) or periodic acid–Schiff stains. *Aspergillus* appears as acute-angle branching septate hyphae. Culture helps to distinguish *Aspergillus* from other filamentous fungi, including *Fusarium* species and *Scedosporium* species.

Aspergillus Culture

The fungal culture has a low yield, and a negative culture does not eliminate the possibility of *Aspergillus* infection. *Aspergillus* grows in 2–5 days at 37°C on fungal culture media. Growth on culture helps in species identification and susceptibility testing (Figs. 17.1 to 17.3).

Aspergillus Polymerase Chain Reaction

Aspergillus polymerase chain reaction (PCR) is not being used as a routine diagnostic test due to lack of conclusive validation of commercially available kits. It has limitations as it cannot

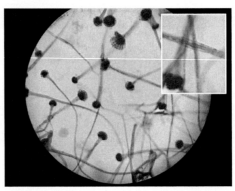

Fig. 17.2: *Aspergillus fumigatus* on (lactophenol cotton blue LPCB) mount.

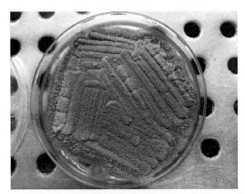

Fig. 17.3: Velvety, smoky-green colonies of *Aspergillus fumigatus* on Sabouraud dextrous agar (SDA).

distinguish colonization from disease. Moreover, PCR cannot distinguish various *Aspergillus* species.

Galactomannan

It is the most important and accurate biomarker for diagnosis of IA and an adjunctive test in high-risk patients, who are not on mold prophylaxis. It can be applied on BAL specimens rather than blood in patients who are on mold-active antifungals. The sensitivity of GM testing is approximately 70% in patients with hematological malignancy and allogeneic HSCT. The sensitivity is lower in SOT recipients, CGD, or non-neutropenic patients. Neutropenic patients may have a higher fungal burden or less robust inflammatory response. The sensitivity in chronic pulmonary aspergillosis and aspergilloma is lower and test can be negative in cystic fibrosis patients colonized with *Aspergillus*. False-positive GM test results are obtained with the use of piperacillin–tazobactam, amoxycillin–clavulanate, neonatal colonization with *Bifidobacterium*, and other fungal infections, including penicilliosis, fusariosis, histoplasmosis, and blastomycosis.

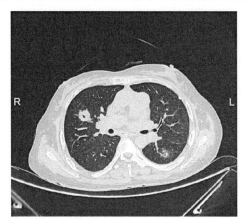

Fig. 17.4: CT scan of chest, axial section, shows irregular nodular opacity in right middle lobe with small area of cavitation in a patient of pulmonary aspergillosis.

A strategy of combining PCR and GM improves sensitivity, aids early diagnosis, and reduces injudicious antifungal use.

β-D-Glucan

This is not a specific investigation for IA. Other fungal infections, including candidiasis, fusariosis, and *P. jiroveci* pneumonia can also give a positive result. It is useful in diagnosing fungal infection in immunocompromised patients. β-D-glucan may be false positive due to various drugs, including ampicillin–sulbactam, cephalosporins, carbapenems, pegylated asparaginase, and glucan-contaminated blood sample collection tubes.

Pulmonary Function Test

Pulmonary function test shows an obstructive pattern with reduced forced expiratory volume 1 (FEV_1). A positive bronchodilator response is seen in less than 50% patients. In the cases with chronic fibrosing pulmonary aspergillosis, vital capacity and diffusion capacity are reduced. Patient has hypoxemia accompanied by hypocapnia or hypercapnia.

Radiographic Diagnosis of Aspergillosis (Figs. 17.4 to 7.8)

The role of radiography in aspergillosis is vital in the following:
- Identifying the site of infection
- Extent of involvement, type and size of lesions
- Spread to contiguous structures
- Decision regarding further diagnostic procedures, including bronchoscopy or computed tomography (CT)-guided biopsy.

Conventional imaging techniques including X-rays may show nonspecific findings, and chest CT is highly recommended if there is strong suspicion of IA. High-resolution CT (HRCT) scan is the

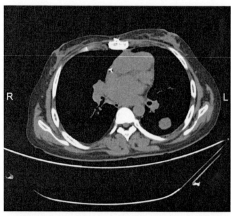

Fig. 17.5: CT scan of chest, axial section, shows a well-defined opacity in left lower lobe due to pulmonary aspergillosis.

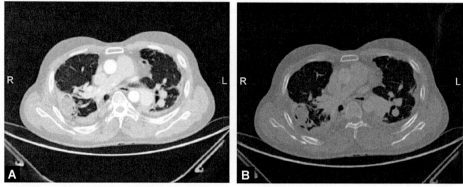

Figs. 17.6 A and B: Chest CT scans, axial sections, show cavitary lesion in right upper lobe with intracavitary soft tissue density and eccentric air in the cavity suggestive of aspergilloma along with bilateral pleural effusion.

preferred modality. CT scan helps in diagnosing the focus of infection in febrile neutropenia. Contrast scan is recommended in cases where a nodule or a mass needs further evaluation. A follow-up scan is ordered 2 weeks after the initiation of treatment if unresponsive to treatment, clinical deterioration or lesion is close to a blood vessel.

The classical findings of IPA on CT scan include nodules, consolidative lesions, or wedge-shaped infarcts. Nodules and a halo sign are indicative of angioinvasion. Involvement of airways and bronchiolar obstruction produces micronodules and tree-in-bud opacities.

Halo sign: A nodule >1 cm in diameter is surrounded by a perimeter of ground-glass opacity consequent to hemorrhage. It is more frequent finding in CT scan in neutropenic patients.

Air crescent sign: A crescent-shaped radiolucency due to air within a consolidation or a nodule is a radiological finding in the late phase of the disease seen during the recovery phase of neutropenia.

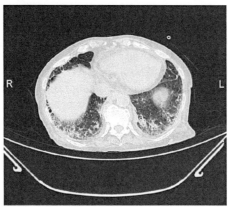

Fig. 17.7: Chest CT scan, axial section, shows patchy interstitial and alveolar opacities in bilateral lower lobes in a patient of febrile neutropenia with IPA.

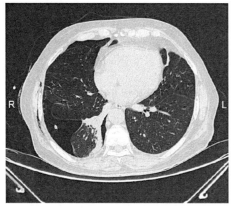

Fig. 17.8: Chest CT scan, axial section, shows sub-segmental atelectasis in right lower lobe with associated pneumothorax with occluded right lower lobe bronchus.

Reverse halo sign is noted more frequently in patients with mucormycosis rather than with IPA. The halo and reverse halo sign are nonspecific and may be seen in TB and noninfectious diseases. The size of pulmonary lesions shows an initial increase and a subsequent decrease on initiation of treatment.

The classical feature of ABPA on imaging is central bronchiectasis affecting the central one half of the lungs. A conventional radiograph shows parenchymal opacities, atelectasis, and various patterns of bronchiectasis. Tram-line shadows appear due to thickened walls of nondilated bronchi, while parallel lines are due to ectatic bronchi. Saccular bronchiectasis produces ring shadows. Mucoid impaction appears as toothpaste shadows. Branched tubular radiodensities varying in length from 2 cm to 3 cm and extending from the hilum are called gloved-finger shadows. These are caused by intrabronchial exudates. HRCT thorax reveals proximal cylindrical bronchiectasis predominantly involving the upper lobes.

Magnetic resonance imaging (MRI) has a role in aspergillosis with CNS, paranasal sinus, and osseous involvement.

Radiological findings of chronic rhinosinusitis include a hyperattenuating soft tissue collection on noncontrast CT within one or more paranasal sinuses. Iso- or hypointense signals are observed on T1-weighted MRI images. CT scan is superior to MRI for evaluating the sinuses, while MRI should be performed to study orbital or intracranial spread. CT scan or MRI images of CNS aspergillosis show ring-enhancing lesions due to brain abscesses, cerebral cortical or subcortical infarcts, leptomeningeal dural enhancement due to contiguous spread from paranasal sinuses.

Ultrasound or CT scan of the kidneys may show filling defects in the renal pelvis with hydronephrosis. Cystoscopy may be useful.

Bronchoscopy

Flexible bronchoscopy and BAL have a definite role in establishing an etiological diagnosis in patients with pulmonary infiltrates in immunocompromised patients, nonresolving pneumonias, and nosocomial pneumonias. BAL is recommended for direct or indirect identification of mold in suspected patients with IPA. Relative contraindications for bronchoscopy include the following:

- Severe hypoxemia and insufficient respiratory capacity
- Bleeding diathesis
- Platelet-transfusion refractory thrombocytopenia.

Bronchoalveolar lavage samples are sent for gross appearance for hemorrhage and alveolar proteinosis, cell count, differential count, Gram stain, fungal stain, including Calcofluor/GMS, antigen or nucleic acid detection, immunohistochemistry, and GM. The optimal threshold for galactomannnan positivity has not been established, and optical density (OD) of 1.0 has been cleared by the Food and Drug Administration.

Lavage is performed from the segmental/subsegmental bronchus most involved on CT scan. Percutaneous or endobronchial lung biopsy is performed for peripheral nodular lesions where BAL has a low yield. Tracheobronchial biopsies are not recommended as a routine due to relative contraindications, including thrombocytopenia and low yield of biopsies.

▨ PROPHYLAXIS

- *In neutropenia:*
  During prolonged neutropenia, there is high risk of IA. Prophylaxis with posaconazole or voriconazole is strongly recommended. Caspofungin and micafungin prophylaxis is a weak recommendation. Itraconazole is effective as a prophylactic antifungal but use is limited by tolerability.
- *In GVHD:*
  Posaconazole prophylaxis is recommended for allogeneic HSCT recipients with GVHD who are at a high risk of IA. Voriconazole has been used but did not show improved

Table 17.3: Prophylaxis of aspergillosis.

Antifungal drug	Dose
Posaconazole (drug of choice)	*Oral suspension*: 200 mg TID Tablet: 300 mg BID on day 1, then 300 mg daily *IV*: 300 mg BID on day 1, then 300 mg daily
Voriconazole	200 mg BID
Itraconazole	*Suspension*: 200 mg PO BID
Micafungin	50–100 mg/day
Caspofungin	50 mg/day

survival in various trials. Itraconazole has tolerability and absorption issues. Prophylaxis is continued in these patients throughout the entire duration of immunosuppression with various agents, including corticosteroids, TNF-α or lymphocyte-depleting agents.

- *In lung transplant recipients:*
  Drugs used for IA prophylaxis in lung transplant include voriconazole, itraconazole, or inhaled AmB for 3–4 months post-transplant. The azoles show better efficacy in transplant recipients with mold colonization pre- or post-transplant, mold infection in explanted lung, single lung recipients, and fungal sinusitis. Prophylaxis needs to be reinitiated in the case of immunosuppression augmentation with thymoglobulin, alemtuzumab, or corticosteroids.

- *Non-lung SOT:*
  Anti-*Aspergillus* prophylaxis is not routinely recommended in patients undergoing non-lung SOT. Factors that make liver transplant recipients more vulnerable to IA include fulminant hepatic failure, retransplantation, and renal failure. Cardiac transplant patients at higher risk of IA include pretransplant colonization, reoperation, CMV infection, renal impairment, and *Aspergillus* outbreaks in institutions. Decision for IA prophylaxis and duration need to be individualized in the above situations (Table 17.3).

■ TREATMENT

Treatment of Invasive Aspergillosis

Triazoles

Azoles are the first-line antifungal agents in the prophylaxis and treatment of IA. Voriconazole is used in a dose of 6 mg/kg IV every 12 h for day 1, followed by 4 mg/kg IV every 12 h. Oral preparation of voriconazole is used at 200–300 mg every 12 h or weight-based dosing on an mg/kg basis. In the cases of endophthalmitis or keratitis, IV or oral voriconazole is combined with intravitreal AmB or voriconazole along with partial vitrectomy surgery.

Isavuconazole is used as an alternative drug. The loading dose is 200 mg every 8 h for six doses, followed by a maintenance dose of 200 mg daily.

Therapeutic drug monitoring (TDM) is recommended for voriconazole, itraconazole, and posaconazole suspension once a steady state has been achieved. This has a threefold advantage:

1. To improve efficacy
2. To evaluate drug failure due to suboptimal drug exposure
3. Reduce toxicity of azoles.

More data is needed regarding TDM for extended release or IV posaconazole and for isavuconazole.

Amphotericin B

Amphotericin B deoxycholate and its lipid formulations are used either as initial treatment or as salvage therapy in patients where voriconazole cannot be used. Lipid formulations are preferred over conventional AmB deoxycholate. The route of administration may be IV, or in some cases, additional/alternative routes include intraperitoneal, intravitreal, intrathecal, bladder irrigation, and aerosolization. The serum levels are not affected by hepatic or renal derangement, and it is a poorly dialyzable drug. It penetrates poorly into intact and inflamed meninges.

The dosage of liposomal AmB (LAmB) is 3–5 mg/kg/day IV as an alternative to primary treatment with voriconazole. Doses of AmB deoxycholate range from 0.1 mg/kg to 1.5 mg/kg daily. Major adverse events include acute infusion reaction with rigors, chills and nausea, administration site phlebitis, and nephrotoxicity.

Aerosolized AmB has been used as prophylaxis in prolonged neutropenia in patients on induction/reinduction therapy for acute leukemia and allogeneic HSCT recipients following conditioning, lung transplant, and recalcitrant fungal infections of the lung.

Echinocandins

Echinocandins are effective in salvage therapy when used alone or in combination against IA. Use as monotherapy for IA is not recommended. Although all three agents have activity against *Aspergillus* species, caspofungin and micafungin have been mainly used as salvage therapy with a variable response rate.

Combination Antifungal Therapy

Combinations of polyenes or azoles with echinocandins suggest synergistic or additive effects in some studies but results are inconsistent.

Antifungal Susceptibility Testing

Routine antifungal susceptibility testing is not recommended for *Aspergillus* isolates. It is used for the following:

- Patients with azole-resistant isolates
- Unresponsive to antifungal agents
- For epidemiological purposes.

Invasive Pulmonary Aspergillosis Treatment

- Voriconazole is recommended as primary antifungal treatment.
- Early initiation of therapy is recommended if index of suspicion is high while diagnostic tests are being conducted.
- Alternative therapy options include liposomal/lipid formulations of AmB, isavuconazole.
- Primary therapy with echinocandins is not recommended.
- Combination antifungal therapy with voriconazole and an echinocandin may be considered in documented IPA.
- Treatment duration is 6–12 weeks depending on the site of disease, level of immuno-suppression, and disease response to therapy.
- Secondary prophylaxis is recommended to prevent recurrence in patients previously treated for IPA who require subsequent immunosuppression.

Role of Surgery in Aspergillosis

Surgery is considered in the cases with localized disease amenable to debridement, e.g. fungal sinusitis or localized cutaneous disease. Patients with endocardial fungal lesions require surgical resection. Pericardiectomy is performed in the cases of *Aspergillus* pericarditis. Surgical resection of devitalized bone is necessary in fungal osteomyelitis. Patients on peritoneal dialysis (PD) should have their PD catheter removed in the case of fungal peritonitis.

Adjunctive Treatment and Measures in Invasive Pulmonary Aspergillosis

- Colony-stimulating factors may be considered in neutropenia. The role of granulocyte-colony-stimulating or granulocyte-macrophage colony-stimulating factor is less well defined.
- Granulocyte transfusions can be considered in neutropenia refractory to standard treatment and for an anticipated duration of more than 1 week.
- Reducing doses of immunosuppressants to minimum feasible dose.
- Recombinant interferon γ is recommended in CGD patients.

Salvage Therapy for Progressive/Refractory Aspergillosis

The principles of salvage therapy include the following:
- Changing the class of antifungal.
- Reducing or reversal of underlying immunosuppression.
- Surgical resection of necrotic tissue.
- Adding an agent from a different class of antifungals to the current therapy, or combination antifungal drugs from different classes other than those used in the initial regimen.
- Agents used for salvage therapy include LAmB, micafungin, caspofungin, posaconazole, or itraconazole.
- In the case of triazole use as salvage, consider prior antifungal use and possibility of drug resistance.

Proceeding with Transplantation/Chemotherapy in a Patient with Invasive Aspergillosis

Invasive aspergillosis is not an absolute contraindication to HSCT or additional chemotherapy. Decision is based on the risk of death from the underlying malignancy if the treatment is further delayed versus risk of progression of aspergillosis.

Biomarkers for Assessing Response to Therapy

Serial monitoring of serum GM can be done in patients who have a baseline elevated level. This can be especially useful in patients with HSCT and hematological malignancy. It helps to monitor therapeutic response, disease progression, and prognosis. β-D-Glucan has not been evaluated adequately in IA as a prognostic marker.

Treatment of Tracheobronchial Aspergillosis in Transplant or Nontransplant Recipients

- Saprophytic forms of TBA do not require antifungal treatment except for symptomatic or immunocompromised patients.
- Treatment options include triazoles or AmB.
- Bronchoscopic removal of mucus plugs.
- Bronchoscopic debridement of airway lesions if feasible.
- Bronchocentric granulomatosis treatment is the same as that of ABPA.
- Minimize/reverse immunosuppression.
- Apart from systemic antifungal, inhaled AmB is to be used for TBA with anastomotic endobronchial ischemia or ischemic reperfusion injury in lung transplant recipients.
- Duration of therapy is till complete resolution or at least 3 months, whichever is longer.

Management of Extrapulmonary Aspergillosis

Central Nervous System Aspergillosis

Voriconazole is a drug of choice. Use LAmB in refractory/intolerant cases. Most successfully treated patients have had open or stereotactic drainage of their cerebral lesions.

Aspergillus Endophthalmitis

Oral or IV voriconazole + intravitreal voriconazole or AmB deoxycholate is to be used. The role of intravitreal corticosteroid remains controversial. For *Aspergillus* keratitis, topical natamycin 5% ophthalmic suspension or topical voriconazole is sufficient. The outcome of treatment of endophthalmitis ranges from death of the patient due to disseminated aspergillosis to enucleation or evisceration of the affected eye to improvement in the clinical condition.

Aspergillus Sinusitis

Systemic voriconazole or LAmB along with surgery has a role in fungal sinusitis. Surgical removal alone may be sufficient to treat fungal ball of the paranasal sinuses. Enlargement of the sinus ostium improves drainage and reduces recurrence. The standard management involves a combination of surgical debridement of necrotic tissue and long-term antifungal treatment to prevent relapse. Patients with granulomatous fungal sinusitis are believed to have a better prognosis than those with invasive fungal rhinosinusitis.

Cardiac Aspergillosis

Surgery of endocardial lesions has a definite role to prevent embolization and valvular decompensation. Following surgical replacement of an infected valve, lifelong antifungal therapy should be considered. Voriconazole or LAmB is recommended as initial therapy.

Aspergillus Osteomyelitis/arthritis

Surgical debridement along with voriconazole is the combined approach for the management of *Aspergillus* osteomyelitis or septic arthritis.

Cutaneous Aspergillosis

Evaluate for a primary site of aspergillosis since skin involvement is secondary to dissemination. Treat the primary infection with voriconazole. Surgical debridement has a role in burns and wounds with secondary fungal infection.

Aspergillus peritonitis

Systemic therapy with voriconazole in addition to the removal of PD catheter is required.

Gastrointestinal Tract and Hepatic Aspergillosis

Surgical consultation is recommended to prevent dreaded complications, including hemorrhage, perforation, obstruction, and infarction.

Voriconazole or LAmB is to be used for gastrointestinal or hepatic aspergillosis. Extrahepatic or perihepatic biliary obstruction or loculated lesions refractory to medical therapy require surgical intervention.

Renal Aspergillosis

Parenchymal disease is treated with voriconazole, itraconazole, or AmB. Obstruction of one or both ureters should be managed with decompression if possible and local instillation of AmB deoxycholate. The management of these cases is challenging since efficacy of antifungal agents is not proven. Endourological access for extraction, lavage, and debulking or nephrectomy is required. Nephrectomy may be lifesaving but not a welcome option for patients with bilateral disease.

Aspergillus Ear Infection

Otomycosis or otitis externa is managed with mechanical cleaning of external auditory canal, followed by topical antifungals or boric acid. IA of the ear is treated with prolonged course of voriconazole in combination with surgery.

Aspergillus Bronchitis in Nontransplant Patient

Diagnosis is confirmed by the identification of *Aspergillus* species in sputum or respiratory secretions and GM rather than by culture. Voriconazole or itraconazole is used as treatment with TDM.

Empiric/Preemptive Strategies in allogeneic Hematopoietic Stem Cell Transplantation Recipients/Acute Myeloid Leukemia

These strategies for "empiric" antifungal therapy are recommended for high-risk patients with prolonged neutropenia who remain persistently febrile despite the use of broad-spectrum antibiotics. It is not recommended if the duration of neutropenia is expected to be less than 10 days, unless there are other evidences of invasive fungal infection.

Drugs used include LAmB, caspofungin, micafungin, or voriconazole. Serum or BAL GM or β-D-glucan helps to choose appropriate antifungal therapy in high-risk asymptomatic or febrile patients. This is called "preemptive" or "biomarker-driven" antifungal therapy. This preemptive approach can be used as an alternative to empiric therapy.

Chronic and Saprophytic Syndromes of *Aspergillus*

Patients with CCPA without pulmonary or systemic symptoms including fatigue or weight loss, no significant decline in lung capacities, may be kept under observation without any antifungal therapy and followed up every 3–6 months.

Candidates for antifungal therapy include the following:
- Pulmonary or systemic symptoms
- Major impairment of lung function
- Radiographic progression.

The duration of therapy is for a minimum of 6 months. Oral voriconazole or itraconazole are first line of therapy. Posaconazole is used as an alternative agent in the cases with clinical unresponsiveness. Hemoptysis can be managed with tranexamic acid, bronchial artery embolization, or surgical resection of involved portion of lung.

Indications for surgery include:
- Localized disease
- Pan-azole-resistant infection
- Hemoptysis despite arterial embolization
- Failure of medical therapy.

In the case of progressive lung disease, antifungal therapy is continued indefinitely or even lifelong.

Aspergilloma

- Patients who have a solitary aspergilloma, nonprogression and are asymptomatic should be evaluated every 6–24 months and may not require initiation of treatment.

- Patients who are symptomatic and have a single aspergilloma causing significant hemoptysis should undergo surgical resection. Lobectomy is the most common procedure followed by wedge resection, segmentectomy, and pleurectomy.
- Peri- or postoperative antifungal therapy is required only in the cases with surgical spillage of the aspergilloma. Voriconazole prevents development of *Aspergillus* empyema. If possible, voriconazole should be given for 1–2 weeks before surgery. In case the aspergilloma has been fully resected without any spillage, 4-week postoperative voriconazole is adequate. If there is a spillage, then a minimum of 12 weeks of therapy is recommended. In addition, pleural washout with AmB is used. Retrospective studies of perioperative adjuvant antifungal therapy have found no long-term survival benefit. Instillation of nystatin and AmB has been tried in some cases.
- The poor response observed with antifungal therapy alone may be explained by the genetic variability exhibited by *Aspergillus* strains within the fungal ball with multiple strains isolated in each patient. These have different azole sensitivity profiles. Moreover, in aspergillomas a typical biofilm is formed where fungal hyphae are surrounded by a thick extracellular matrix containing polysaccharides, such as GM.
- Embolization of the bleeding artery may be performed for patients with large volume hemoptysis. A skilled interventional radiologist is required.
- Approximately, 10% of aspergillomas resolve spontaneously.

Allergic Bronchopulmonary Aspergillosis

Acute exacerbations are best treated with systemic corticosteroids. Patients in remission require no therapy. ABPA in asthmatic patients with bronchiectasis and mucoid impaction who do not improve with oral or inhaled corticosteroid therapy may benefit from the use of itraconazole. Cystic fibrosis patients with declining FEV_1 and/or frequent exacerbations are prescribed itraconazole to reduce steroid dependence.

Allergic Rhinosinusitis

Patients have thick eosinophilic mucus containing fungal hyphae, nasal polyposis, and positive *Aspergillus* IgE serum antibody assay. Sinus washout and polypectomy induce remission but relapses are frequent. Topical steroids used postoperatively reduce frequency and intensity of relapse. Oral antifungals are reserved for rapidly relapsing or refractory patients. Viral and/or bacterial infections precipitate relapse in a patient of allergic fungal rhinosinusitis (AFRS) who is in remission. Omalizumab has been shown to be promising in asthma with AFRS. Management protocols are still evolving in patients with AFRS.

▨ CLINICAL PEARLS

- Voriconazole is essential therapy for aspergillosis. Monitor serum voriconazole trough concentrations 5–7 days into therapy and target serum concentrations >1 and <5.5 µg/mL.

- In patients intolerant to voriconazole, use LAmB or isavuconazole. Consider isavuconazole in patients with renal dysfunction.
- Combination of voriconazole and an echinocandin may be used in severe invasive disease.
- Surgical debridement of necrotic tissue wherever feasible.
- Allergic bronchopulmonary aspergillosis presents as asthma with recurrent exacerbations-specific serum IgE, precipitins to *Aspergillus*, and eosinophil count help in diagnosis.

SUGGESTED READING

1. Agarwal R, Chakrabarti A, Shah A, et al. Allergic bronchopulmonary aspergillosis: review of literature and proposal of new diagnostic and classification criteria, ABPA Complicating Asthma ISHAM Working Group. Clin Exp Allergy. 2013;43:850-73.
2. Chowdhary A, Agarwal K, Kathuria S, et al. Allergic bronchopulmonary mycosis due to fungi other than *Aspergillus*: a global overview. Crit Rev Microbiol. 2014;40:30-48.
3. Denning DW, Cadranel J, Beigelman-Aubry C et al. Chronic pulmonary aspergillosis: rationale and clinical guidelines for diagnosis and management, European Society for Clinical Microbiology and Infectious Diseases and European Respiratory Society. Eur Respir J. 2016;47:45-68.
4. Herbrecht R, Patterson TF, Slavin MA, et al. Application of the 2008 definitions for invasive fungal diseases to the trial comparing voriconazole versus amphotericin B for therapy of invasive aspergillosis: a collaborative study of the Mycoses Study Group (MSG 05) and the European Organization for Research and Treatment of Cancer Infectious Diseases Group. Clin Infect Dis. 2015;60:713.
5. Kosmidis C, Denning DW. The clinical spectrum of pulmonary aspergillosis. Thorax. 2015;70:270-7.
6. Limper AH, Knox KS, Sarosi GA, et al. An official American Thoracic Society statement: treatment of fungal infections in adult pulmonary and critical care patients. Am J Respir Crit Care Med. 2011;183:96.
7. Marr KA, Schlamm HT, Herbrecht R, et al. Combination antifungal therapy for invasive aspergillosis: a randomized trial. Ann Intern Med. 2015;162:81.
8. Page ID, Richardson MD, Denning DW. Comparison of six *Aspergillus*-specific IgG assays for the diagnosis of chronic pulmonary aspergillosis (CPA). J Infect. 2016;72: 240-9.
9. Patterson TF, Thompson GR 3rd, Denning DW, et al. Practice guidelines for the diagnosis and management of aspergillosis: 2016 update by the Infectious Diseases Society of America. Clin Infect Dis. 2016;63:e1.

18

Mucormycosis

Monica Mahajan

INTRODUCTION

Mucormycosis is a spectrum of diseases caused by filamentous fungi belonging to the order *Mucorales*. The importance of *Mucorales* has grown recently as a rare but emerging lethal fungal infection since the number of patients with predisposing factors for mucormycosis has increased dramatically. It is an angioinvasive fungus with nearly 100% mortality in case treatment is delayed. There is paucity of data to provide guidance for clinical decisions. The third European Conference on Infections in Leukemia has developed guidelines for the diagnosis and treatment of mucormycosis. These guidelines are applicable to patients with other underlying diseases also apart from leukemia patients.

TAXONOMY

Recent reclassification based on molecular techniques has abolished the class Zygomycetes and placed the order *Mucorales* in the subphylum *Mucoromycotina*. The *Entomophthorales* have been accommodated in a separate subphylum *Entomophthoromycotina*. These cause infection in immunocompetent hosts and occur predominantly in tropical and subtropical areas. Earlier all these fungi had been grouped together under the class Zygomycetes.

EPIDEMIOLOGY

These molds are ubiquitous saprophytic fungi. Being thermotolerant, they are found on decaying organic debris, food items, such as fruits and bread, and in the soil. They release large number of spores and spread by the airborne route.

The most common causes of infections in humans are *Rhizopus oryzae* (*Rhizopus arrhizus*) and *Rhizopus microsporus*. Other etiological agents include *Mucor*, *Cunninghamella*, *Apophysomyces*, *Lichtheimia* (formerly *Absidia*), *Saksenaea*, *Rhizomucor*, and *Cokeromyces*. Although these fungi are found worldwide, some of them have specific geographic distributions. For example, *Apophysomyces elegans* caused necrotizing soft tissue infections during the Joplin tornado. *Saksenaea vasiformis elegans* has been isolated from combat victims in Afghanistan. Seasonal variations in *Mucorales* are known with more cases reported in autumn.

All humans are exposed to *Mucorales* on a day-to-day basis. Yet, mucormycosis is a rare infection. In healthy population the inhaled sporangiospores are transported by the cilia into the pharynx and then cleared by the gastrointestinal tract. The immune system is easily able to combat the fungus.

In immunocompromised host, *Mucorales* cause angioinvasion and infarction of the infected tissue associated with a very high mortality rate. The management of the patient involves therapy with liposomal amphotericin B, aggressive surgery, and correction of the precipitating factors. Mucormycosis is the second most frequent infection seen in the immuno-compromised host.

Arnold Paltauf reported the first histologically proven case of *Mycosis mucorina* in Austria in 1885.

■ RISK FACTORS

Mucorales have a propensity to affect the immunocompromised host. Very few patients may have no identifiable risk factors. The classic risk factors include the following:

- *Uncontrolled diabetes mellitus with ketoacidosis*: Diabetes has been identified as a risk factor for mucormycosis in 36–88% of cases. It can be the first manifestation in an undiagnosed diabetic, especially in the developing countries. It is rare in well-controlled diabetics. The growth of the fungus is promoted by elevated concentration of free iron in the serum. An acidic pH increases free serum iron. This can explain the association of diabetic ketoacidosis with mucormycosis. Moreover, there is impairment of macrophage and neutrophil function in diabetics leading to fulminant course of the disease. *Rhizopus* has an enzyme ketone reductase that allows it to grow in high glucose acidic conditions.
- Patients on corticosteroids and immunosuppressive agents are at high risk. Neutropenia increases the risk manifold.
- Among patients with hematological malignancy, those with acute myelogenous leukemia are at the highest risk of mucormycosis. Hematopoietic stem cell transplant patients are more prone to mucormycosis due to graft-versus-host disease (GVHD), use of immunosuppressive agents, breakthrough mucormycosis in the setting of antifungal prophylaxis with voriconazole since it is effective against most fungi, such as *Aspergillus*, but *Mucorales* are intrinsically resistant to it. There is emergence of rare fungi in the late posttransplant phase.
- *Solid organ transplant (SOT) patients*: The predisposing reasons for mucormycosis in these patients include hyperglycemia, renal failure, and prior use of voriconazole or caspofungin rather than neutropenia. In contrast, tacrolimus use has been associated with a reduced risk. Liver transplant recipients are more likely to have disseminated disease and earlier development of mucormycosis versus other SOT recipients.
- Persistent metabolic acidosis due to renal disease, diarrhea, or multiorgan failure.
- *Iron chelation therapy with deferoxamine (DFO)*: DFO has been traditionally used for aluminum chelation in renal failure patients and iron overload in patients receiving multiple blood transfusions. The DFO-iron chelate, called feroxamine, is a siderophore for the fungus. It increases iron uptake by the fungus and promotes fungal growth

leading to angioinvasive disease. Up to 78% of dialysis recipients with mucormycosis received DFO. Fortunately, DFO is no longer used. Newer agents for chelation, such as deferasirox and deferiprone, do not act as siderophores and therefore do not increase risk of mucormycosis. Instead, these agents cause iron starvation. In addition to DFO, iron overload due to transfusion or dyserythropoiesis is associated with increased risk of mucormycosis.

- Healthcare associated/nosocomial use of contaminated medical supplies, including nonsterile dressings, wooden splints, and bandages, is associated with nosocomial outbreaks. Renovation work in hospitals is more often associated with aspergillosis rather than mucormycosis.
- Low-birth-weight and malnourished babies.
- Natural disasters including tsunamis, tornadoes, and volcanic eruptions.
- Combat-associated injuries and outbreaks in soldiers require frequent debridements and amputations.
- *Others*: Postsplenectomy, intravenous (IV) drug users, peritoneal dialysis patients, burns, and road accidents.

PATHOPHYSIOLOGY

The spores are introduced into the body by:
- Inhalation
- Ingestion of contaminated food and nonnutritional substances (pica)
- Traumatic inoculation
- Wound infections
- Catheter insertion or injections.

The *Mucoraceae* are molds in the environment, which become hyphae forms in tissues. The hyphae are broad (5–15 µm diameter), irregularly branched and have rare separation. This is in contrast to the hyphae of *Aspergillus*, which are narrower, septate, and exhibit regular acute angle branching. The hallmark of *Mucoraceae* is angioinvasion leading to thrombosis and infarction of tissue. There is necrosis of surrounding tissue.

The proliferation of the fungus happens due to:
- Defects in phagocytic activity due to neutropenia.
- Functional defects due to hyperglycemia, acidosis, and steroid use promote germination of fungal spores.

Two-thirds of cases of mucormycosis occur in males. The reason for this unequal sex distribution is poorly understood.

CLINICAL FEATURES (BOX 18.1)

Mucormycosis is associated with a spectrum of syndromes depending on the portal of entry of the spores and the underlying disease factors. The poor outcomes of the disease can be attributed to its pleiotropic clinical manifestations and delay in diagnosis.

Box 18.1: Clinical manifestations of mucormycosis.

- Rhinocerebral
- Pulmonary
- Gastrointestinal
- Cutaneous
- Disseminated
- Unusual presentations

The most common reported sites of invasive mucormycosis are sinuses (39%), lungs (24%), and skin (19%). The skin and gut are affected more frequently in children than in adults. The clinical hallmark of mucormycosis is tissue necrosis resulting from angioinvasion and subsequent thrombosis. The infection is rapidly progressive and associated with high mortality if left untreated.

Rhinocerebral Mucormycosis

It is also referred to as rhino-orbital-cerebral mucormycosis or craniofacial mucormycosis.

The infection begins with the inhalation of fungal sporangiospores. It starts in the paranasal sinuses and on germinating, the invading fungus then contiguously involves the orbit, face, palate, and brain. The fungus invades the cranium through either the orbital apex or cribriform plate of the ethmoid bone. If untreated, it can be fatal within 1 week of onset. Early symptoms of the disease mimic sinusitis. Patients present with fever, nasal stuffiness, facial pain and numbness, retro-orbital headache, hyposmia, and blood-tinged black discharge. The late symptoms include diplopia, visual loss, and altered sensorium. Most patients have history of diabetes, malignancy, corticosteroid use, neutropenia, or recent use of broad-spectrum antibiotics.

Necrotic black eschar on the nasal mucosa or hard palate is characteristic. The involved tissue is initially red and then violaceous and finally black. The eschar is a classic diagnostic but unfortunately late visible sign of the disease. Its absence should not exclude the possibility of mucormycosis. There is perinasal and periorbital swelling with the destruction of facial tissue. Facial numbness is due to infarction of sensory bundles of fifth cranial nerve. Eye involvement manifests as proptosis, chemosis, diplopia, blepharoptosis, progressive external ophthalmoplegia, eyelid gangrene, retinal detachment, and endophthalmitis. Retinal artery thrombosis may occur. Symptoms may range from headache to acute visual loss.

Infection progresses to the cavernous sinus and internal carotid artery causing thrombosis. Frontal lobe involvement causes obtundation and altered consciousness. There can be bone destruction, epidural and subdural abscesses, and basilar artery aneurysm. Imaging studies and nasal endoscopy should be ordered early in the course of the disease.

Pulmonary Mucormycosis

This is the second most common clinical manifestation of mucormycosis. Infection may reach the lungs through inhalation, aspiration of infectious material, hematogenous, or lymphatic spread. Infection occurs more often in patients with underlying malignancies, stem cell transplant or SOT, and neutropenia. The clinical features are nonspecific. Symptoms include prolonged high-grade fever that is unresponsive to broad-spectrum antibiotics, nonproductive cough, dyspnea, pleuritic chest pain, and massive, potentially fatal hemoptysis. Hemoptysis is due to the invasion of major pulmonary blood vessels by fungal hyphae.

Physical examination reveals fever, diminished breath sounds, and rales. Spread to the adjacent structures including the chest wall, pleura, or diaphragm occurs. Chest wall cellulitis demonstrates the ability of the fungus to cross tissue planes.

Mucorales can form mycetomas in lung cavities. Sawmill workers may suffer from allergic alveolitis due to *Rhizopus*, which is also known as "wood trimmer's disease".

Rarely, mucormycosis may manifest as endobronchial lesions causing airway obstruction, lung collapse, or fatal hemoptysis.

Pulmonary mucormycosis can be indistinguishable from pulmonary aspergillosis. Subtle clues favoring mucormycosis include the following:

- Pansinusitis
- Absence of detectable galactomannan antigen in serum
- Use of voriconazole or echinocandins for *Aspergillus* prophylaxis or treatment.

The infection may prove fatal in 2–3 weeks, especially if the patient is on voriconazole for suspected aspergillosis since it lacks activity against *Mucorales*.

Cutaneous Mucormycosis

Skin and soft tissue mucormycosis can occur in victims of severe skin or muscular injury, traumatic inoculation of spores, burns, spider bites, or seemingly innocuous insults, such as insulin injections or catheter insertion.

The clinical course can be gradual, slowly progressive, or fulminant. The skin lesion starts with erythematous macule, induration at the puncture site and black eschar formation. The margins are sharply demarcated. It extends onto the deeper fascia and muscle layers causing cellulitis. Necrotizing fasciitis is rare. Less common manifestations include targetoid plaques with erythematous rims and necrotic centers. Skin lesions may resemble pyoderma gangrenosum. Cutaneous mucormycosis can disseminate although the reverse is very rare.

Likelihood of other molds, such as *Fusarium* and *Scedosporium* species, involving the skin is much more than cutaneous mucormycosis. In the cases of suspected mucormycosis, the patient should be investigated for possible dissemination of the disease.

Gastrointestinal Mucormycosis

Gastrointestinal mucormycosis affects low-birth-weight premature neonates, malnourished patients, and diabetics. Infection is acquired from contaminated food, bread, fermented porridges, and alcoholic drinks derived from corn, herbal, and homeopathic remedies contaminated with spores. Gastrointestinal mucormycosis transmitted from contaminated tongue depressors has been reported. It is a rare condition with death within several weeks of onset. The diagnosis is mostly established postmortem.

The most common sites of infection are the stomach, ileum, and colon. The symptoms are nonspecific and include fever, abdominal pain and distension, nausea, vomiting, hematemesis, hematochezia, melena, and obstruction. Clinical examination may reveal diffuse tenderness, appendiceal, ileal, or cecal mass, or signs of peritonitis. Premature infants may have necrotizing enterocolitis. Massive gastrointestinal hemorrhage is the most common cause of death. Some cases of liver abscess following ingestion of herbal products contaminated by *Mucor indica* have been described.

Disseminated Mucormycosis

Disseminated mucormycosis results from hematogenous spread of *Mucor* from one organ to other organs and is seen in patients with prolonged neutropenia, GVHD, or DFO therapy. It has an extremely high mortality rate and diagnosis requires a very high index of suspicion. The most common organ as a source of dissemination is the lungs, and the most common site of spread is the brain. Dissemination can also occur from the gastrointestinal tract, burns, or extensive cutaneous lesions. Virtually all organs, including the brain, kidneys, heart, and bones, can be involved in disseminated mucormycosis. Patients develop metastatic necrotic lesions. A metastatic cutaneous lesion is an important hallmark and may offer a clue to the diagnosis. Vascular infarction may be associated with endocarditis, pyelonephritis, or osteomyelitis.

Rare Presentations of Mucormycosis

Isolated organ involvement due to mucormycosis has been reported in patients with malignancy, renal transplant, ambulatory peritoneal dialysis, IV, drug use, or head trauma.

Cerebral mucormycosis manifests as lethargy, confusion, obtundation, and focal neurological signs and symptoms. Brain abscesses involving the basal ganglia and cranial nerve involvement without rhino-orbital involvement have been described.

Mucormycosis can cause perirenal abscess and renal infarction. Patients have fever, loin pain, oliguria, anuric renal failure, hematuria, and unilateral or bilateral renal involvement. Isolated renal mycormycosis has been reported in IV drug users as well as renal transplant recipients in the developing countries with warm climate, including India, Egypt, and Kuwait. Peritonitis has been reported in patients undergoing continuous ambulatory peritoneal dialysis.

Mucormycosis can be a rare cause of prosthetic or native valve endocarditis and can cause aortic thrombosis. IV drug use is a predisposing factor. Catheter-related mucormycosis mandates removal of catheter.

Mucormycosis can involve other structures including the mediastinum, trachea, bone, heart, cornea, mastoid, ear, and bladder.

▦ DIFFERENTIAL DIAGNOSES

Refer to Table 18.1 for differential diagnoses of mucormycosis.

▦ DIAGNOSTIC WORKUP

It is challenging to establish a clinical diagnosis of mucormycosis. A high index of suspicion is necessary to reduce mortality in the cases of mucormycosis. No serologic laboratory findings

Table 18.1: Differential diagnoses of mucormycosis.	
Rhinocerebral	▪ Aspergillosis ▪ Cavernous sinus thrombosis ▪ Pseudallescheriasis (*Pseudallescheria boydii* infection) ▪ Orbital cellulitis of bacterial origin ▪ Orbital tumor
Pulmonary	▪ Aspergillosis ▪ Gram-negative bacterial pneumonia ▪ *Pseudallescheria boydii* infection ▪ Pulmonary embolism ▪ Nocardiosis ▪ Wegener granulomatosis ▪ Tuberculosis
Cutaneous	▪ Aspergillosis ▪ Anthrax ▪ Ecthyma gangrenosum (*Pseudomonas aeruginosa*)
Gastrointestinal	▪ Intestinal obstruction ▪ Appendicular lump ▪ Bacterial peritonitis ▪ Ileocecal tuberculosis

are diagnostic. The following two important issues need to be kept in mind while diagnosing the condition:

1. Tissue swabs and cultures of sinus secretions, sputum and bronchoalveolar lavage fluid are usually nondiagnostic.
2. Growth on cultures may not always represent true invasive mucormycosis as spongio-spores are airborne and can contaminate clinical samples. The culture results need to be interpreted in the context of the patient's disease.

Laboratory Investigations

▪ *Routine investigations* including complete blood count to assess the degree of neutropenia, blood glucose, electrolytes, arterial blood analysis, and iron studies may be routinely conducted.
▪ *Blood and cerebrospinal fluid (CSF) culture* are usually negative. CSF examination reveals mononuclear pleocytosis and elevated protein levels. Mucormycosis is rarely present in the CSF even during central nervous system (CNS) infections.
▪ The *Mucorales* lack β-D-glucan and galactomannan in their cell wall, and both tests are negative in patients of mucormycosis.
▪ *Polymerase chain reaction* for detecting DNA of *Mucorales* is only available for investigational purposes. At present, there are no standardized methods available for commercial use.
▪ *Matrix-assisted laser desorption/ionization time-of-flight mass spectrometry* is used for species identification from the cultures. However, there is sparse evidence that the

identification of the causative species of *Mucorales* would alter the course of treatment or choice of antifungal agent. More data is needed to validate this technique.

Radiological Examination

Mucormycosis may have subclinical involvement of multiple organ systems. Hence, it is advisable to do imaging studies or computed tomography (CT) scan of the brain, sinuses, chest, and abdomen even if subclinical disease is present.

- *Radiography/X-rays:*
  Plain films of the sinuses may reveal mucosal thickening, air–fluid levels, and/or bony erosions. Chest radiographs show areas of consolidation.
- *Computed tomography scan:*
  Computed tomographic images of the sinuses may show ethmoid and sphenoid sinusitis with a clear unilateral predilection. With the progression of the disease, there is bony erosion, orbital involvement, thrombosis of internal carotid artery and cavernous sinus, epidural and subdural abscesses and/or basilar artery aneurysm, frontal lobe necrosis.
  Computed tomography scan in the case of pulmonary disease reveals predilection of the fungus for the upper lobe. Later on, there can be multilobar bilateral involvement with the areas of consolidation. Frequent findings include infiltration, consolidation, nodules, cavitation, effusion, atelectasis, hilar, and mediastinal lymphadenopathy. Patterns of radiological involvement seen on the CT scan, which may suggest a fungal involvement, include the following:
  - *Halo sign:* A ring of ground-glass opacity surrounding a nodular infiltrate.
  - *Air crescent sign:* A crescent-shaped or circumferential area of radiolucency within a parenchymal consolidation or nodular opacity.
  - *Reversed halo sign (inversed halo sign or atoll sign):* An area of ground-glass opacity surrounded by a ring of consolidation.
  - These radiological signs do not distinguish mucormycosis from aspergillosis. Patients with more than 10 nodules on CT scan and a reversed halo sign are more likely to have mucormyosis than aspergillosis as per one case series. Pleural effusion may be present.
  Computed tomography scans of gastrointestinal tract show a mass, perforation, or peritonitis.
- *Magnetic resonance imaging:*
  Magnetic resonance imaging is better than CT scans in assessing the full extent of structural involvement and also assessing the need for surgery. It can be a better option in patients with deranged renal function tests.

Biopsy and Histology

Every effort has to be made to obtain tissue biopsies for culture and histopathology. This can be difficult in patients with severe thrombocytopenia. Ear, nose, and throat endoscopy; bronchoscopy; and CT-guided or surgical biopsy should be performed based on the radiological findings. The biopsy material from necrotic tissue may be obtained from the following:

- Nasal turbinates
- Palatine tissue

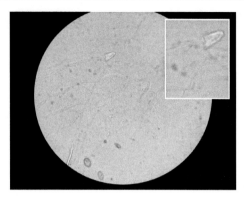

Fig. 18.1: Aseptate fungal hyphae on potassium hydroxide (KOH) mount.

- Lung by bronchoscopy
- Skin/abscess wall
- Gastrointestinal tract by esophagogastroduodenoscopy.

Fungal hyphae can be examined directly by using a potassium hydroxide preparation. Fixed tissues can be examined with hematoxylin and eosin, Grocott-Gomori methenamine-silver, or periodic acid–Schiff stain. Direct microscopy of clinical specimens, preferably using optical brighteners, allows a rapid diagnosis. Calcofluor binds to chitin and cellulose and fluoresces on ultraviolet light.

In contrast to the other molds, *Mucorales* are broad-based 3–25-μm diameter, ribbon-like, aseptate, or pauciseptate hyphae with irregular branching that may occur at right angles (Fig. 18.1).

The biopsy tissue shows neutrophil infiltration, vascular invasion, and infarction, which are characteristic features of the infective process. Perineural invasion may be observed. A granulomatous reaction may also occur.

Most of these fungi grow rapidly on Sabouraud dextrose agar on incubation at 25–37°C for 24 hours. For fungal culture, it is better to mince rather than homogenize tissue specimens and then culture them in semianaerobic conditions. Excessive tissue manipulation damages the friable hyphae, and the fungal culture will be negative. Fungal growth occurs in 2–3 days, and the fungal morphology is then determined by microscopic examination.

Despite their predilection for hematogenous dissemination, blood cultures in all forms of mucormycosis are always negative. On the other hand, culture of specimens is considered an essential investigation, which allows identification and susceptibility testing of the isolate in the case of growth. Identification of the species is of interest for studying epidemiology of mucormycosis and to investigate any outbreaks. It is not necessary to guide treatment.

TREATMENT OF MUCORMYCOSIS (BOX 18.2)

Treatment of mucormycosis needs a multimodal, multidisciplinary involvement. The combined approach to treatment involves the following:
- Antifungal therapy

Box 18.2: Treatment.

Antifungal therapy:
- AmB—liposomal, ABLC, ABCD, deoxycholate
- Posaconazole—not recommended as initial monotherapy
- Combination therapy

Second-line/salvage therapy:
- Posaconazole/isavuconazole
- Combination lipid AmB and posaconazole
- Combination lipid AmB and caspofungin

Maintenance therapy:
- Posaconazole

Surgery:
- Rhino-orbito-cerebral
- Soft tissue
- Localized pulmonary lesion

Adjunctive therapy:
- Hyperbaric oxygen therapy
- Deferasirox
- Colony-stimulating factors (G-CSF, GM-CSF)
- Metabolic acidosis/DKA management
- Withdrawing immunosuppressive drugs/corticosteroids

ABCD, amphotericin B colloidal dispersion; ABLC, amphotericin B lipid complex; AmB, amphotericin B; DKA, diabetic ketoacidosis; G-CSF, granulocyte-colony stimulating factor; GM-CSF, granulocyte-macrophage colony-stimulating factor.

- Early surgical debridement of involved tissue
- Correction/elimination of predisposing factors.

Antifungal Treatment

Early initiation of antifungal therapy improves the outcomes in this otherwise fatal fungal infection. Although there are no randomized trials on the efficacy of various antifungal drugs due to the rarity of the disease, amphotericin B is the drug of choice. Posaconazole and isavuconazole are used in the following scenarios:

- Salvage therapy in patients unresponsive to amphotericin B
- Combination therapy with amphotericin B
- Patients intolerant to amphotericin B
- Step-down therapy after initial treatment with amphotericin B.

Mucorales are resistant to many antifungals, including flucytosine, ketoconazole, fluconazole, voriconazole, and the echinocandins.

Minimum inhibitory concentration (MIC) of antifungal drugs for mucormycosis is inconsistent and difficult to interpret. There is a relative lack of clinical breakpoints and insufficient data to correlate MIC and clinical outcomes. Use of antifungal susceptibility testing for *Mucorales* is only marginally recommended. No clinical trial has been conducted evaluating the timing of fever-driven treatment directed against mucormycosis. In general, a diagnosis-driven treatment is preferable.

Amphotericin B: Amphotericin B is the gold standard for the treatment of mucormycosis. Liposomal amphotericin B at a dose of 5 mg/kg/day is preferred over conventional amphotericin B. Higher doses of up to 10 mg/kg/day have been used in CNS mucormycosis, but the risk of nephrotoxicity may outweigh the benefits. Amphotericin B deoxycholate in doses of 1–1.5 mg/kg/day is used in the setting of cost constraints. There is major concern about renal toxicity as many of these patients may have preexisting kidney involvement. Careful monitoring of kidney function test and electrolytes is required while on treatment.

Posaconazole: Posaconazole is a triazole used as step-down therapy or as salvage therapy after the failure of amphotericin B. Compared with itraconazole and isavuconazole on an mg:mg basis, posaconazole has enhanced in vitro activity with 90% MIC ranging from 1 μg/mL to ≥4 μg/mL. While fungicidal activity of posaconazole has been demonstrated against *Rhizopus* and *Mucor* spp., amphotericin B was more rapidly fungicidal, with 95% killing noted as early as 6 hours and 99.9% killing at 24 hours. For comparison, posaconazole showed less than 70% killing at 6 hours and 99.9% killing at 48 hours. Posaconazole monotherapy cannot be recommended as primary treatment of mucormycosis.

    The IV and delayed release oral formulations are given as a loading dose of 300 mg every 12 hours on the first day. The consequent maintenance dose is 300 mg every 24 hours. The oral suspension is dosed at 200 mg (5 mL) per os ter in die. The IV formulation is avoided in patients with moderate-to-severe renal impairment (creatinine clearance <50 mL/min). This is due to the nephrotoxicity associated with the carrier vehicle betadex sulfobutyl ether sodium. Administration of the oral formulations improves with acidic beverages or a fatty meal. Coadministration of antacids, such as proton-pump inhibitors, is avoided with posaconazole. Therapeutic levels of the drug should be monitored if the integrity of the gastrointestinal tract is disrupted in patients with mucositis or GVHD. A serum trough concentration of posaconazole should be checked after 1 week of initiating therapy. A goal trough concentration of >1 μg/mL should be achieved, but higher levels are preferred. The benefit of dual antifungal therapy with amphotericin B and posaconazole needs more robust data to endorse it.

Isavuconazole: Isavuconazole is the active moiety of the drug isavuconazonium sulfate. The loading dose of 200 mg or two capsules of oral isavuconazole (372-mg isavuconazonium sulfate) are given every 8 hours for a total of 6 doses over 48 hours. The maintenance dose is 200 mg orally once daily starting 12–24 hours after the last loading dose. An IV formulation of isavuconazole has also been introduced. The drug was approved for the treatment of mucormycosis in 2015 but lacks controlled clinical trials.

Other antifungals: Since *Rhizopus* expresses the target enzyme for echinocandins, there can be some clinical utility of echinocandins in mucormycosis, but their role remains questionable. Fluconazole and voriconazole have no clinical efficacy against mucormycosis.

Duration of Therapy

The total duration of therapy may vary from several weeks to several months till there is full clinical recovery and complete resolution of signs and symptoms. The radiographic studies should show no disease activity.

Surgical Management

Aggressive adjunctive surgical debridement of devitalized tissue is lifesaving as tissue infarction and necrosis may impair the penetration of antifungal agents to the site of infection. Timely debridement of all devitalized tissue may reduce the mass of infecting molds and prevent the extension of mucormycosis to adjacent structures. It may not be feasible in patients with profound thrombocytopenia. Surgery is considered on a case-by-case basis according to the site and extension of the disease. In rhinocerebral mucormycosis, it involves drainage of sinuses, removal of palate, orbital contents, and involved area of the brain. Surgery is disfiguring, and multiple debridements may be required. Patients with pulmonary mucormycosis localized to a single lobe may require wedge resection, lobectomy, or pneumonectomy. Multilobar involvement precludes surgical resection. Resection of gastrointestinal masses and nephrectomy improves survival rates. Surgical debridement may have to be repeated, and amputation may be required if limb involvement is extensive.

Adjunctive Therapy

- *Hyperbaric oxygen therapy:*
  Hyperbaric oxygen therapy has been used with the assumption that it will improve wound healing by increased tissue concentration of oxygen and increased neutrophil antifungal activity. It inhibits the growth of *Mucorales*. Its benefits have not been fully established for this indication, and the efficacy of this expensive intervention has not been fully defined in mucormycosis.
- *Deferasirox:*
  It is an oral iron-chelating agent. Unlike DFO that increases the risk of mucormycosis by acting as a siderophore for *Mucorales*, deferasirox, and deferiprone do not have xenosiderophore activity. So it may cause iron starvation that reduces the fungal growth and could be useful adjunctive therapy. There is insufficient evidence to recommend the role of these agents as rational adjuncts to antifungal agents.
- *Colony-stimulating factors:*
  Granulocyte colony-stimulating and granulocyte-macrophage colony-stimulating factors shorten the duration of neutropenia and may improve outcomes. Their use in non-neutropenic patients is not recommended.
- *Diabetic ketoacidosis management:*
  Rehydration, insulin, and sodium bicarbonate reduce morbidity and mortality.
- *Withdrawing drugs:*
  Withdrawing corticosteroids and immunosuppressants improve outcomes.

▉ PREVENTION

- *High-efficiency particulate air filters:*
  High-efficiency particulate air filters in rooms where patients with prolonged neutropenia are managed may reduce risk of disease.

- *Examining wounds:*
  Examining wounds to detect any worsening in preexisting wounds, avoiding use of contaminated biomedical equipment and nonsterile surgical bandages is important to reduce the incidence of mucormycosis.
- *Reducing environmental exposure:*
  Remove plants and flowers from vicinity of patient. Avoid serving stale bread and fruits potentially contaminated with *Mucor*.

PROPHYLAXIS

There is currently no effective antifungal prophylaxis recommended for mucormycosis.

PROGNOSIS

Case fatality rates are higher in disseminated disease, renal failure, and infection with *Cunninghamella* species. Mortality rates for rhinocerebral mucormycosis are 25–62% with better outcome if disease is only confined to the sinuses. Pulmonary disease has a mortality rate of 76–87% in various studies. Gastrointestinal mucormycosis is associated with 85% mortality, whereas disseminated disease has worst prognosis with 90–100% mortality.

CLINICAL PEARLS

- Mucormycosis may be considered a fungal emergency due to the aggressive nature of the disease and there is a need for multidisciplinary intervention.
- Diagnosis is made on direct microscopy, histopathology, and culture of tissue.
- Blood culture, galactomannan, and β-D-glucan are negative and help to rule out invasive aspergillosis, the most frequent differential diagnosis.
- Minimum inhibitory concentration values for guiding treatment have not yet been standardized.
- Reverse halo sign on CT scan can be a clue to diagnosis.
- Surgical debridement can be lifesaving.
- Liposomal amphotericin B is the first-line antifungal.
- Posaconazole and isavuconazole are useful step-down or salvage therapy.
- Reversing predisposing factors is important.
- Metabolic acidosis and iron overload are important predisposing factors.
    Previous voriconazole prophylaxis, paranasal sinus involvement, diabetes mellitus, and more than 10 pulmonary nodules on CT scan favor mucormycosis rather than aspergillosis. These need prospective validation.

SUGGESTED READING

1. Boelaert JR, Van Cutsem J, de Locht M, et al. Deferoxamine augments growth and pathogenicity of *Rhizopus*, while hydroxypyridinone chelators have no effect. Kidney Int. 1994;45:667.
2. Green JP, Karras DJ. Update on emerging infections: news from the Centers for Disease Control and Prevention. Notes from the field: fatal fungal soft-tissue infections after a tornado—Joplin, Missouri, 2011. Ann Emerg Med. 2012;59:53.

3. Kontoyiannis DP, Lewis RE. How I treat mucormycosis. Blood. 2011;118:1216.

4. Kontoyiannis DP, Lionakis MS, Lewis RE, et al. Zygomycosis in a tertiary-care cancer center in the era of *Aspergillus*-active antifungal therapy: a case-control observational study of 27 recent cases. J Infect Dis. 2005;191:1350.

5. Lanternier F, Sun HY, Ribaud P, et al. Mucormycosis in organ and stem cell transplant recipients. Clin Infect Dis. 2012;54:1629.

6. Marty FM, Ostrosky-Zeichner L, Cornely OA, et al. Isavuconazole treatment for mucormycosis: a single-arm open-label trial and case-control analysis. Lancet Infect Dis. 2016;16:828.

7. Rammaert B, Lanternier F, Zahar JR, et al. Healthcare-associated mucormycosis. Clin Infect Dis. 2012;54(Suppl 1):S44.

8. Roden MM, Zaoutis TE, Buchanan WL, et al. Epidemiology and outcome of zygomycosis: a review of 929 reported cases. Clin Infect Dis. 2005;41:634.

9. Spellberg B, Ibrahim A, Roilides E, et al. Combination therapy for mucormycosis: why, what, and how? Clin Infect Dis. 2012;54(Suppl 1):S73.

10. Spellberg B, Walsh TJ, Kontoyiannis DP, et al. Recent advances in the management of mucormycosis: from bench to bedside. Clin Infect Dis. 2009;48:1743.

11. Wahba H, Truong MT, Lei X, et al. Reversed halo sign in invasive pulmonary fungal infections. Clin Infect Dis. 2008;46:1733.

12. Walsh TJ, Gamaletsou MN, McGinnis MR, et al. Early clinical and laboratory diagnosis of invasive pulmonary, extrapulmonary, and disseminated mucormycosis (zygomycosis). Clin Infect Dis. 2012;54(Suppl 1):S55.

19

Pneumocystis Jirovecii Pneumonia

Monica Mahajan

INTRODUCTION

Pneumocystis jirovecii pneumonia (PJP) is the most common opportunistic infection in HIV patients. It was first described in 1909 by Carlos Chagas who mistook the cysts for the sexual state of *Trypanosoma cruzi*. The Delamoes, a husband and wife team, realized that the cysts were a separate entity when they found them in the lungs of sewer rats. They named the organism in the honor of Dr Antonio Carini. Since Dr Otto Jrovec was the first to isolate the organism from humans, so the organism was renamed after him. The strains that infect humans have been redesignated *P. jirovecii*, whereas *Pneumocystis carinii* and *Pneumocystis muris* infect rats and mice, respectively. There is antigenic, karyotypic, and genetic heterogeneity between these species, and there is no cross infection.

TAXONOMY

Pneumocystis genus was initially classified as a trypanosome and then as a protozoan. Genetic studies have shown that it is a unicellular fungus. It has some unique characteristics. It has only a single copy of nuclear RNA locus, whereas most fungi contain hundreds of loci. Its plasma membrane does not contain ergosterol. However, its genes contain elongation factor 3 that is unique to fungi and not found in the protein synthesis machinery of protozoa.

LIFE CYCLE

The life cycle and transmission of *Pneumocystis* is not fully established due to the inability to successfully culture it. It has three morphologic stages:
1. Trophic form—Trophozoite (2–6 μm in diameter)
2. Precystic form—Sporozoite
3. Intracystic bodies or spore-bearing form—Cyst/Asci (6–8 μm in diameter)

There is no zoonotic phase of PJP life cycle. There is accumulating evidence supporting sexual phase in the life cycle.

■ TRANSMISSION

Pneumocystis is a ubiquitous organism found worldwide. It is found in the lungs of healthy individuals. About 85% of healthy children have antibodies to *pneumocytes* by 3 years of age. Molecular analysis of *Pneumocystis* isolates from case clusters in hospitals suggests that transmission is airborne.

Studies are ongoing to determine the relative importance of latency versus reinfection in patients. There may be de novo infection or reactivation of latent disease acquired in childhood, especially in older children and adults. Reinfection model is supported by the fact that genotypical different strains may be found in the same patient during different episodes.

■ PATHOPHYSIOLOGY

The trophozoites of *Pneumocystis* attach to the Type 1 *pneumocytes* of the alveolar wall and increase alveolar capillary permeability. Activated macrophages are unable to clear the organisms in the presence of cellular and humoral immune defects. This results in hypoxemia and increased alveolar–arterial oxygen gradient.

Staining with hematoxylin and eosin demonstrates an acellular, foamy eosinophilic, and intra-alveolar exudate with mild plasma cell interstitial inflammation. In the later stage of the disease, hyaline membrane formation and interstitial as well as intraluminal fibrosis develops. Electron micrographs reveal that the exudate is composed almost entirely of *Pneumocystis* organisms.

■ SUSCEPTIBLE PATIENT POPULATION

Various congenital and acquired diseases predispose to PJP.
- HIV infection with CD4+ cell count less than 200/µL (80–90% cases) and not receiving PJP prophylaxis. High viral load, oral thrush, and previous episode of pneumonia increase the risk of PJP regardless of CD4 count.
- Primary immune deficiencies including X-linked hyperimmunoglobulin, M syndrome and severe combined immunodeficiency (SCID).
- Patients with hematologic and nonhematologic malignancies.
- Patients on long-term immunosuppressive drugs for connective tissue disorder, vasculitides or solid-organ transplantation. Corticosteroids and cyclosporine are most closely associated with PJP since these agents have inhibitory effects on T lymphocytes. In addition tacrolimus and monoclonal anti-T-cell antibodies, e.g. OKT3 and alefuzamab also make a patient susceptible to PJP.
- Protein-calorie malnutrition, premature or debilitated infants.
- Cases have been reported in patients with chronic granulomatous disease (CGD).

■ EPIDEMIOLOGY

Pneumocystis jirovecii pneumonia is a ubiquitous organism found worldwide. It is found in 80% of infants with pneumonia who have HIV infection. *Pneumocystis* was detected on postmortem studies in 52% HIV-positive infants who died of pneumonia in a series in South

Africa and 67% in a series in Zimbabwe. The incidence of PJP is reducing with the increasing use of highly active antiretroviral therapy (HAART) and PJP prophylaxis. Still PJP remains the most common opportunistic infection in patients with HIV. The lower incidence recorded in the developing countries may be due to lack of diagnostic facilities. Tuberculosis may be a common coinfection with PJP.

CLINICAL FEATURES

There is no classical clinical presentation pathognomonic of PJP. Patients with HIV may have a smouldering subacute presentation over several weeks. Other patients may have a more acute presentation.

The symptoms of PJP include a progressively worsening dyspnea, especially on exertion, fever, substernal chest tightness and cough, which is typically nonproductive. Patients may experience weight loss.

The physical examination may be normal in up to half of the patients and chest examination findings may be slight or disproportionate to the degree of illness. Other patients may have nonspecific findings including fever, tachycardia, tachypnea and mild bibasilar crackles. Patients with severe disease may have cyanosis and signs of respiratory distress. Patients may develop acute respiratory distress syndrome (ARDS). Purulent sputum, hemoptysis, and pleuritic chest pain are atypical for PJP.

Pneumocystis can disseminate to virtually any site including meninges, cerebral cortex, eye, bone marrow, thyroid, lymph nodes, liver, spleen and gastrointestinal (GI) tract. These organs can be involved in the absence of lung involvement.

Extrapulmonary manifestations are more common in patients, if they are:
- Receiving aerosolized pentamidine
- Not on PJP prophylaxis.

DIFFERENTIAL DIAGNOSES

- Viral pneumonia including cytomegalovirus (CMV) and adenovirus
- Fungal pneumonia including aspergillosis, cryptococcosis and histoplasmosis
- Mycoplasma infection
- Tuberculosis
- Legionellosis
- *Mycobacterium avium* complex
- Acute respiratory distress syndrome
- Nonspecific interstitial pneumonia
- Radiotherapy and chemotherapy-induced pneumonia
- Kaposi's sarcoma
- Congestive heart failure
- Pulmonary embolism.

▨ INVESTIGATIONS

- Laboratory studies
- Radiological examination
- Invasive diagnostic procedures.

Laboratory Studies

- *Lactate dehydrogenase (LDH)*:
  - ◆ Usually elevated (>220 U/L) in PJP
  - ◆ High sensitivity (78–100%)
  - ◆ A normal LDH does not exclude the diagnosis of PJP.
  - ◆ Gradual decreases in serial measurements predict survival while rising values predict mortality.
  - ◆ It may be elevated in other diseases too.
- β-D-*Glucan (BDG)*:
  - ◆ Elevated in fungal infections including PJP, *Candida* and *Aspergillus.*
  - ◆ Quantitative polymerase chain reaction (PCR) for PJP
  - ◆ On bronchoalveolar lavage (BAL), fluid or induced sputum can be done but it is not widely available.
- *Analysis of induced sputum*:
  - ◆ Expectorated sputum has very low sensitivity as patients with PJP have a nonproductive cough.
  - ◆ For processing a sample of induced sputum, the patient is nebulized with 3% hypertonic saline for 15–30 minutes and then asked to cough. The sample thus obtained is subject to histopathologic testing. It has a sensitivity ranging from 50% to 90% but a specificity which can be as high as 100%. HIV-positive patients have the highest alveolar load of *Pneumocystis.*
- *Arterial blood gas analysis and pulse oximetry*:
  - ◆ Pulse oximetry at rest and exercise pulse oximetry on room air demonstrate the degree of hypoxemia. If the oxygen saturation is less than 90% then arterial blood gas analysis should be done.
  - ◆ The ABGA abnormalities serve as a marker of the severity of the disease and help in evaluating the need for introducing corticosteroids in therapy. However, hypoxemia on ABGA cannot be used to rule in or rule out PJP.
- *Pulmonary function test*:
  - ◆ Pulmonary function test (PFT) may demonstrate a reduced diffusion capacity of carbon monoxide (DLCO) of less than 75% predicted. PFT is nonspecific for PJP but a normal DLCO makes the diagnosis of PJP unlikely.
- *HIV testing*:
  - ◆ Testing for HIV is recommended if not already done.

Radiological Examination

- *Chest radiography (Fig. 19.1)*:
  - ◆ May be normal in patients with mild disease.

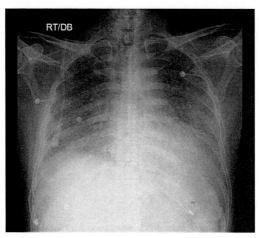

Fig. 19.1: Chest X-ray film reveals diffuse ground-glass opacities and reticular shadows in bilateral mid and lower zones.

- Symmetrical diffuse infiltrates extending from the perihilar region are seen in most of the patients of PJP.
- Atypical findings include pneumatoceles, pneumothorax and asymmetrical infiltrates.
- Pleural effusion, consolidation, mediastinal lymphadenopathy, nodular lesions and cavitation are rare.
- Spontaneous pneumothorax in HIV patients should be presumed to be PJP unless proved otherwise.
- Patients on aerosolized pentamidine are more likely to have pneumothorax and apical disease.
- On clinical recovery the chest radiograph may remain abnormal for many months. Later on, bronchiectasis or fibrosis can occur.
- *Computed tomography (CT) scan (Figs. 19.2A to C):*
  - High-resolution CT should be done if the chest radiography findings are inconclusive.
  - Computed tomography scan shows patchy areas of ground-glass attenuation along with interlobular septal thickening.
- *Gallium scintigraphy:*
  - Gallium-67 citrate concentrates in the areas of inflammation, infection and tumor which may not be visible in a radiograph.
  - Diffuse radionuclide uptake in the lungs in PJP
  - Expensive and nonspecific
  - Using monoclonal antibodies directed against PJP may increase specificity.
  - Limited utilization presently.
- *Diethylenetriamine pentaacetic (DTPA) scan:*
  - Measuring the lung clearance of aerosolized DTPA labeled with radioactive Technetium^{99m} to study alveolar damage.
  - Sensitive but expensive.

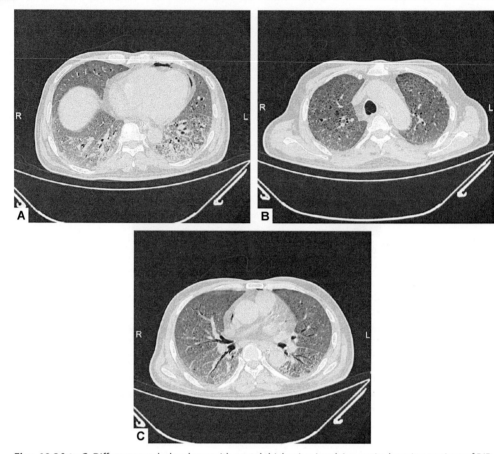

Figs. 19.2A to C: Diffuse ground-glass haze with septal thickening involving entire lung in a patient of PJP. Small cystic areas are noted in upper lobes. Patchy peribronchial opacities are noted in bilateral lower lobes.

Invasive Diagnostic Procedures

- *Bronchoalveolar lavage:*
    - Bronchoalveolar lavage has a sensitivity of 85–98% in patients of PJP.
    - It is the most invasive procedure used in the diagnosis of PJP.
    - In patients on aerosolized pentamidine prophylaxis, BAL should include at least one upper lobe.
    - Useful in the cases where induced sputum is negative, patient is uncooperative or PJP relapse is suspected.
    - A patient with confirmed PJP failing to improve after 4–8 days of therapy needs to undergo a repeat bronchoscopy to look for undiagnosed pathogens, including CMV.

- *Lung biopsy:*
  - ◆ Open lung biopsy 100% sensitive and specific
  - ◆ Video-assisted thoracoscopic surgery (VATS) may be useful in peripheral lesions.
  - ◆ Computed tomography-guided biopsy is less invasive but provides smaller sample.
  - ◆ Multiple samples can be obtained by transbronchial lung biopsy (TBLB). Contraindications to TBLB are as follows:
    - • Mechanical ventilation
    - • Bleeding diathesis
    - • Pulmonary hypertension.

Histology

Since PJP cannot be cultured, it is vital to demonstrate *Pneumocystis* by special stains for establishing a definite diagnosis. Three groups of stains are used:

1. *Indirect stains:* These stains are taken up by the noncyst forms—sporozoites and extracystic trophozoites. They do not stain the cyst wall. These stains include crystal violet, Giemsa, Wright and Diff-Quik stains.
2. *Cyst wall stains:* These stains selectively stain the walls of *Pneumocystis* cysts. These include Gomori's methenamine silver, toluidine blue, periodic acid–Schiff, Gram-Weigert, and calcofluor white.
3. *Direct and indirect fluorescent antibody stains:* These use monoclonal and polyclonal antibodies, respectively. All the developmental stages, including cysts and trophozoites, can be seen with these stains. These are more sensitive than the histologic staining.

▨ TREATMENT (TABLE 19.1)

General Principles

- Although PJP is a fungus, it does not respond to antifungal treatment. Few case reports have shown efficacy of caspofungin in salvage therapy of PJP due to its activity on BDG but it needs more robust data to be included in the treatment protocols.

Table 19.1: Treatment of PJP.	
Drug	*Dosage*
TMP–SMX	TMP–SMX (15–20 mg/kg/day of TMP component) orally or IV in three or 4 divided doses
TMP plus dapsone	TMP 5 mg/kg orally three times daily; dapsone 100 mg orally once daily
Primaquine plus clindamycin	Primaquine 30 mg base orally once daily; clindamycin 600–900 mg daily IV or orally three to four times daily
Pentamidine	4 mg/kg IV or IM once daily
Atovaquone	750 mg orally twice daily with fatty meal
IM, intramuscular; IV, intravenous; TMP–SMX, trimethoprim–Sulfamethoxazole.	

- Trimethoprim–sulfamethoxazole (TMP–SMX) is the drug of choice. Second-line agents include pentamidine, dapsone with pyrimethamine, atovaquone.

Empirical Therapy

- Do not delay treatment in high-risk patients even if the workup is incomplete. Since PJP persists for days to weeks in the host, workup may be continued even after the initiation of treatment.
- Indications for hospitalization are based on the degree of hypoxemia and the need for corticosteroids. Based on the alveolar–arterial gradient, the severity of the disease is graded as:
    - Mild (<35 mm Hg)
    - Moderate (35–45 mm Hg)
    - Severe (>45 mm Hg)
- Response to therapy should begin between 4 days and 8 days of initiating treatment.
- The Centers for Disease Control and Prevention (CDC) recommends that a PJP patient should not have direct contact with other immunocompromised patients.
- Patients should receive 21 days of therapy.

Trimethoprim–Sulfamethoxazole (Table 19.2)

This is the treatment of choice for PJP. The dose of TMP–SMX in patients with normal renal function is 15–20 mg/kg/day. Dosing is based upon the TMP component and expressed as mg/kg/day of TMP. It is given in three to four divided doses for 14–21 days.

Since oral bioavailability is excellent, oral administration is better in patients with normal functioning GI tract. The parenteral route is preferred in severe disease or in patients suffering from vomiting or intractable diarrhea.

Trimethoprim–sulfamethoxazole is as effective as intravenous (IV) pentamidine and more efficacious than other alternative regimens.

For patients with allergy to TMP–SMX, desensitization should ideally be performed unless there is a history of Stevens-Johnson syndrome (SJS).

Desensitization of the patient may be done with a gradual dose escalation using TMP–SMX pediatric suspension (TMP 8 mg/mL and SMX 40 mg/mL) (Table 19.2).

Table 19.2: Proposed desensitization regimen for TMP/SMX.

Day	Dose
1	1.25 mL once
2	1.25 mL twice
3	1.25 mL thrice
4	2.5 mL twice
5	2.5 mL thrice
6	One single strength (SS) tablet

One single strength tablet can be used for prophylaxis. For treatment, the dose is gradually doubled.

Side effects with TMP–SMX are common and include rash, fever, GI intolerance, elevation in transaminases, photosensitivity, hyperkalemia, increased serum creatinine, and rarely SJS.

Recommendations to discontinue TMP–SMX include persistent rash and fever for more than 5 days, hypotension, absolute neutrophil count <500 cell/mm^3, intractable hyperkalemia, and features of SJS, including desquamation of skin and mucous membrane involvement.

There are reports of TMP–SMX resistance mediated by mutations in the *DHPS* and *DHFR* genes but the clinical implications for these are unclear.

Minor reactions with TMP–SMX may be managed with hydration, antihistamines, antiemetics and antipyretics.

Alternative Regimens

- *Dapsone and trimethoprim:* In patients intolerant to sulfa drugs, TMP may be combined with dapsone to achieve similar efficacy with lesser side effects.

  Trimethoprim is used at 5 mg/kg orally three times daily, whereas dapsone is given 100 mg orally once per day. Dose of TMP needs to be modified in renal insufficiency.

  Check for glucose-6-phosphate dehydrogenase (G6PD) deficiency before starting dapsone. The side effects of dapsone include rash, fever, lymphadenopathy, elevation in transaminases (sulfone hypersensitivity syndrome), methemoglobinemia, hemolytic anemia and GI upset.

- *Primaquine and clindamycin:* Primaquine as 30 mg base orally once per day is used along with oral or IV clindamycin 600 mg three or four times per day. It has superior results when compared with pentamidine.

  Glucose-6-phosphate dehydrogenase deficiency must be ruled out before using primaquine.

  Side effects of primaquine include rash, fever, GI distress, leukopenia, neutropenia, hemolytic anemia and methemoglobinemia.

  Clindamycin has significant GI side effects including abdominal pain, rash, diarrhea and *Clostridium difficile* colitis.

- *Pentamidine isethionate:* With the use of better alternative regimens, the use of pentamidine has reduced. It is administered IV or intramuscular as a single dose of 4 mg/kg once daily. It should be used in patients hospitalized with severe disease. Half of the patients on pentamidine experience side effects including nephrotoxicity, infusion reactions, hyperkalemia, pancreatitis, hyperglycemia, cardiac arrhythmias, including torsades de pointes, deranged liver function test, hypotension, hypokalemia, hypocalcemia and hypoglycemia. Nephrotoxicity and azotemia may be delayed. Certain adverse effects, including hypotension and hypoglycemia, may be life-threatening.

  Aerosolized pentamidine should not be used to treat PJP due to limited efficacy and higher chances of relapse.

  Patients may develop permanent insulin requiring diabetes with pentamidine.

- *Atovaquone:* It is approved for use in mild-to-moderate disease in patients intolerant to TMP–SMX or pentamidine. Atovaquone suspension is used 750 mg orally twice daily along with a fatty meal. Side effects are mild and few and include GI distress, fever, elevated transaminases, and rash. Failure of treatment is noted in 15–30% cases.

Adjunctive Corticosteroid Therapy

Indications for the use of adjunctive corticosteroids in HIV patients who have PJP are as follows:
1. Room air arterial oxygen pressure <70 mm Hg
2. Arterial–alveolar oxygen gradient exceeding 35 mm Hg.

Resting room air oxygen saturation <92% may also be used as a criteria.

The role of steroids in non-HIV patients with PJP is unclear.

Steroids reduce the inflammatory response generated by the clearance of *Pneumocystis* by the antimicrobials. Therefore the probability of respiratory failure reduces.

Dosage: Prednisone is used as follows:
- 40 mg orally twice daily for 5 days, followed by
- 40 mg orally once daily for 5 days, followed by
- 20 mg orally once daily for 11 days

Intravenous methylprednisolone can be administered as 75% of prednisone dose.

Initiating Antiretroviral Therapy in a Patient of *Pneumocystis jirovecii* Pneumonia (Highly Active Antiretroviral Therapy)

If a patient of PJP is not already on highly active antiretroviral therapy (HAART), it should be started within 2 weeks of PJP treatment. The advantages of early therapy over deferred ART are as follows:
- Reduced risk of acquired immune deficiency syndrome progression
- Reduced mortality
- No significant increased risk of adverse events or immune reconstitution inflammatory syndrome (IRIS)

Treatment Failure

Lack of improvement or further worsening of respiratory functions as documented by arterial blood gas analysis constitutes clinical treatment failure after at least 4–8 days of PJP treatment has been given to the patient.

Reasons for clinical failure include the following:
- Lack of drug efficacy.
- Treatment-limiting toxicities of drugs being used
- Other concomitant infections, including CMV and tuberculosis, which may or may not have been diagnosed.
- Immune reconstitution inflammatory syndrome due to lysis of organisms by the antimicrobials
- *P. jirovecii* pneumonia may develop resistance to sulfa drugs.

Management of treatment failure includes the following:
- Repeat bronchoscopy and BAL to rule out concomitant infections.
- Oral primaquine with IV clindamycin is the most effective salvage regime.
- Adjunctive corticosteroids to be used wherever indicated.

Pneumocystis jirovecii Pneumonia during Pregnancy

Diagnostic workup and indications for therapy in pregnant women with PJP are the same as for nonpregnant women. There are no large, well-controlled trials on impact of pregnancy on the course of illness or prognosis in patients with PJP. TMP–SMX is the drug of choice. PJP may increase the chances of preterm labor and delivery. Women on PJP prophylaxis should be counseled about deferring pregnancy till their CD4+ cell count is more than 200 cells/μL for 3 months, and PJP prophylaxis can be discontinued (Table 19.3).

Role of Folic Acid in Pregnant Pneumocystis jirovecii Pneumonia Patient

Folic acid is supplemented in all pregnant women to reduce the chances of congenital anomalies. There is inadequate data to support the use of higher levels of folic acid in pregnant women on TMP–SMX in the first trimester to prevent congenital anomalies. However, supplementing folinic acid in patients on TMP–SMX for PJP may result in treatment failure and death. Therefore, folic acid use in PJP patients should be restricted to the first trimester.

Adjunctive Corticosteroids in Pregnant Pneumocystis jirovecii Pneumonia Patients

The use of adjunctive corticosteroids in a pregnant woman with PJP is the same as in nonpregnant adults. The problems associated with steroid use in these women include the following:
- Increased risk of cleft palate in the baby
- Increased risk of hypertension, gestational diabetes and infections in the mother

Table 19.3: Treatment of *Pneumocystis jirovecii pneumonia* in pregnancy.

Drug	Special considerations
Trimethoprim	Associated with an increased risk of neural tube defects and cardiovascular, urinary tract and multiple congenital anomalies after first trimester exposure. ART and folate antagonist combination has more chances of birth defects than ART or TMP alone. The benefits of TMP–SMX outweigh the risks in the first trimester
Sulfamethoxazole	Increased risk of neonatal kernicterus on sulfonamide use near delivery
Dapsone	Crosses placenta, mild maternal hemolysis, and potential low risk of hemolytic anemia in newborn with G6PD deficiency exposed to the drug
Clindamycin	Crosses placenta, considered safe for use throughout pregnancy
Primaquine	Generally not used in pregnancy due to risk of maternal and fetal hemolytic anemia
Atovaquone	Limited data
Pentamidine	Embryotoxic

ART, antiretroviral therapy; G6PD, glucose-6-phosphate dehydrogenase; TMP–SMX, trimethoprim–sulfamethoxazole.

However, adjunctive corticosteroids should not be withheld from the treatment plan as these improve the treatment outcomes for the mother. An extra stress dose of corticosteroid may be required to be administered at the time of delivery.

Chemoprophylaxis for *Pneumocystis jirovecii* Pneumonia (Table 19.4)

Chemoprophylaxis for PJP may be:
- Primary chemoprophylaxis in immunocompromised patient with no prior history of PJP
- Secondary chemoprophylaxis in patients with a prior bout of PJP.

Indications for Chemoprophylaxis

- In patients with HIV infection
- In patients without HIV infection.

Indications in Human Immunodeficiency Virus Patients

- CD4+ cell count less than 200 cells/µL.
- Oropharyngeal candidiasis
- Unexplained fever for more than 2 weeks
- Prior episode of PJP regardless of CD4+ count
- Children born to mothers with HIV infection should receive prophylaxis with TMP-SMX beginning at age 4–6 weeks if HIV infection has not been ruled out by two negative HIV DNA PCRs done at birth and at 4 weeks.
- All children determined to be HIV infected should receive prophylaxis through the first year of life.

Indications in Non-HIV Patients

- Primary immunodeficiency
- Solid-organ transplant recipients

Table 19.4: Chemoprophylaxis regimens.	
Drug	*Dosage*
TMP–SMX	1 SS or DS PO daily (cross protection against *Toxoplasma gondii*)
Dapsone	100 mg PO daily or 50 mg PO BID
Dapsone + (pyrimethamine + leucovorin)	Dapsone 50 mg PO daily + (pyrimethamine 50 mg + leucovorin 25 mg) PO weekly
Aerosolized pentamidine	300 mg via nebulizer every month
Atovaquone	1,500 mg PO daily with food
BID, bis in die/twice daily; DS, double strength; PO, per os/orally; SS, single strength.	

- Hematopoietic stem cell transplant recipients
- Patients with cancer, vasculitides or collagen vascular disorders on cytotoxic drugs or corticosteroids.

Indications for Discontinuing Primary Prophylaxis

CD4 cell count >200 cells/µL for at least 3 months in response to ART.

Indications for Restarting Primary Prophylaxis

CD4 cell count <200 cells/µL.

Secondary Chemoprophylaxis

- After a bout of PJP, chemoprophylaxis with TMP–SMX is given for life unless the CD4 cell count increases to >200 cells/µL for at least 3 months as a result of ART.
- If an episode of PJP occurs at a CD4 cell count of more than 200 cells/µL, continue prophylaxis for life irrespective of CD4 cell count.

▓ PROGNOSIS

Mortality rates of 10–20% are reported in PJP infection. Patients without HIV infection have a worse prognosis. On biopsy, greater degree of neutrophils was found in the lungs of these patients without HIV. This causes more severe inflammation and respiratory impairment resulting in worse prognosis.

Factors associated with poor prognosis include the following:
- Severe hypoxia on presentation
- Intensive care unit admission and mechanical ventilation
- Pneumothorax
- Low CD4+ cell count
- Coinfection with CMV
- Delay in diagnosis and initiating therapy.

  Administering ART early improves prognosis.

▓ CLINICAL PEARLS

- The most common opportunistic infection in HIV and potentially life-threatening in immunocompromised host.
- Start empirical treatment with TMP–SMX, if PJP is suspected. If diagnosis is established, continue treatment for 21 days.
- In patients with allergy to TMP–SMX, perform desensitization. Otherwise, use alternative regimens.
- Primary and secondary chemoprophylaxis are recommended.
- Prognosis is worse in non-HIV immunocompromised patients.

■ SUGGESTED READING

1. Alanio A, Hauser PM, Lagrou K, et al. ECIL guidelines for the diagnosis of *Pneumocystis jirovecii* pneumonia in patients with haematological malignancies and stem cell transplant recipients. J Antimicrob Chemother. 2016;71:2386.

2. Barreto JN, Ice LL, Thompson CA, et al. Low incidence of *Pneumocystis pneumonia* utilizing PCR-based diagnosis in patients with B-cell lymphoma receiving rituximab-containing combination chemotherapy. Am J Hematol. 2016;91:1113.

3. Edman JC, Kovacs JA, Masur H, et al. Ribosomal RNA sequence shows *Pneumocystis carinii* to be a member of the fungi. Nature. 1988;334:519.

4. Ewald H, Raatz H, Boscacci R, et al. Adjunctive corticosteroids for *Pneumocystis jirovecii* pneumonia in patients with HIV infection. Cochrane Database Syst Rev. 2015(4):CD006150.

5. Hidalgo A, Falcó V, Mauleón S, et al. Accuracy of high-resolution CT in distinguishing between *Pneumocystis carinii* pneumonia and non-*Pneumocystis carinii* pneumonia in AIDS patients. Eur Radiol. 2003;13:1179.

6. Huang L, Morris A, Limper AH, et al. An official ATS workshop summary: recent advances and future directions in *Pneumocystis pneumonia* (PCP). Proc Am Thorac Soc. 2006;3:655.

7. Kovacs JA, Gill VJ, Meshnick S, et al. New insights into transmission, diagnosis, and drug treatment of *Pneumocystis carinii* pneumonia. JAMA. 2001;286:2450.

8. Limper AH. *Pneumocystis* nomenclature. Clin Infect Dis. 2006;42:1210.

9. Mocroft A, Reiss P, Kirk O, et al. Opportunistic Infections Project Team of the Collaboration of Observational HIV Epidemiological Research in Europe (COHERE). Is it safe to discontinue primary *Pneumocystis jirovecii* pneumonia prophylaxis in patients with virologically suppressed HIV infection and a CD4 cell count <200 cells/microL? Clin Infect Dis. 2010;51:611.

10. Overgaard UM, Helweg-Larsen J. *Pneumocystis jirovecii* pneumonia (PCP) in HIV-1-negative patients: a retrospective study 2002-2004. Scand J Infect Dis. 2007;39:589.

11. Panel on Opportunistic Infections in HIV-infected Adults and Adolescents. Guidelines for the prevention and treatment of opportunistic infections in HIV-infected adults and adolescents: Recommendations from the Centers for Disease Control and Prevention, the National Institutes of Health, and the HIV Medicine Association of the Infectious Diseases Society of America 2018. [online] Available at http://aidsinfo.nih.gov/contentfiles/lvguidelines/adult_oi.pdf.

12. Rodriguez M, Fishman JA. Prevention of infection due to *Pneumocystis* spp. in human immunodeficiency virus-negative immunocompromised patients. Clin Microbiol Rev. 2004;17:770.

13. Sassi M, Ripamonti C, Mueller NJ, et al. Outbreaks of *Pneumocystis pneumonia* in 2 renal transplant centers linked to a single strain of *Pneumocystis*: implications for transmission and virulence. Clin Infect Dis. 2012;54:1437.

20

Histoplasmosis

Monica Mahajan

INTRODUCTION

Histoplasmosis is a pulmonary and hematogenous infection caused by the dimorphic fungus *Histoplasma capsulatum*. The species include *Histoplasma capsulatum* and *Histoplasma duboisii*. *Histoplasma* grows as a yeast at body temperature in humans and as a mycelial form in soil at ambient temperatures. The fungus causes a nonspecific chronic illness that is diagnosed on the basis of isolation of fungus in sputum or using serum and urine antigen tests.

MORPHOLOGY

Histoplasma capsulatum is a dimorphic fungus. It grows as a mold in nature or at room temperature. On invading the host cells, it converts to 1-5-μm-diameter yeast cell at body temperature of 37°C. Spores of *H. capsulatum* are oval and have two sizes. Macroconidia are large with a diameter of 8-15 μm; while microconidia are 2-5 μm in diameter. Inhalation of airborne conidial spores from the contaminated soil causes outbreaks of the disease.

EPIDEMIOLOGY

Histoplasma capsulatum is found worldwide in areas with temperate climate. The river valleys with damp soil and high organic decaying matter are ideal for growth of the fungus. The Ohio River Valley and the lower Mississippi River Valley are the endemic areas in the United States. The fungus has also been isolated along the Rio Grande and St. Lawrence rivers. Other areas for histoplasmosis include river valleys in North and Central America, Eastern and Southern Europe, East Asia, Australia, and Africa. The other habitat is soil near bat caves and chicken coops. Bats suffer from the disease and transmit the disease through their droppings. Paradoxically, birds do not suffer from histoplasmosis, but bird droppings act as manure for the soil by increasing nitrogen content, thereby promoting fungal growth. The active and inactive roosts of blackbirds—starlings, grackles, cowbirds, red-winged blackbirds—have been found to be heavily contaminated. The fungus can survive in the contaminated soil for many years. Any sort of construction or renovation activities disrupt the soil and cause an outbreak to occur. *H. duboisii* has a more limited distribution along the Tropics of Cancer and Capricorn and Madagascar. Positive histoplasmin test is found in 90% residents of highly endemic areas.

Histoplasmosis is not contagious. Most cases are sporadic although large outbreaks have also been reported. There is no predisposition to sex, race, or ethnicity.

PREDISPOSING FACTORS

- Infants and adults >55 years of age
- Prolonged and heavy exposure
- Defects in T-cell-mediated immunity—HIV, solid-organ transplant recipients in endemic areas, corticosteroid use or tumor necrosis factor-α antagonists (etanercept, infliximab) use, diabetes, chronic lung disease including emphysema
- Certain occupations including construction workers, gardeners, microbiology laboratory workers, pest control workers, spelunkers (cave explorers)

Disseminated histoplasmosis is common in acquired immunodeficiency syndrome (AIDS) defining opportunistic infection (OI).

PATHOPHYSIOLOGY

The aerosolized conidia and mycelial fragments from contaminated soil are inhaled and deposit in the alveoli. The mycelia convert into yeast intracellularly. The yeast is phagocytosed by the macrophages and starts to replicate in 15–18 hours. The yeast produces proteins that inhibit lysosomal proteases.

The host defense mechanisms rely on the fungistatic activity of neutrophils and macrophages. T-lymphocytes limit the infection, and cell-mediated immune response prevents dissemination of disease. A delayed-type hypersensitivity to histoplasmal antigens develops 3–6 weeks after exposure, resulting in a positive skin antigen test. Gradually, patients develop calcified fibrinous granulomas with caseous necrosis. Reactivation, reinfection, and complications of histoplasmosis are determined by the immune status of the individual.

CLINICAL MANIFESTATIONS

Histoplasmosis is also called *cave disease/caver's disease; Darling's disease; Ohio Valley disease; reticuloendotheliosis; and spelunker's lung.*

The clinical features of the disease depend on:
- The immunity of host
- The intensity of exposure—low versus high level.

The spectrum of the disease may range from asymptomatic to severe histoplasmosis. The illness is labeled acute if symptoms develop within 1 month, subacute within 1–3 months, or chronic if >3 months duration.

Acute Primary Histoplasmosis

Although exposure is common in histoplasmosis endemic areas, 90% individuals are asymptomatic, have a positive skin test, or have a mild, self-limiting disease. Acute illness due to heavy exposure develops 2–4 weeks after exposure and manifests as fever, cough, breathlessness, headache, chest pain, myalgias, arthralgia, pericarditis, and in some cases, erythema nodosum or erythema multiforme. Patients may develop significant mediastinal lymphadenopathy causing bronchial compression or dysphagia due to esophageal compression. In endemic areas, most people either have positive skin tests or typical radiological features of lymph node or diffuse or multifocal parenchymal calcification, signifying prior exposure. About 10% patients may have symptomatic pleural effusions. Complications of pulmonary histoplasmosis include the following:

- Mediastinal lymphadenopathy
- Mediastinal granuloma—3–10 cm caseous masses of mediastinal lymph nodes that coalesce into a single encapsulated lesion in paratracheal or subcarinal region
- Chronic cavitary disease (more often in patients with emphysema)
- Broncholithiasis—spitting of chalk-like material or lithoptysis due to erosion of calcified lymph nodes into a bronchus leading to hemoptysis and intense cough
- Fibrosing mediastinitis—invasive fibrosis encases mediastinal or hilar lymph nodes and causes occlusion of central airways and vessels, including superior vena cava (SVC) syndrome as a manifestation.
- Pulmonary nodules—infection sites contract and persist indefinitely.
- Progressive disseminated histoplasmosis by hematogenous dissemination if host suffers from defects in cell-mediated immunity.

Chronic Cavitary Histoplasmosis

Chronic cavitary histoplasmosis is seen most often in patients with underlying emphysema. Patients experience progressively worsening cough, dyspnea, and respiratory compromise. The lung lesions are typically apical, near emphysematous bullae, with surrounding inflammation and mimic cavitary pulmonary tuberculosis. There is no dissemination of the disease.

Progressive Disseminated Histoplasmosis

There is subacute or chronic involvement of the reticuloendothelial system. The patient presents with fever, fatigue, weight loss, or other nonspecific symptoms. Clinical signs comprise lymphadenopathy, hepatosplenomegaly, or oral/mucosal ulcerations. Central nervous system (CNS) involvement results in meningitis or focal brain lesions that cause altered sensorium, cranial nerve deficits, ataxia, or focal neurological deficits. Adrenal involvement causes Addison disease. HIV patients may develop severe pneumonia and acute respiratory distress syndrome resembling *Pneumocystis jiroveci infection*. Extrapulmonary involvement may also include gastrointestinal ulcerations, pancytopenia, elevation in liver enzymes, coagulopathy, obtundation, endocarditis, rhabdomyolysis, and hypotension.

Presumed Ocular Histoplasmosis Syndrome

There can be chronic chorioretinitis and unexplained visual loss due to macular involvement in endemic areas since *H. capsulatum* has not been isolated from ocular lesions, and patient can be unresponsive to amphotericin B treatment. This may be a hypersensitivity reaction to *H. capsulatum.*

Fibrosing Mediastinitis

It is a rare complication that leads to circulatory compromise.

Pericarditis

It occurs as a complication of inflammation in adjacent mediastinal lymph nodes in patients with acute pulmonary histoplasmosis. It is an inflammatory response rather than a true infection of the pericardium. Large pericardial effusions impair cardiac output and require emergency drainage of fluid. Pericardial constriction is rare. The pericardial fluid is generally exudative.

Rheumatologic Syndromes

Bone and joint involvement represents a systemic inflammatory response rather than infection and manifests as arthralgia, arthritis, or erythema nodosum. It occurs in 5–10% of the cases and is more frequent in females.

Central Nervous System Histoplasmosis

Central nervous system involvement causes meningitis, parenchymal involvement of brain or spinal cord, or both. Patients complain of headache, visual or gait disturbances, confusion, seizures, neck stiffness, and altered sensorium.

DIFFERENTIAL DIAGNOSES

- Aspergillosis
- Blastomycosis
- Tuberculosis
- Sarcoidosis
- *Pneumocystis jiroveci* infection
- Chlamydial pneumonia
- *Legionella* pneumonia
- Lymphoma
- Malignancy lung
- Carcinoid lung
- Viral pneumonias.

MANAGEMENT OF HISTOPLASMOSIS

Diagnosis

Complete Blood Count

Anemia or pancytopenia in disseminated histoplasmosis.

Alkaline Phosphatase

Elevated in chronic pulmonary and progressive disseminated histoplasmosis.

Lactic Dehydrogenase

Lactate dehydrogenase is elevated in patients with HIV with disseminated histoplasmosis.

Histopathology

Histoplasma capsulatum is seen as an intracellular yeast in Wright- or Giemsa-stained buffy coat or peripheral blood specimens. Using the Grocott–Gomori methenamine silver stain, yeast may be detected in caseous material. Hematoxylin and eosin staining may also be used. Bronchoalveolar lavage or tissue biopsy specimens may be required.

Culture

Since culture of *H. capsulatum* may pose a biohazard, the laboratory personnel need to be aware of the suspected diagnosis. The yield of blood culture improves by lysis centrifugation or culture of buffy coat. Positive cultures are seldom obtained during acute illness and are more likely to be positive in progressive disseminated disease.

Antigen Testing

H. capsulatum antigen test is quite specific and sensitive. *H. capsulatum* antigen is detected in serum in 80% and in urine in 90% patients with disseminated histoplasmosis. Serum and urine specimens should be simultaneously tested. A radioimmunoassay is used to measure *H. capsulatum* polysaccharide antigen levels in the sample. It is a rapid and accurate method for early diagnosis of disseminated disease. There can be cross-reactivity with other fungi, including *Blastomyces dermatitidis*, *Coccidioides immitis*, *Paracoccidioides brasiliensis*, and *Penicillium marneffei*. Antigenemia and antigenuria decrease during successful therapy. Failure of levels to fall can be indicative of treatment failure. Antigen levels should be measured:

- Before initiation of treatment
- At 2 weeks
- At 1 month
- Every 3 months during therapy
- For at least 6 months after treatment has been stopped.

Complement-fixing antibodies: Titer is considered positive at reciprocal dilutions >1:8. Active histoplasmosis results in titers >1:32 after 3 weeks from exposure. Results normalize with resolution of the infection in the next few months in acute infection; whereas they remain positive for long periods in chronic pulmonary and progressive disseminated disease. False-positive results are seen in *B. dermatitidis* and *C. immitis* infections, tuberculosis, sarcoidosis, and lymphoma.

Immunoprecipitating antibodies: These are antibodies to two glycoproteins, H and M.

Anti-H antibodies: These are more specific for active histoplasmosis, detected in only 20% patients and disappear within 6 months in the absence of an ongoing infection.

Anti-M antibodies: These are detected in 50–80% patients and remain positive for many years.

Polymerase Chain Reaction for Histoplasmosis

Polymerase chain reaction provides rapid detection of *H. capsulatum* in clinical samples.

Radiology

Chest X-ray in acute pulmonary histoplasmosis can be normal or may show patchy infiltrates in lower lung fields, hilar or mediastinal lymphadenopathy, and reticular or miliary pattern. Chronic cavitary histoplasmosis presents as upper lobe infiltrates and thick-walled cavities. There can be evidence of fibrosis and scarring. Healed pulmonary lesions appear as residual nodules. These can be coin-shaped 1–4-cm lesions that need to be differentiated from malignant lesions. Underlying emphysematous changes can be noted.

Computed tomography (CT) scan and magnetic resonance imaging are useful for diagnosing CNS histoplasmosis. Echocardiography is helpful for diagnosing pericarditis or endocarditis. CT abdomen is useful in the cases with suspected adrenal involvement.

Pulmonary Function Test

Restrictive defect, small airway involvement, and diffusion defects are determined.

Diagnostic procedures: These include bronchoscopy, lumbar puncture, tissue biopsy, pericardiocentesis, and thoracocentesis.

Treatment

General Principles

Asymptomatic individuals need no treatment. The only definite indications for antifungal therapy with proven or probable efficacy are:
- Acute diffuse pulmonary infection with moderately severe to severe symptoms
- Chronic cavitary pulmonary infection
- Progressive disseminated infection
- Central nervous system infections.

Drugs that are used are amphotericin B deoxycholate (AmBd), liposomal amphotericin B (LAmB), amphotericin B lipid complex, and itraconazole.

The oral capsule or solution of itraconazole may be used. To maximize absorption, itraconazole capsules should be taken with food or cola, which produce high gastric acidity. Solution formulation is preferred on an empty stomach. Blood concentration levels achieved are approximately 30% higher with the solution compared with the capsule formulation. Drug levels are measured only after the use of the drug for at least 2 weeks. It has a long half-life of 24 hours so samples can be drawn any time irrespective of timing of last dose administered. Avoid use of proton-pump inhibitors or antacids. The response rate to oral itraconazole in mild cases of pulmonary or disseminated disease may range from 80% to 100%.

In patients intolerant to itraconazole, fluconazole may be used but has lower efficacy. It is used in a dose of 200–800 mg daily. Ketoconazole use is associated with increased adverse events. Posaconazole and voriconazole are also used as second-line alternative therapy. Therapeutic drug monitoring is recommended for voriconazole and posaconazole but not for fluconazole. Monitor for hepatotoxicity and drug interactions while the patient is on azoles. There is insufficient data to recommend the use of echinocandins in histoplasmosis.

Therapy is not recommended or is ineffective in mediastinal fibrosis, pulmonary nodule, broncholithiasis, or presumed ocular histoplasmosis syndrome. Calcified healed lesions do not require treatment.

Role of granulocyte macrophage colony-stimulating factor, interferon-γ, or antibodies to *H. capsulatum* cell surface proteins are unknown.

Acute Primary Histoplasmosis

- Patients may show a spontaneous improvement over 1 month.
- Use itraconazole 200 mg thrice daily for 3 days, followed by 200 mg once daily for 6–12 weeks in patients with mild-to-moderate disease who continue to be symptomatic for >1 month. Fluconazole is less efficacious.
- Manage severe cases of pneumonia with amphotericin B. LAmB in doses of 3–5 mg/kg/day or AmBd 0.7–1.0 mg/kg/day intravenous (IV) for 1–2 weeks, followed by itraconazole, is recommended. Itraconazole is used 200 mg thrice daily × 3 days, followed by 200 mg twice daily for a total of 12 weeks.
- Methylprednisolone is added to the treatment regime in a dose of 0.5–1 mg/kg/day IV in patients with severe hypoxia or respiratory distress. These patients need to be hospitalized.
- Antifungal therapy should be continued till there is complete resolution of pulmonary infiltrates on chest X-ray.
- Persistent fever, fatigue, or weight loss may indicate development of progressive disseminated histoplasmosis.

Chronic Cavitary Histoplasmosis

- For chronic cavitary histoplasmosis, itraconazole is used in a loading dose of 200 mg thrice daily for 3 days, followed by a maintenance dose of 200 mg once or twice daily for 12–14 months. Blood levels of itraconazole need to be measured in patients who have received the drug for at least 2 weeks to ensure adequate drug exposure.
- Use amphotericin B for severe disease.

- Therapy is continued until pulmonary imaging shows no further improvement when monitored at 4–6-month intervals. Chest radiograph is sufficient for monitoring, and patients need to be monitored for at least 1 year after stopping therapy to detect any relapse.
- Antigen tests are generally negative in chronic cavitary histoplasmosis and have a limited role in assessing response to therapy.
- Relapse occurs in approximately 15% cases.

Progressive Disseminated Histoplasmosis

- Progressive disseminated histoplasmosis is fatal if left untreated. LAmB in a dose of 3 mg/kg/day IV or AmBd 0.7–1 mg/kg/day IV is used till the patient starts showing signs of clinical improvement and then switch to oral itraconazole 200 mg thrice daily for 3 days, followed by twice daily for 12 months after fever resolves, and the patient is hemodynamically stable.
- For HIV-positive patients, itraconazole is continued till CD4 cell count is >150 cells/mm^3 or indefinitely to prevent relapse. Timing of initiation of highly active antiretroviral therapy is a dilemma as early therapy entails improvement in cell-mediated immunity but also put the patient at risk of immune-reconstitution inflammatory syndrome (IRIS). IRIS in histoplasmosis is usually mild.
- Lifelong therapy is recommended for immunosuppressed patients.
- For mild-to-moderate disseminated disease, itraconazole alone used in abovementioned doses for 12 months can be sufficient.
- Blood levels of itraconazole should be monitored during therapy.
- Serum and urine antigen levels are measured during the therapy, and for 12 months after therapy for relapse. In the cases where patient has fully recovered yet low-level antigenemia persists, there is no reason to prolong the therapy.

Mediastinal Lymphadenitis

- Treatment is usually unnecessary.
- In patients who are symptomatic for >1 month, itraconazole is used for 6–12 weeks in standard doses along with tapering doses of steroids.
- Prednisone 0.5–1 mg/kg/day is used in tapering doses over 1–2 weeks in case the lymph nodes are causing compressive symptoms over adjacent structures.

Mediastinal Fibrosis

- Antifungal therapy is not recommended for established mediastinal fibrosis unless erythrocyte sedimentation rate is high, and complement fixation antibodies for *H. capsulatum* are positive. In these cases, antifungal therapy may be tried for 12 weeks if mediastinal granuloma cannot be entirely ruled out.
- Corticosteroid therapy is discouraged.
- Intravascular stents may be placed in pulmonary vasculature, including SVC, pulmonary artery, or pulmonary vein in appropriate patients.
- Surgery should be avoided.

- Occlusion of the SVC or loss of function of one lung causes chest pain, hemoptysis, or significant morbidity, whereas occlusion of vessels/airways of both lungs may prove fatal
- Stents may get obstructed due to granulation tissue.

Mediastinal Granuloma

- Antifungal treatment is not recommended unless symptomatic.
- Itraconazole is used 200 mg thrice daily for 3 days, followed by once or twice daily for 6–12 weeks.
- Surgery may be required to relieve obstruction or in the cases where adjacent esophagus or SVC get involved.
- The caseous center of the granuloma can spontaneously drain via a fistula or sinus tract to the bronchus, skin, or esophagus.
- Antibiotics may be required for secondary bacterial infection.
- Mediastinal granuloma does not progress into mediastinal fibrosis.

Broncholithiasis

- Bronchoscopically or surgically remove the broncholith.
- There is no role of antifungals.

Pulmonary Nodules of Histoplasmosis

- Calcification occurs in the center or in concentric rings in the nodule.
- No role of antifungals. It needs to be distinguished from malignancy.

Pericarditis

- In the case of hemodynamic compromise or tamponade, pericardiocentesis relieves the symptoms.
- Prednisone 0.5–1 mg/kg/day is recommended for symptoms unremitting with nonsteroidal anti-inflammatory drugs or patients showing hemodyamic compromise.
- Itraconazole is recommended for 6–12 weeks if corticosteroids are administered.
- Nonsteroidal anti-inflammatory drugs alone are used in mild cases.

Rheumatologic Syndromes

Nonsteroidal anti-inflammatory drugs, tapering doses of steroids along with 6–12 weeks of itraconazole are used.

Central Nervous System Histoplasmosis

- Liposomal amphotericin B (5 mg/kg daily for a total of 175 mg/kg) given over 4-6 weeks, followed by itraconazole 200 mg two or three times daily for at least 1 year until resolution of cerebrospinal fluid abnormalities, including *Histoplasma* antigen levels, is recommended. Monitor blood levels of itraconazole.

- Combination therapy is not recommended.
- Surgery is rarely needed.

Histoplasmosis in Pregnancy

- Liposomal amphotericin B 3–5 mg/kg daily is used for 4–6 weeks. AmBd is used as an alternative.
- Neonate with signs of infection is treated with LAmB.
- The placenta should be examined for granulomas and for organisms resembling *H. capsulatum.*
- Azole therapy is associated with teratogenic complications.

Histoplasmosis in Children

- Progressive disseminated disease with meningitis occurs in children less than 2 years of age due to relatively immature cell-mediated immunity.
- Recommendations same as that for adults except that AmBd is well tolerated and the lipid preparations are not preferred.
- Itraconazole dose in children is 5–10 mg/kg daily in two divided doses.

Prophylaxis in Immunosuppressed Patients

- Itraconazole prophylaxis is indicated in HIV if CD4 cell count <150 cells/mm^3 and endemicity >10 cases per 100 patient years.
- Itraconazole 200 mg/day is recommended in immunocompromised patients.

Reducing Exposure to Histoplasma capsulatum

- Excluding a colony of bats or a flock of birds from a building by sealing all entry points. When openings are inaccessible, installing and maintaining lights in a roosting area will force bats to seek another daytime roosting site. Mechanical anti-roosting systems include angled and porcupine wires made of stainless steel.
- Posting health-risk warnings for anyone who enters the roosting areas.
- Communicating health risk to workers.
- Controlling aerosolized dust when removing bat or bird manure from a building by wetting it with water spray, vacuum systems.
- Inform travelers to endemic areas how to reduce exposure.
- Workers involved in high-risk activities should wear respirators.

Prognosis

Acute primary histoplasmosis is mild, self-limiting, and very rarely fatal. Chronic cavitary histoplasmosis causes progressive respiratory failure and death. Cure rates in meningitis are

50% with a high rate of relapse. Untreated progressive disseminated histoplasmosis has a high mortality rate of >90%.

Clinical Pearls

- Histoplasmosis is a dimorphic fungal infection, especially in residents in river valleys in endemic areas. Check for travel to endemic areas or exposure to bats.
- It results in acute primary pulmonary involvement, chronic cavitary infection, or progressive disseminated disease.
- Extrapulmonary involvement includes pericarditis, meningitis, ocular involvement, and rheumatologic symptoms.
- Urine and serum antigen tests are useful in diagnosis and follow-up.

▧ SUGGESTED READING

1. Bahr NC, Antinori S, Wheat LJ, et al. Histoplasmosis infections worldwide: thinking outside of the Ohio River Valley. Curr Trop Med Rep. 2015;2:70.
2. Benedict K, Derado G, Mody RK. Histoplasmosis-associated hospitalizations in the United States, 2001–2012. Open Forum Infect Dis. 2016;3:ofv219.
3. Benedict K, Mody RK. Epidemiology of histoplasmosis outbreaks, United States, 1938–2013. Emerg Infect Dis. 2016;22:370.
4. Kauffman CA. Histoplasmosis: a clinical and laboratory update. Clin Microbiol Rev. 2007;20:115.
5. Panackal AA, Hajjeh RA, Cetron MS, et al. Fungal infections among returning travelers. Clin Infect Dis. 2002;35:1088.
6. Richer SM, Smedema ML, Durkin MM, et al. Improved diagnosis of acute pulmonary histoplasmosis by combining antigen and antibody detection. Clin Infect Dis. 2016;62:896.
7. Wheat LJ, Connolly P, Smedema M, et al. Emergence of resistance to fluconazole as a cause of failure during treatment of histoplasmosis in patients with acquired immunodeficiency disease syndrome. Clin Infect Dis. 2001;33:1910.
8. Wheat LJ, Freifeld AG, Kleiman MB, et al. Clinical practice guidelines for the management of patients with histoplasmosis: 2007 Update by the Infectious Diseases Society of America. Clin Infect Dis. 2007;45:807.
9. Wheat LJ. Approach to the diagnosis of the endemic mycoses. Clin Chest Med. 2009;30:379.

21

Blastomycosis

Monica Mahajan

INTRODUCTION

Blastomycosis refers to disease caused by the dimorphic fungus *Blastomyces dermatitidis*. It is also known as Chicago disease, Gilchrist's disease, and North American Blastomycosis. It is endemic in certain areas of the United States. Some autochthonous cases have been reported from Africa and India. Infection is caused by the inhalation of conidia of *Blastomyces*. Blastomycosis commonly affects the lungs and skin. The spectrum of illness ranges from asymptomatic state to fulminant multilobar pneumonia. It causes skin lesions and abscesses that heal with disfiguring scars. It is a common infection among dogs, particularly in areas where it is prevalent.

ETIOLOGY

Blastomyces dermatitidis is the asexual form of *Ajellomyces dermatitidis*. It belongs to the phylum Ascomycota. Phylogenetic analysis shows the *B. dermatitidis* comprises two species: *B. dermatitidis* and *B. gilchristii*. It is a thermal dimorphic fungus since it has both a mold and a yeast phase. At body temperature (37°C), colonies appear as wrinkled and folded, smooth, and yeast like. When grown on Sabouraud's dextrose agar at 25°C, the colonies have variable morphology and growth rate. The rapidly growing colonies produce a fluffy white mycelium, whereas the slow growth produces tan-colored, smooth, and nonsporulating colonies. Growth is promoted by nitrogenous substances, including yeast extract and Starling dung. Strains are pleomorphic.

The typical yeast form of the fungus is characterized by a thick wall and a single bud with a wide base. The yeast cells are 12–15 µm in diameter. The yeast converts to the mycelial form when incubated at 25°C for a few days to a few weeks. Similarly, the mycelial form can be converted to yeast when incubated at 37°C. Since the mycelial form is easier to grow, deoxyribonucleic acid (DNA) probes can identify the fungus early from the mycelial growth. The conidia are round in shape and 2–10 µm in diameter. Inhaled conidia result in pulmonary infection.

EPIDEMIOLOGY

Certain areas that are endemic for blastomycosis include midwestern, south central, and south-eastern states of the United States. These areas surround the Ohio and Mississippi River valleys, the Great Lakes, and the Saint Lawrence River. Parts of Canada that are endemic include Ontario, Quebec, and Manitoba. Autochthonous (indigenous) cases have also been reported from India and Africa. Residential areas near rivers and waterways have a higher incidence of blastomycosis.

The fungus is found in soil containing decaying organic matter, such as leaves, rotting wood, and animal droppings. Exposure to soil is the predisposing factor. Blastomycosis infects people engaged in outdoor activities, such as collecting firewood, fishing, hunting, and tearing down old buildings or construction of highways. The disease can affect any age, sex, race, or occupation but there is a slight male preponderance due to these outdoor activities. Blastomycosis is found in dogs, cats, horses, cows, bats, and lions but animal-to-human transmission or human-to-human transmission does not occur except in bite wounds. Canine blastomycosis should raise suspicion of human blastomycosis in a particular area.

PATHOPHYSIOLOGY

Once the soil containing the spores is disturbed, the airborne spores are inhaled and reach the lungs. The neutrophils, monocytes, and macrophages present in the respiratory tract phagocytose and kill most of the pathogens explaining why approximately 50% of cases are asymptomatic. At body temperature the mycelial form undergoes a phase transition to the larger yeast form. The yeast form is sturdier due to its larger diameter and thick cell wall. It is more resistant to phagocytosis.

BAD-1 is an immune-modulating glycoprotein expressed on the cell surface and released into the extracellular matrix. BAD-1 promotes the binding of *B. dermatitidis* to macrophages. Subsequently, the yeast form disseminates to other organs through the blood stream and lymphatics. This leads to the influx of neutrophils and macrophages leading to granuloma formation. This pyogranulomatous systemic response is a hallmark of blastomycosis.

CLINICAL FEATURES

The incubation period is variable and can range from 3 weeks to 6 weeks. Half of the patients remain asymptomatic.

Pulmonary Blastomycosis

Pulmonary involvement is seen in the majority of the patients. The spectrum of pulmonary manifestations is wide and nonspecific. Reactivation of infection can occur even when blastomycosis has resolved (Table 21.1).

Extrapulmonary Blastomycosis

Extrapulmonary manifestations of blastomycosis are present in approximately 25–40% of symptomatic patients. These manifest as cutaneous, osteoarticular, genitourinary, or central nervous system (CNS) disease (Table 21.2).

Table 21.1: Pulmonary manifestations of blastomycosis.

Pulmonary manifestation	Clinical features
Flu-like illness	- Fever, chills, headache, myalgia, nonproductive cough Generally self-limiting - D/D-influenza
Acute pneumonitis	- High-grade fever, chills, cough, productive cough, mucopurulent or purulent sputum, pleuritic chest pain - D/D-bacterial pneumonia
Acute respiratory distress syndrome	High-grade fever, tachypnea, tachycardia, respiratory distress
Chronic pulmonary involvement	- Low-grade fever, night sweats, productive cough, weight loss - D/D-TB, lymphoma, malignancy

ARDS, acute respiratory distress syndrome; TB, tuberculosis.

Table 21.2: Extrapulmonary manifestations of blastomycosis.

Extrapulmonary manifestation	Clinical features
Cutaneous lesions	Most common site of extrapulmonary involvement. Papules or pustules leading to ulcers with granulomatous or verrucous borders, plaques with serpiginous borders, wart-like scars, facial disfigurement Laboratory workers develop chancriform lesions
CNS	Intracranial or epidural abscesses, meningitis
Osteoarticular	Bone or joint pain or swelling, osteomyelitis, draining abscess Vertebrae and pelvis most frequently involved
Genitourinary	Prostatitis or epididymoorchitis—asymptomatic pyuria or dysuria
Other organs	Ocular, thyroid, adrenal, liver, breast, or lymph nodes involvement

CNS, central nervous system.

Immunocompromised patients have more frequent dissemination, larger pleural effusions, and severe disease resulting in respiratory failure.

DIFFERENTIAL DIAGNOSES

- *Pulmonary blastomycosis:*
    - Influenza
    - Bacterial pneumonia
    - Tuberculosis (TB)
    - Viral pneumonia
    - Sarcoidosis
    - Acute respiratory distress syndrome (ARDS)
    - Metastatic cancer
    - Aspergillosis

- ◆ Cryptococcosis
- ◆ Histoplasmosis
- ■ *Cutaneous blastomycosis:*
  - ◆ Tuberculosis verrucosa cutis
  - ◆ Atypical mycobacterial infection
  - ◆ Lupus vulgaris
  - ◆ Pyoderma gangrenosum
  - ◆ Squamous cell carcinoma
  - ◆ Basal cell carcinoma
  - ◆ Keratoacanthoma
- ■ *Central nervous system blastomycosis:*
  - ◆ Pyogenic abscesses
  - ◆ Tuberculomas and tubercular meningitis
  - ◆ Neoplasms
- ■ *Osteoarticular blastomycosis:*
  - ◆ Septic arthritis and osteomyelitis
  - ◆ Tuberculosis
  - ◆ Bony metastasis.

DIAGNOSIS

Laboratory Investigations

- ■ *Sputum examination:* Sputum analysis is simple, inexpensive, sensitive, and rapid. Sputum sample should be processed with 10% potassium hydroxide or a fungal stain. Yeast can be identified by direct visualization in sputum, tissue, or respiratory secretions. It appears as 12–15-µm diameter yeast with double refractile walls, multiple nuclei, and single broad-based bud. Calcofluor white stain binds to chitin in cell wall and produces fluorescence. It is especially useful when the organisms in the specimen are sparse. Wet mounts of bronchoalveolar lavage (BAL), cerebrospinal fluid (CSF), urine, and pus or skin scrapings can also be examined.
- ■ *Culture:* Sputum, tracheal aspirate, BAL, CSF, and urine or tissue biopsy samples may be used for culture. Urine sample may be obtained after prostatic massage, and the sediment is cultured after centrifuging the sample. Culture is the gold standard for diagnosis. The pathogen can be cultured on sabouraud dextrose agar, brain–heart infusion, or potato dextrose agar at room temperature. To prevent bacterial contamination, chloramphenicol is added to the culture medium. Growth occurs in 5–30 days. The colonies are creamy white, which change to brown–gray when hyphal growth occurs. The mold has a lollipop appearance with oval, spherical, or pyriform conidia at the tip of a thin conidiophore. They also have thin septate hyphae. Colonization and contamination with *Blastomyces* is not known. A DNA probe allows rapid identification of the pathogen.
- ■ *Antigen detection:* Enzyme immunoassay is performed on urine or serum but can also be used on BAL. Cross-reaction can occur with histoplasmosis, penicilliosis, paracoccidioidomycosis, and other fungal diseases.

- *Antibody detection tests*: Immunodiffusion and complement fixation have low sensitivity and specificity.
- *Polymerase chain reaction (PCR)*: PCR for detecting blastomycosis directly from specimens is still experimental.
- There can be a nonspecific leukocytosis with left shift. Arterial blood gas analysis shows hypoxemia.

Radiology Studies

- *Chest radiography*: X-ray findings are nonspecific and include lobar or segmental airspace opacities, focal mass, miliary or reticulonodular patterns, pleural effusion, or pleural thickening. Cavitary lesions and diffuse interstitial infiltrates are more common in immunocompromised patients. Lymphadenopathy is infrequent. ARDS changes on X-ray are associated with poorer outcomes. In the cases with osteomyelitis, well-circumscribed osteolytic lesion is the most common radiological finding.
- *Computed tomography (CT chest)* helps in identifying nodular lesions, consolidation with or without cavitation, mediastinal abnormalities, and loculated pleural effusions. Unlike TB and histoplasmosis, hilar lymphadenopathy is rare in blastomycosis.
- CT head is useful in detecting brain abscesses.
- *Magnetic resonance imaging* and radionuclide bone scans identify skeletal involvement due to blastomycosis.

Diagnostic Procedures

- Bronchoscopy and BAL are indicated in the absence of sputum, especially in pediatric patients, mass lesions, and patients with hemoptysis.
- Lung, skin, or bone biopsy reveals broad-based budding yeasts typical of *Blastomyces*, granuloma formation, suppuration, and/or necrosis. Methenamine silver stain or the periodic acid–Schiff stain is better than hematoxylin and eosin for detecting the fungus.

▨ TREATMENT

Amphotericin B (AmB) is used in the treatment of severe blastomycosis and for CNS involvement due to blastomycosis. Clinical data regarding the use of newer azoles and echinocandins is insufficient. Itraconazole levels should be measured during therapy (Table 21.3).

Disseminated Blastomycosis

- *Moderately severe-to-severe disseminated blastomycosis*: Treatment recommendations are same as for moderately severe-to-severe pulmonary blastomycosis.
- *Mild-to-moderate disseminated blastomycosis*: Treatment is same as for mild-to-moderate pulmonary blastomycosis (Tables 21.3).

Table 21.3: Treatment of pulmonary blastomycosis.

Manifestation	Initial therapy	Step-down therapy
Moderately severe-to-severe disease	LAmB 3–5 mg/kg/day or AmBd 0.7–1 mg/kg/day for 1–2 weeks	Itraconazole 200 mg 3 times/day for 3 days and then twice daily for 6–12 months
Mild-to-moderate disease	Itraconazole 200 mg once/twice daily for 6–12 months	–

LAmB, liposomal amphotericin B; AmBd, amphotericin B deoxycholate.

◼ TREATMENT OF CENTRAL NERVOUS SYSTEM BLASTOMYCOSIS (TABLE 21.4 AND 21.5)

Table 21.4: Treatment of central nervous system blastomycosis.

Initial therapy	Step-down therapy
LAmB 5 mg/kg/day for 4–6 weeks	Fluconazole 800 mg/day or itraconazole 200 mg 2–3 times/day or voriconazole 200–400 mg twice daily for at least 1 year

LAmB, liposomal amphotericin B.

Table 21.5: Treatment of blastomycosis in immunosuppressed patients.

Initial therapy	Step-down therapy
LAmB 3–5 mg/kg/day or AmBd 0.7–1 mg/kg/day for 1–2 weeks	Itraconazole 200 mg thrice daily for 3 days and then 200 mg twice daily for 12 months or lifelong

LAmB, liposomal amphotericin B; AmBd, amphotericin B deoxycholate.

Osteoarticular Disease

Itraconazole 200–400 mg/day is used for 12 months.

Pregnant Women

Pregnant women are more likely to have disseminated disease than nonpregnant women. Perinatal transmission may occur due to aspiration of infected vaginal secretion or transplacental transmission. Liposomal AmB 3–5 mg/kg/day intravenous is the only treatment recommended in pregnancy. Azoles are contraindicated.

◼ PROGNOSIS

Most immunocompetent patients recover fully. ARDS and respiratory failure can prove fatal. The mortality rate is higher in human immunodeficiency virus–positive patients and can range from 30% to 40%.

CLINICAL PEARLS

- *Blastomyces* is an endemic fungus that causes a spectrum of illnesses ranging from asymptomatic infection, pulmonary infection to extrapulmonary disease.
- Definitive diagnosis requires culture of the organism.
- Amphotericin B and itraconazole are the mainstay of treatment.

SUGGESTED READING

1. Bariola JR, Hage CA, Durkin M, et al. Detection of *Blastomyces dermatitidis* antigen in patients with newly diagnosed blastomycosis. Diagn Microbiol Infect Dis. 2011;69:187.
2. Bariola JR, Perry P, Pappas PG, et al. Blastomycosis of the central nervous system: a multicenter review of diagnosis and treatment in the modern era. Clin Infect Dis. 2010;50:797.
3. Chapman SW, Dismukes WE, Proia LA, et al. Clinical practice guidelines for the management of blastomycosis: 2008 update by the Infectious Diseases Society of America. Clin Infect Dis. 2008;46:1801.
4. Martynowicz MA, Prakash UB. Pulmonary blastomycosis: an appraisal of diagnostic techniques. Chest. 2002;121:768-73.
5. McTaggart LR, Brown EM, Richardson SE. Phylogeographic analysis of *Blastomyces dermatitidis* and *Blastomyces gilchristii* reveals an association with North American freshwater drainage basins. PLoS One. 2016;11:e0159396.
6. Pappas PG, Threlkeld MG, Bedsole GD, et al. Blastomycosis in immunocompromised patients. Medicine (Baltimore). 1993;72:311.
7. Proia LA, Harnisch DO. Successful use of posaconazole for treatment of blastomycosis. Antimicrob Agents Chemother. 2012;56:4029.
8. Saccente M, Woods GL. Clinical and laboratory update on blastomycosis. Clin Microbiol Rev. 2010;23:367.

22

Coccidioidomycosis

Monica Mahajan

■ INTRODUCTION

Coccidioidomycosis is also known as San Joaquin fever or Valley fever. It is a disease caused by the fungi *Coccidioides immitis* and *Coccidioides posadasii*. The two species are genetically distinct but produce the same manifestations. The disease has protean manifestations ranging from self-limiting respiratory disease to nonspecific disseminated disease secondary to hematogenous spread. Antifungals used in treatment include amphotericin B, itraconazole, fluconazole, and the newer triazoles.

■ ETIOLOGY

Coccidioides immitis is a dimorphic saprophytic fungus. It grows as a mycelium in the soil and as a spherule form in the host organism.

■ LIFE CYCLE

The life cycle of the fungus starts with the growth of fungus in the mycelial form, a few inches underneath the soil. Heavy rain promotes the growth of the fungus. The hyphae grow in both the vertical and horizontal directions. During the prolonged dry spell or drought-like conditions, the cells within the hyphae degenerate to form alternating barrel-shaped cells called anthroconidia. Any activity, such as farming or construction, which disturbs the soil, causes these lightweight conidia to be dispersed by the wind. The anthroconidia can remain suspended in the air for prolonged periods. Earthquakes and windstorms can result in outbreaks. These spores are inhaled by humans and reach the alveoli. The anthroconidia turn into larger tissue invasive double-walled spherules and develop internal septations. Endospores form within the spherules within 48–72 hours. The human body temperature is ideal for the formation of endospore. Rupture of spherules releases thousands of smaller sized endospores that repeat the cycle to form more spherules and also disseminate into the infected individual's tissues. A very low dose of inoculum of anthroconidia can be sufficient to produce the disease. Inhalation of even a single anthroconidium may result in the disease.

Rare cases of infection by direct inoculation from contaminated sharp objects, transplantation of infected tissues, and sexual transmission have been documented. A rare instance of coccidioidomycosis transmitted by cat bite has been recorded.

EPIDEMIOLOGY

Coccidioidomycosis is most commonly found in the southwestern United States, including California and Arizona. It is also found in northern Mexico, Central and South America. The resident population in these endemic areas has an exposure rate of 30–60% during their lifetime. Cases may be noted in nonendemic areas due to travel and windstorms.

PATHOPHYSIOLOGY

The inhaled endospores transform into spherules and lead to the activation of complement pathway, release of cytokines, and an acute inflammatory response mediated by neutrophils and eosinophils. The macrophages engulf some of the endospores. Th-1 cytokines promote macrophage activity. If the infection is not cleared during this acute phase, a more chronic inflammatory process sets in. The lymphocytes and histiocytes form granulomas with giant cells. There is formation of nodules, cavitation, and fibrosis. The patient may have an acute, subacute, or chronic illness. Dissemination occurs to skin, subcutaneous tissue, brain, bones, and joints. The endospores travel from the bronchioles into the lung parenchyma and then spread to distant organs through lymphatics via the lymph nodes and thoracic duct and through the vascular supply.

The pathogenicity of the fungus is mainly because of the resistance offered by the spherules to attack by the recruited neutrophils and macrophages. Cell-mediated immunity and T-cell response are important host defense mechanisms for killing the pathogen. Giant cell formation is mainly to attack the spherules. Patients with impaired cell-mediated immunity have more severe disseminated disease. Antigen overload and formation of immune complexes may impair cell-mediated immune responses.

PREDISPOSING FACTORS

The conditions that predispose to progressive disease include the following:
- Human immunodeficiency virus (HIV)
- Immunosuppressants and corticosteroids use
- Pregnancy
- Old age
- Certain ethnicities, including Filipinos, African Americans, Hispanics, and Asians.

CLINICAL FEATURES

The incubation period for the disease is 1–3 weeks. Most patients are asymptomatic. About 30–40% patients develop symptoms ranging from a flu-like illness to community-acquired pneumonia. It is important to take a detailed exposure history of travel or residence in an endemic area. Exposure can be as short as a car drive or a transit flight or it can be a significant dust exposure during construction, farming, or archaeological dig. Patient is suspected to be suffering from coccidioidomycosis in the case of fever with respiratory symptoms and a lower limb rash (erythema nodosum or erythema multiforme).

"San Joaquin Valley fever" or "desert rheumatism" refers to a constellation of symptoms, including fever, chest pain, arthralgias, erythema nodosum, or erythema multiforme.

Primary Coccidioidomycosis

Majority of the patients are asymptomatic. Others may present with flu-like symptoms, community-acquired pneumonia, bronchitis, or pleural effusion. The symptoms include fever, chills, cough, expectoration, hemoptysis, dyspnea, and pleuritic chest pain. Physical signs can be minimal and include rales, rhonchi, bronchial breath sounds, diminished breath sounds, or a dull/stony dull note on percussion. Respiratory failure is rare. A hypersensitivity response to the pulmonary involvement may manifest as erythema nodosum, erythema multiforme, or reactive arthritis.

Nodular involvement of the lung may resemble tumors, tuberculosis, or other granulomatous lesions. The nodules can either resolve or degenerate into thin-walled cavities. These may rupture causing hemoptysis or pneumothorax.

Progressive Coccidioidomycosis

Symptoms develop and persist for few weeks to few years and are nonspecific in nature. These include low-grade fever, anorexia, malaise, night sweats, urticaria, and weight loss. Progression of pulmonary disease results in increasing dyspnea and cough with mucopurulent phlegm. Chronic fibrosis may ensue. Extrapulmonary involvement includes draining sinuses, arthritis, osteomyelitis, and meningitis. A hepatopulmonary syndrome due to coccidioidomycosis is a combination of hepatitis due to hepatic granulomas and pneumonitis.

Skin involvement is a hypersensitivity reaction. It begins as urticaria or diffuse maculopapular rash. This progresses to erythema nodosum or erythema multiforme. The latter is more common in children. Erythema nodosum develops on the skin as 1–2 cm, tender and erythematous nodules. Erythema multiforme presents as symmetric, erythematous macules, or papules that change to target lesions. Differential diagnoses include streptococcal infection, tuberculosis, sarcoidosis, histoplasmosis, and drug hypersensitivity reaction. Ocular involvement as a hypersensitivity response includes scleritis, episcleritis, and phlyctenular conjunctivitis. Hypersensitivity manifestations indicate a good cell-mediated immune response.

Cutaneous infectious involvement due to coccidioidomycosis needs to be distinguished from hypersensitivity since the fungus can be isolated from an infected site. It is as a consequence of hematogenous spread or direct inoculation. Patients develop granulomatous papule or nodules on the head, which ulcerate or form abscesses/draining sinuses. Complications include osteomyelitis and associated coccidioidal meningitis. Cervical lymphadenopathy is secondary to pulmonary involvement. Some patients may develop generalized lymphadenopathy.

Musculoskeletal involvement due to hematogenous dissemination includes monoarticular arthritis, tenosynovitis, and lytic/sclerotic bone lesions. Arthritis predominantly involves the large joints and can be migratory in nature. An exudative effusion may develop. Osteomyelitis can involve the long bones, skull, vertebrae, hands, and feet. Draining sinus or fistulae may form in patients with chronic osteomyelitis. Paraspinal abscess formation can lead to cord compression.

Other systemic manifestations include pericardial effusion, myocarditis, peritonitis, obstructive jaundice, thyroiditis, prostatitis, pyelonephritis, or a lacrimal gland mass.

Central nervous system (CNS) involvement occurs in half of the patients with disseminated disease. It is an insidious onset, chronic granulomatous meningitis with basilar involvement, abscesses, and/or hydrocephalus.

Fungemia and septicemic shock develops in immunocompromised hosts. Disseminated coccidioidomycosis and meningitis may prove fatal if untreated. Mortality rates are higher in HIV-positive patients.

DIFFERENTIAL DIAGNOSES

- Histoplasmosis
- Paracoccidioidomycosis
- Blastomycosis
- Tuberculosis
- *Mycoplasma pneumoniae* infection
- Sarcoidosis
- Babesiosis
- *Pneumocystis jiroveci* pneumonia
- Wegener granulomatosis
- Viral pneumonia
- Malignancy
- Lymphoma
- Pulmonary infarct
- Bullae and pneumatoceles.

DIAGNOSIS

Laboratory Studies

- Microscopic examination of specimens, including sputum, cerebrospinal fluid (CSF), pleural fluid, bronchoalveolar lavage (BAL), pus from draining sinuses, or biopsy specimens by Gomori methenamine silver stain, periodic acid-Schiff, calcofluor white, or hematoxylin & eosin stain for the presence of spherules and endospores of *C. immitis*. Spherules are 20–80 μm in diameter, thick walled, and filled inside with 2–4-μm endospores. The ruptured spherules may release endospores into the tissues.
- Fungal culture for *C. immitis* is a biohazard, and laboratory workers must be warned about the suspected diagnosis. Culture is performed in a biosafety level-3 laboratory. Growth

appears on fungal media in 3–5 days as white or cottony colonies Anthroconidia can be present. Nucleic acid probes confirm the identity of the pathogen.

- Serological tests include detection of *C. immitis* antibodies by:
    - Enzyme immunoassay: Most commonly used technique as a screening test. Titers ≥1:4 indicate recent infection. Higher titers are seen in disseminated disease. Highly sensitive but lacks specificity, and results need to be verified by immunodiffusion tube precipitin.
    - Immunodiffusion tube precipitin techniques for IgM antibodies are more specific but require longer time to perform than enzyme immunoassay.
    - Complement fixation for IgG antibodies: These are positive in 90% of patients by 3 months after the onset of infection and persist for 6 months. Higher titers indicate more severe disease. Meningitis is diagnosed by the presence of complement-fixing antibodies in CSF.
    IgM quantification has no clinical significance, whereas higher IgG levels indicate progression and dissemination of disease. IgG titers are low during successful therapy or in immunosuppressed patients. Response to therapy is monitored by measuring coccidioidal complement fixation titers in serum or CSF.
- Urine antigen test for *C. immitis* is positive in disseminated extrapulmonary disease and in immunocompromised patients with HIV or single organ transplant (SOT).
- *Polymerase chain reaction (PCR) test*: Polymerase chain reaction amplification and gene identification in serum for *C. immitis* and *C. posadasii* is highly sensitive and specific. It is safer and faster than the culture techniques.
- *Skin testing*: Hypersensitivity response to coccidioidin or spherulin antigen preparations, following an intradermal injection, is positive in all residents in endemic areas within 2–3 weeks of exposure. The induration (not erythema) is measured at 24 and 48 hours after the injection. An induration greater than 5 mm is considered positive. This test has epidemiological implications and is now obsolete.
- Eosinophilia can be present.

Imaging Studies

Chest radiography can be normal or show nonspecific changes, including unilateral infiltrates with ipsilateral lymphadenopathy, pulmonary cavities and nodules, parapneumonic effusion. Computed tomography, magnetic resonance imaging, and positron emission tomography scans are important for diagnosing extrapulmonary manifestations.

Diagnostic Procedures

- *Lumbar puncture*: It is performed if patient has fever, headache, obtundation, and nuchal rigidity. It may also be performed if complement fixation titers for IgG are significantly high. CSF examination reveals lymphocytic and eosinophilic pleocytosis, elevated protein levels, hypoglycorrhachia, and complement-fixing antibodies.
- *Bronchoscopy*: The procedure is performed in a patient with parenchymal infiltrates and cavitary lesions if the sputum examination is not diagnostic. It is more useful in establishing

diagnosis for endobronchial lesions. BAL, needle aspiration, and/or lung biopsy may be performed.

- *Biopsy*: Lung, pleura, lymph node, skin, or synovial biopsies may be obtained to establish diagnosis. Histological findings include the presence of spherules and endospores and granuloma formation.

TREATMENT

The antifungal drugs used for the treatment of coccidioidomycosis include amphotericin B, itraconazole, and fluconazole. There is a lack of consensus amongst treating physicians regarding which patient deserves to be treated, choice of antifungal and duration of treatment. Certain guiding principles have been published by the Infectious Diseases Society of America to assess the severity of the illness and the risk of dissemination (Boxes 22.1 and 22.2).

Choice of Antifungals

Amphotericin B deoxycholate (AmBd) [0.5–1 mg/kg/day intravenous (IV)] or liposomal amphotericin B (LAmB) (3–5 mg/kg/day IV) is used for the treatment of severe

---

Box 22.1: Indicators for severe coccidioidomycosis

- >10% loss of body weight
- Continuous fever for >1 month
- Night sweats for >3 weeks
- Pulmonary infiltrates involving more than half of one lung or portions of both lungs
- Prominent or persistent hilar lymphadenopathy
- Anticoccidioidal complement fixation immunoglobulin G (IgG) titers of 1:16 or higher
- Inability to work
- Symptoms persisting for >2 months

Box 22.2: Risk factors for dissemination of coccidioidomycosis

- Immunosuppressed patients—HIV, SOT recipients, high-dose glucocorticoid use (≥20-mg prednisone or its equivalent per day), antitumor necrosis factor therapy, chemotherapy
- Lymphoma
- Pregnancy especially when disease develops in the third trimester
- Diabetes mellitus with pulmonary cavitation
- Pre-existing cardiopulmonary conditions
- Elderly, frail patients
- Africans, Filipinos, and Hispanics
- Thymectomy
- HIV: human immunodeficiency virus; SOT: solid-organ transplant.

coccidioidomycosis, worsening disease, CNS or spinal involvement, or in a pregnant patient since azoles are contraindicated in pregnancy.

Azoles are the first line of therapy and also used as step-down therapy. Itraconazole (200 mg twice or thrice daily) and fluconazole (400–800 mg/day) are the agents recommended. Ketoconazole is no longer used. There is no comparative data of amphotericin B versus azoles in the treatment of coccidioidomycosis. Data regarding the use of voriconazole, posaconazole, and caspofungin is limited, and these agents have been tried in a few cases refractory to first-line therapy. Itraconazole is preferred for skeletal lesions, while fluconazole has better efficacy in pulmonary and soft tissue involvement. Therapeutic drug levels for itraconazle need to be monitored.

There is no consensus regarding duration of therapy, but it should be at least 6 months in all patients. Patients should be monitored every 2–4 weeks initially, and later on, every few months for systemic signs and serial serologic testing for complement-fixing anticoccidioidal antibodies. The antigen testing is used to confirm a response to treatment. It should not be used to determine timing of discontinuation of therapy. Patients may require continuation of therapy even after the titers become negative. Immunocompromised patients including HIV, SOT recipients, and patients with meningitis need lifelong therapy.

Pulmonary Coccidioidomycosis

There is no role of antifungal therapy in uncomplicated acute pulmonary coccidioidomycosis in healthy individuals. Most patients will have a spontaneous resolution of symptoms. Regular follow-up is required for 1 year to confirm complete recovery. Treatment is reserved for patients at high risk of dissemination and with high titers of complement fixation antibodies. Treatment with itraconazole or fluconazole causes early resolution of symptoms and reduces chances of hematogenous spread. Therapy should be continued for at least 6 months.

Patients with reticulonodular infiltrates or miliary involvement should be treated with AmBd or LAmB for few weeks. Alternatively, high-dose fluconazole may be used. Once the patients start showing clinical improvement, oral azoles may be used. Therapy must be continued for 1 year or longer.

Chronic progressive fibrocavitary pneumonia is treated with itraconazole 200 mg twice daily or fluconazole 400 mg/day continued for at least 1 year.

Asymptomatic nodules do not require treatment in immunocompetent patients and need follow-up for at least 2 years. The indications for therapy include an enlarging nodule and rising complement fixation antibody titers during serial follow-up. Surgical resection is recommended if there is a suspicion of the nodule being malignant.

Small thin-walled pulmonary cavities resolve spontaneously and may be left untreated. These need follow-up for at least 2 years. Azole therapy is recommended in case the cavities are producing symptoms, including chest pain, hemoptysis. Amphotericin B is used in patients requiring surgery.

Indications for surgery include:
- Cavities refractory to azole therapy
- Large or enlarging cavities >5 cm in diameter with impending rupture into pleural space
- Persistent or massive hemoptysis

- Empyema
- Hydropneumothorax
- Ruptured nodules
- Bronchopleural fistula closure.

  A video-assisted thoracoscopic surgery should be attempted.

Extrapulmonary Nonmeningeal Coccidioidomycosis

Severe infection is treated with AmBd 0.5–1 mg/kg/day IV over 4–12 weeks till a cumulative dose of 1–3 g is reached. LAmB is preferred due to lesser nephrotoxicity. Amphotericin B is continued till there is clinical, radiological, and complement fixation IgG titers improvement. Step-down therapy is with azoles. Mild-to-moderate disease is managed with itraconazole 200 mg twice daily or fluconazole 400 mg once daily. Therapy for HIV-positive patients is continued till CD4+ cell count is ≥250/μL.

Itraconazole is better than fluconazole in bone disease. Surgical management includes incision and drainage, synovectomy, drainage of sequestrum, debridement of wound, arthrodesis, and surgical stabilization of the spine.

Meningeal Coccidioidomycosis

Fluconazole is used 800–1,200 mg/day as lifelong therapy. It has excellent penetration in CSF. Alternatively, itraconazole may be used in a dose of 400–600 mg/day. Discontinuation of therapy results in relapse. Intrathecal amphotericin B may be administered in severe cases. Ventriculoperitoneal shunt is needed in the cases with hydrocephalus. Corticosteroids are used for CSF vasculitis associated with coccidioidomycosis.

▩ COMPLICATIONS

- *Prolonged fatigue*: Extreme lethargy may persist for many weeks or months after resolution of all other symptoms. There is no role of antifungals in improving the energy levels. Patient needs a structured physical rehabilitation program.
- Pulmonary complications include nodules, cavities, progressive fibrosis, hemoptysis, and pneumothorax.
- Extrapulmonary complications include involvement of CNS, skin, bone, and joints.

▩ CLINICAL PEARLS

- Coccidioidomycosis is caused by a dimorphic fungus (*C. immitis* or *C. posadasii*) due to inhalation of endospores.
- It is endemic to the southwestern United States and northern Mexico.
- Most patients are asymptomatic or have a subclinical illness.
- Hypersensitivity response includes symmetrical arthralgia, erythema nodosum, or erythema multiforme.

- Serologic testing is diagnostic.
- Patients with severe, CNS, or disseminated disease require treatment with azoles or amphotericin B.

SUGGESTED READING

1. Crum NF, Lederman ER, Stafford CM, et al. Coccidioidomycosis: a descriptive survey of a reemerging disease. Clinical characteristics and current controversies. Medicine (Baltimore). 2004;83:149.

2. Galgiani JN, Ampel NM, Blair JE, et al. 2016 Infectious Diseases Society of America (IDSA) clinical practice guideline for the treatment of coccidioidomycosis. Clin Infect Dis. 2016;63:e112.

3. Galgiani JN, Catanzaro A, Cloud GA, et al. Comparison of oral fluconazole and itraconazole for progressive, nonmeningeal coccidioidomycosis. A randomized, double-blind trial. Mycoses Study Group. Ann Intern Med. 2000;133:676.

4. Litvintseva AP, Marsden-Haug N, Hurst S, et al. Valley fever: finding new places for an old disease: *Coccidioides immitis* found in Washington State soil associated with recent human infection. Clin Infect Dis. 2015;60:e1.

5. Saubolle MA, McKellar PP, Sussland D. Epidemiologic, clinical, and diagnostic aspects of coccidioidomycosis. J Clin Microbiol. 2007;45:26.

6. Singh VR, Smith DK, Lawerence J, et al. Coccidioidomycosis in patients infected with human immunodeficiency virus: review of 91 cases at a single institution. Clin Infect Dis. 1996;23:563.

7. Stevens DA, Clemons KV, Levine HB, et al. Expert opinion: what to do when there is *Coccidioides* exposure in a laboratory. Clin Infect Dis. 2009;49:919.

23

Paracoccidioidomycosis

Monica Mahajan

■ INTRODUCTION

Paracoccidioidomycosis is a progressive systemic mycosis of the lungs, skin, mucous membranes, and lymph nodes caused by dimorphic fungi of the genus *Paracoccidioides*. It is also known as South American blastomycosis and Lutz's mycosis. Adolfo Lutz discovered the mycosis in Brazil in 1908. This endemic fungus is limited to coffee growers of Colombia, Argentina, Venezuela, and Brazil but has a high incapacitating potential. It is caused by two distinct species: *Paracoccidioides brasiliensis* and *Paracoccidioides lutzii*. Treatment is with azoles, amphotericin B, or sulfonamides.

■ ETIOLOGY

The genus *Paracoccidioides* belongs to phylum Ascomycota and family Ajellomycetaceae. This is the same as *Histoplasma capsulatum*, *Blastomyces dermatitidis*, *Coccidioides immitis*, and *Coccidioides posadasii*. These are all thermally dimorphic fungi, produce arthroconidia, and are endemic in a geographically restricted habitat.

Paracoccidioides brasiliensis* and *P. lutzii* are thermally dimorphic fungi. These lack a sexual stage or teleomorph. The fungi exist as filamentous mycelial form with septate hyphae with occasional chlamydospores and conidia at 25°C and as an oval or round budding yeast-like form at 37°C. At body temperature (37°C), the colonies are white or cream in color and have a variable texture. The spherical cells produce pyriform microconidia by synchronous budding. This produces the characteristic *steering wheels* or *pilot's wheel* appearance.

At 25°C, the mycelial form produces white to brownish colonies. Conidia are usually absent. Intercalary chlamydospore cells might be present. If present, conidia are barrel shaped.

Paracoccidioides brasiliensis* is a complex of four cryptic species, whereas *P. lutzii* appears to be a single species. Sequencing of the internal transcribed spacer (ITS) fragment is the best technique for species identification.

■ EPIDEMIOLOGY

Paracoccidioidomycosis is restricted to certain areas of Central and South America. Countries where it has been diagnosed include Brazil, Argentina, Colombia, Uruguay, Peru, Ecuador, and Venezuela. In endemic areas, 50–75% of adult population may be infected. Brazil has the highest annual incidence estimated in 1–3 cases/10,000 inhabitants.

The disease is much more frequent in males, with a male:female ratio of ~20:1. In the chronic form, it is most prevalent between 30 and 60 years of age. Estradiol can be protective in adult females. The high male preponderance is not seen in the juvenile/prepubescent form of the disease. Smoking and alcoholism seem to be risk factors.

Although the disease is noted to occur mostly in humans, cases have been reported in nine-banded armadillos, Brazilian guinea pigs, spiny tree porcupine, ferrets, and dogs. Certain ecological features that favor paracoccidioidomycosis include tropical forests, heavy rainfall, rivers, mild temperature, and coffee and tobacco plantations. Use of plant pesticides, fungicides and plant burning are reducing the incidence of the disease in certain regions.

PATHOGENESIS

The fungus is a soil saprophyte. Farmers get exposed to the fungus in the soil primarily while working in coffee, cotton, and tobacco fields. Following inhalation of the conidia, the fungus is targeted by the neutrophils and macrophages as host defense mechanisms. The T helper (Th) 1 response helps to curtail the fungal infection, whereas Th 2 cell response increases the host susceptibility to the disease. The initial response is a granuloma formation at the primary site. The fungus may remain dormant at a metastatic site for many years and then activate to result in chronic form of the disease and its sequelae. In some cases, there can be no gap between the primary focus and progression of the disease, resulting in acute/subacute manifestations. Although cell-mediated immunity plays a major role in host defense, the prevalence of disease amongst solid-organ transplant recipients, hematological malignancies, or human immunodeficiency virus (HIV) is not majorly increased.

CLINICAL FEATURES

Majority of the patients will have asymptomatic pulmonary infection with positive intradermal paracoccidioidin skin testing. The acute/subacute form manifests within 45 days of inhalation of conidia. The chronic form represents reactivation of the disease and occurs over months or years.

Acute/Subacute Juvenile Paracoccidioidomycosis

It is observed in children, adolescents, and young adults below 30 years of age. Unlike the chronic form, males and females are equally affected. It represents fewer than 10% of the cases. Patients present with fever, weight loss, malaise, and abdominal pain. Involvement of the reticuloendothelial system causes hepatosplenomegaly, lymphadenopathy, and bone marrow involvement.

Superficial lymphadenopathy involves the cervical, axillary, or inguinal lymph nodes. These may develop suppuration, sinus tracts, and draining fistulae. Abdominal lymphadenopathy manifests as pain in abdomen, obstructive jaundice, or intestinal obstruction or abdominal masses. Patients may have multiple papular or acneiform skin lesions with sinus tracts. However, pulmonary and mucous membrane involvements are unusual. Bone marrow involvement results in anemia/aplastic anemia. The sequelae of the infection are few and include malabsorption due to fibrosis of mesenteric and peritoneal lymph nodes.

Adult Paracoccidioidomycosis

Chronic form of paracoccidioidomycosis is seen in adults, represents reactivation of disease, and can be unifocal or multifocal. About 90% of the cases of paracoccidioidomycosis are chronic and develop months or years after exposure to the fungus. Males between the ages of 30 and 60 years are predominantly involved since this is the age group involved in agrarian activities. The fungus disseminates by the hematogenous or lymphatic route to any organ of the body. The lungs are the organ most frequently involved. The spectrum of illness may range from mild upper respiratory symptoms to fatal disease. Patients present with cough, expectoration, dyspnea, fever, weight loss, and occasional hemoptysis. Some patients may develop extensive pulmonary fibrosis with little pulmonary symptoms. Mucosal involvement of the oral cavity, especially the lower lips and the gums, is in the form of painful ulcers with microgranules and hemorrhagic dots classically called *moriform stomatitis of Aguiar Pupo* or mulberry stomatitis. Face and nasal mucosa involvement presents as slowly expanding ulcers with a granular base. Genital and ocular lesions may also develop. Regional lymph nodes may be enlarged and necrotic. Patients may complain of hoarseness and odynophagia. Skin lesions are caused by hematological dissemination from the lungs or rarely from direct inoculation. The lesions can be papular, nodular, ulcerated, papillomatous, tuberous, verrucous, or plaque like. Lytic lesions in the bones are more frequent in the ribs, humeri, and clavicles. Central nervous system (CNS) involvement includes meningoencephalitis or spinal cord lesions. Intestinal involvement can be a consequence of mesenteric lymphadenopathy. Genital involvement may involve glans and scrotum or cause urethral obstruction. The sequelae of the infection include obstructive lung disease, emphysema, bullae, fibrosis, airway/tracheal stenosis, cor pulmonale, pulmonary hypertension, and adrenal insufficiency.

▦ DIFFERENTIAL DIAGNOSES

- Lymphoma
- Leukemia
- Tuberculosis
- Histoplasmosis
- Coccidioidomycosis
- Cat-scratch disease
- Infectious mononucleosis
- Cytomegalovirus infection
- Toxoplasmosis
- Syphilis
- Leprosy
- Leishmaniasis
- Wegener granulomatosis

- Sarcoidosis
- Systemic lupus erythematosus
- Idiopathic pulmonary fibrosis
- Carcinoma Lung

▓ DIAGNOSTIC APPROACH

Laboratory Workup

- Direct examination of wet mounts of sputum or aspirate from lesions/enlarged lymph nodes for microscopic visualization of paracoccidioidomycosis reveals large budding yeasts with pilot's wheel or mariner's wheel appearance. Sometimes the mother cell may have only two daughter cells attached appearing like "Mickey Mouse head."
- Culture of specimens for paracoccidioidomycosis is a biohazard, and the laboratory personnel need to be intimated about the provisional diagnosis. It may take 3–4 weeks for the growth of the mold form of the fungus on Sabouraud dextrose agar or yeast agar medium containing chloramphenicol at room temperature. The conversion to yeast form at 37°C confirms diagnosis.
- Serologic testing by double agar gel immunodiffusion: Antibody titers ≥ 1:32 are seen in patients with acute paracoccidioidomycosis. This is the most frequently used test for diagnosis and follow-up. Tests can be negative in *P. lutzii* infection. Counter-immunoelectrophoresis is also useful in diagnosis in endemic areas. There can be cross-reactivity with *H. capsulatum*. HIV-positive patients can be negative on serologic testing.
- Solid-phase immunoassays, including enzyme-linked immunosorbent assay, detect circulating antibodies to glycoprotein (gp) 43 with high sensitivity and specificity. Monoclonal antibodies to antigenic compounds of *P. brasiliensis* are being developed to increase sensitivity.
- Western blot test detects antibodies to gp43 and gp70.
- Polymerase chain reaction (PCR)-based techniques and matrix-assisted laser desorption/ ionization–time-of-flight (MALDI-TOF) are experimental.
- Laboratory investigations reveal anemia, eosinophilia, deranged liver function test with hypoalbuminemia, hypergammaglobulinemia, and raised transaminases.
- Adrenal functions, including serum cortisol levels and response to exogenous 8-adrenocorticotropic (ACTH) hormone injection, are checked for adrenal insufficiency.
- Bone marrow examination helps to evaluate for bone marrow infiltration, aplastic anemia, and to rule out lymphoma.
- Paracoccidioidin skin test is a useful tool for epidemiological studies.

Imaging Studies

Conventional X-rays, ultrasonography, and computed tomography demonstrate mediastinal and abdominal lymphadenopathy. They may also reveal possible compression or obstruction due to lymphadenopathy. Chest images may show nodular, interstitial, or diffuse lung infiltrates; masses; cavities; septal or interlobular thickening; centrilobular or paraseptal emphysema; or lung fibrosis. Reversed halo sign may be present. These also help to rule out other diagnosis, including tuberculosis, lymphoma, and malignancy. Gallium-67 scan is useful for imaging of bony lesions. Imaging of other organs, including brain, adrenals, and joints, depends on the symptoms of the patient. CNS scans reveal ring-enhancing lesions, meningoencephalitis, or hydrocephalus. Joint effusion, reduction in joint space, and bony erosions can be present.

Histopathology

Biopsy specimens show mixed granulomas (epithelioid and suppurative). There are large yeasts with pilot wheel appearance of budding daughter cells within the giant cells or free in the inflammatory infiltrate. Lymph nodes may show caseous necrosis similar to tubercular lymph nodes.

Pulmonary Function Test

These may reveal an obstructive pattern.

▨ TREATMENT (TABLE 23.1)

Azoles are highly effective, and itraconazole is the drug of choice. Fluconazole is not as effective as itraconazole but has the advantage of being available as a parenteral preparation. Few randomized controlled trials have evaluated the role of voriconazole.

Amphotericin B use is reserved for severe cases or in pregnant patients. Liposomal amphotericin B is less nephrotoxic than amphotericin B deoxycholate (AmBd).

Sulfonamides suppress growth of the fungus and cause regression of lesions when used continuously for up to 2–5 years but may not be curative. Trimethoprim–sulfamethoxazole (TMP–SMX) or sulfadiazine is used because of the low cost of treatment. Side effects include nausea, vomiting, rash, and Stevens-Johnson syndrome.

Patients on itraconazle therapy may develop hepatotoxicity, hypokalemia, or rarely heart failure. The capsule formulation is better absorbed in an acidic gastric pH when administered concomitantly with food. Suspension works better on an empty stomach. Dose used is 100 mg twice daily.

Patients who are HIV positive may have an overlap of acute and chronic features and a more rapid progression of the disease. Use of TMP–SMX for *Pneumocystis jiroveci* prophylaxis and azoles for oropharyngeal candidiasis in patients with HIV is likely to reduce the incidence of paracoccidioidomycosis. Moreover, acquired immunodeficiency syndrome is predominantly an urban disease, whereas paracoccidioidomycosis is more rampant in rural areas.

Surgery has a role in reconstruction, cord compression, or hydrocephalus. Supportive treatment includes correction of anemia and advising patients to quit smoking and alcohol. No vaccine is available against paracoccidioidomycosis.

Relapses occur within 3 years and are because of sustained alcohol abuse or because of incomplete/irregular treatment. Paradoxical reaction may be considered in patients who remain symptomatic despite therapy. Re-evaluation must be performed once a month for the first 3 months and subsequently once every quarter.

Table 23.1: Treatment of paracoccidioidomycosis		
Disease severity	*Drug*	*Dose*
Mild to moderate	Itraconazole capsule Itraconazole solution	100 mg once or twice daily 5 mg/kg once daily
Mild to moderate	TMP/SMX	10 mg/kg of trimethoprim component in two divided doses
Severe	LAmB AmBd	3–5 mg/kg/day IV 0.7–1 mg/kg/day IV
Severe	TMP–SMX IV	10 mg/kg TMP IV in three divided doses

AmBd, amphotericin B deoxycholate; IV, intravenous; LAmB, liposomal amphotericin B; TMP–SMX, trimethoprim–sulfamethoxazole

For CNS disease, AmBd or intravenous TMP-SMX may be used. The exact duration of treatment for paracoccidioidomycosis is not well determined. Therapy is continued till complete clinical and radiological improvement and normalization of antibody titers (Table 23.1).

CLINICAL PEARLS

- Paracoccidioidomycosis is a systemic endemic disease limited to Central and South America.
- The thermally dimorphic fungus may cause acute juvenile or chronic form of the disease.
- Itraconazole 100–200 mg/day is the drug of choice.
- Amphotericin B deoxycholate is used for severe disease or in pregnancy.
- Sulfonamides are an alternative but require longer duration of therapy.

SUGGESTED READING

1. Almeida FA, Neves FF, Mora DJ, et al. Paracoccidioidomycosis in Brazilian Patients with and without human immunodeficiency virus infection. Am J Trop Med Hyg. 2017;96:368.
2. Bellissimo-Rodrigues F, Machado AA, Martinez R. Paracoccidioidomycosis epidemiological features of a 1,000-case series from a hyperendemic area on the southeast of Brazil. Am J Trop Med Hyg. 2011;85:546.
3. Menezes VM, Soares BG, Fontes CJ. Drugs for treating paracoccidioidomycosis. Cochrane Database Syst Rev. 2006:CD004967.
4. Peçanha PM, de Souza S, Falqueto A, et al. Amphotericin B lipid complex in the treatment of severe paracoccidioidomycosis: a case series. Int J Antimicrob Agents. 2016;48:428.
5. Queiroz-Telles F, Goldani LZ, Schlamm HT, et al. An open-label comparative pilot study of oral voriconazole and itraconazole for long-term treatment of paracoccidioidomycosis. Clin Infect Dis. 2007;45:1462.
6. Travassos LR, Taborda CP, Colombo AL. Treatment options for paracoccidioidomycosis and new strategies investigated. Expert Rev Anti Infect Ther. 2008;6:251.

24

Mycetoma

Monica Mahajan

INTRODUCTION

Mycetoma is defined as a localized, suppurative, deforming granulomatous infection characterized by a painless yet progressively debilitating soft tissue swelling, underlying sinus tracts, and production of grains/granules. It is caused by a number of bacteria and fungi. Low-income agrarian populations in the tropical countries are primarily affected by the disease.

Mycetoma caused by bacteria is called actinomycetoma, whereas mycetoma caused by fungi is called eumycetoma. A definite microbiological and histopathological diagnosis is a must since the treatment of the two entities is entirely different. Actinomycetoma is treated with the prolonged use of antibiotics. Eumycetoma requires surgical management, followed by antifungal therapy.

HISTORICAL BACKGROUND

Atharva Veda makes reference to *padavalmikam* meaning "anthill." Gill described mycetoma in 1842 in the Indian province of Madura. This lead to the initial name *Madura foot*. The term mycetoma was proposed by Carter. It literally means "a fungal tumor." Chalmers and Archibald divided mycetomas into two groups.
1. *Group 1*: Maduramycosis—caused by true fungi
2. *Group 2*: Actinomycosis—caused by *Actinomyces* (bacteria).

ETIOLOGY

The fungi and bacteria that cause mycetoma are saprophytic in nature. The different species produce grains of different color.

EPIDEMIOLOGY

Mycetoma occurs worldwide. It is endemic in tropical and subtropical regions collectively called the "mycetoma belt" lying between 15°S and 30°N. The countries within this belt include Sudan, Somalia, Senegal, India, Yemen, Mexico, Venezuela, Columbia, and Argentina. The maximum cases are reported from Sudan.

The etiological agent varies from country to country. The pathogen most frequently causing eumycetoma is *Madurella mycetomatis*. The etiological agents responsible for infection in the drier regions include *Actinomadura madurae*, *M. mycetomatis*, and *Streptomyces somaliensis*.

Pathogens implicated in the rainy areas include *Pseudallescheria boydii*, *Nocardia species*, and *Actinomadura pelletieri*.

In India, the most common pathogens responsible for mycetoma are *Nocardia* and *Madurella grisea*.

Eumycetoma is more prevalent in areas where rainfall is scarce, whereas actinomycetoma is more common in areas with abundant rainfall.

The incidence is higher in males since they are frequently involved in agricultural activities. The incidence is lower in children and old age.

PATHOGENESIS

Host Factors

In tropical regions, agricultural workers tend to work barefoot. The pathogens enter through pre-existing abrasions or through a penetrating injury. Predisposing factors include malnutrition and diabetes.

The fungal and bacterial pathogens induce complement-dependent chemotaxis of polymorphs.

The host reaction to mycetoma may have three distinct patterns:

1. *Type I*: A typical granuloma formation with grain in the center, a layer of polymorphs invading the grain and surrounded by plasma cells, macrophages, and lymphocytes with an outermost layer of fibrosis.
2. *Type II*: The macrophages and multinucleated giant cells may replace the neutrophils. Fragments of broken-down grains can be visible within the giant cells.
3. *Type III*: There are organized epithelioid granulomas with Langerhans giant cells. No grains are visible.

Pathogen Virulence Factors

The pathogens have a variety of adaptation mechanisms to evade the immune attack. Cell wall thickening and melanin production are some of the escape mechanisms.

Human-to-human or animal-to-human transmission has not been described for eumycetoma. Nosocomial transmission of *Nocardia farcinica* has been reported.

CLINICAL FEATURES

Mycetoma is a chronic, progressive granulomatous disease with an inflammatory response. Repetitive skin trauma and exposure to bacteria or fungi in the soil will result in the infection. However, majority of patients do not remember the preceding trauma since there is a long incubation period of months or years.

Eumycetomas occur primarily on the extremities with 70% of the patients having foot involvement. The dorsal aspect of the forefoot is typically involved. Actinomycetomas are seen more frequently on the chest, abdomen, and head. The clinical triad of mycetoma comprises:

- Painless, firm, subcutaneous mass
- Multiple sinus formation
- A purulent or seropurulent discharge containing sand-like particles called "grains." The grains are of different colors, sizes, and consistency depending on the etiological pathogen.

The lesion starts as a small, painless, subcutaneous nodule that slowly progresses over time. It softens and ulcerates to form draining sinuses with a serosanguineous or purulent discharge containing grains. At any given point of time, there will be both active and old healed sinuses visible. The overlying skin is fixed to the underlying tissues, hypo- or hyperpigmented and may demonstrate hyperhidrosis. Over the course of years, mycetoma progresses from small nodules to large, bone-invasive lesions. The gradually worsening swelling, induration, fibrosis, sinus formation, and involvement of muscle and bone lead to disfigurement and deformity. Involvement of nerves and tendons is a late feature. The condition becomes painful when osteomyelitis appears. Actinomycetomas are characterized by both osteolytic and osteosclerotic lesions, whereas eumycetomas tend to have punched-out lytic lesions. Actinomycetoma is more rapidly progressive. Lymphatic spread leads to lymphadenopathy, and the lymph nodes may suppurate. Nodal involvement is more frequent in actinomycetoma. There may be superadded bacterial infection (Fig. 24.1 and Table 24.1).

Late presentation and diagnosis is a norm due to painless nature of the disease, low socioeconomic standards, lack of health education, and scarce healthcare facilities in the endemic areas. In 2016, the World Health Organization added mycetoma to the list of 18 priority neglected tropical disease.

COMPLICATIONS

- Disfigurement/Deformity
- Abscess
- Cellulitis
- Ankylosis
- Bacterial superinfection/osteomyelitis
- May be potentially fatal in the late stages.

DIFFERENTIAL DIAGNOSIS

- Bacterial osteomyelitis
- Tuberculosis
- Nontuberculous mycobacterial infection [mycobacteria other than tuberculosis (MOTT)]
- Actinomycosis
- Chromoblastomycosis
- Blastomycosis
- Sporotrichosis
- Aspergillosis
- Pseudomycetomas due to dermatophytes
- Botryomycosis

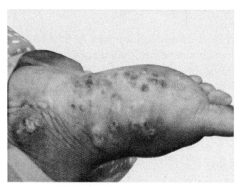

Fig. 24.1: Mycetoma with multiple discharging sinuses.

Table 24.1: Grains produced by different agents causing mycetoma.	
Grain color	*Agent causing mycetoma*
	Eumycetoma
Black to brown	*Madurella mycetomatis*
Black to brown	*Madurella grisea*
Black	*Leptosphaeria senegalensis*
Black	*Curvularia lunata*
Yellow	*Neotestidina rosatii*
White to yellow	*Acremonium* spp.
White to pale yellow	*Fusarium* spp.
White to pale yellow	*Scedosporium apiospermum*
	Actinomycetoma
White	*Nocardia asteroides*
White	*Nocardia brasiliensis*
White	*Nocardia otitidiscaviarum*
Pale white/Yellow	*Actinomadura madurae*
Red to pink	*Actinomadura pelletieri*
White to yellow/Brown	*Streptomyces somaliensis*

- Mossy foot/Podoconiosis
- Sarcoma including Kaposi sarcoma.

DIAGNOSIS

Laboratory Diagnosis

It is very important to establish the correct etiological diagnosis of mycetoma and distinguish actinomycetoma from eumycetoma. Different diagnostic tools have been developed to establish the identity of the causative organism.

Examination of Mycetoma Grains

Grains should be obtained by deep surgical biopsies or aspiration of grains directly from an unopened sinus tract. The grains obtained from the surface are nonviable and contaminated. Grains have different morphological features. The size of the grains varies from microscopic to 1–2 mm in diameter. The grains of *M. mycetomatis* and *A. madurae* are larger in size. The color of the grains may vary—black, white, red, pink, or yellow. Most eumycetoma pathogens produce black or pale grains. The actinomycetoma organisms produce yellow, white, or red grains. Most species produce soft grains. *M. mycetomatis* and *S. somaliensis* are exceptions as grains are quite hard.

Direct Microscopy of Grains

A 10% potassium hydroxide (KOH) mount is made, which digests the mucus and keratin. It can rule out actinomycotic bacteria, but other tests are required to reach a definite diagnosis. Parker ink is used to examine the crushed grains under the light microscope for hyphae and spores. These usually appear dark blue against a light blue cellular background. Actinomycetes show branching filaments with aerial mycelia and chains of spores.

On Gram stain, actinomycetoma organisms are gram-positive, fine, branching filaments that are 1-μm thick. The eumycetoma pathogens are gram-negative, septate hyphae which are 4–5-μm thick. On Ziehl–Neelsen (ZN) stain, *Nocradia* is ZN positive, while *A. madurae* and *S. somaliensis* are ZN negative.

Culture of Grains

Several grains are soaked and stored in saline for culture, washed with saline and inoculated onto a suitable culture media. Modified Sabouraud agar is supplemented with 0.5% yeast extract, blood agar, and brain–heart infusion agar. Kimmig's agar is the other commonly used medium. Culture media recommended for actinomycetes include Lowenstein–Jensen media, thioglycollate broth, Columbia agar, and brain–heart infusion agar. Actinomycetes require a culture media which is antibiotic-free, while fungi need a culture media containing antibiotics, such as gentamycin, streptomycin, penicillin G, or chloramphenicol. Morphological features of pathogens causing mycetoma vary. *Madurella* produces fruiting bodies. *Streptomyces* lacks aerial hyphae and forms a yellowish substrate mycelium. *Nocardia* produces both substrate hyphae and aerial hyphae that appear as rods and coccoid structures. The phenotypic characteristics are different for various causative pathogens and include degradation of adenine, casein, and hypoxanthine; production of β-glucuronidase; growth on adonitol; aesculin hydrolysis, L-aspartic acid, etc.

The culture of these organisms is time-consuming and may take up to 4–6 weeks. The first growth of colonies may not be visible before 10–15 days of cultivating. The samples may grow contaminants.

Fine-needle Aspiration Cytology

Fine-needle aspiration cytology (FNAC) performed under aseptic conditions is examined for suppurative granulomas surrounding the characteristic grains of a causative organism. Various stains including hematoxylin and eosin (H&E), Giemsa, Papanicolaou, and periodic acid–Schiff (PAS) stains are used. The technique is inexpensive and rapid and helps in establishing an early diagnosis.

The core of the granuloma is the grains with a neutrophilic infiltrate. This is surrounded by palisading histiocytes. The outer region of the granuloma is a mixed inflammatory infiltrate comprising lymphocytes, macrophages, plasma cells, eosinophils, and a fibrotic reaction. Multinucleated giant cells are present in the granuloma. The presence of grains is mandatory to establish a diagnosis.

When the smears are stained with H&E, the grains of actinomycetes are homogeneously eosinophilic. On Giemsa stain, the grains are homogeneously blue in the center, while the periphery has fine granules and radiating pink filaments.

The *M. mycetomatis* grains are of two types when smears are stained with H&E. The solid granular grains are more frequent and do not demonstrate septate hyphae since they are embedded in the hard, brown cement matrix. The vesicular type of grains are the swollen fungal cells that appear as vesicles.

The *A. pelletieri* grains are eosinophilic and semilunar in shape.

Surgical Biopsy

Trucut biopsies are fixed and stained for histopathological examination. Actinomycetes grains are stained with Gram and ZN stain. The fungal grains and hyphae are identified using H&E, PAS, and Grocott's methenamine silver. The fungi have broad, septate, or branching hyphae that can be hyaline or pigmented. The grain cement may or may not be visible. The cement contains melanin, proteins, lipids, and heavy metals.

Serodiagnosis

Various serodiagnostic tests have evolved over the years which include enzyme-linked immunosorbent assay (ELISA), immunoblots, immunodiffusion, counterimmunoelectrophoresis, and indirect hemagglutination assays. *Nocardia brasiliensis* is diagnosed by ELISA. *M. mycetomatis* tests include immunodiffusion assay and counterimmunoelectrophoresis using crude cytoplasmic antigens. Since the crude antigens are used, there is cross-reactivity. An ELISA was developed using pure antigens of *M. mycetomatis* but was unsuitable for diagnostic purposes since it also detected antibodies in healthy controls. An immunoblotting technique with high sensitivity and specificity is being used for *M. mycetomatis*. For *P. boydii* an immunodiffusion assay and an indirect hemagglutination assay are in use. All these techniques are time-consuming and show cross-reactivity since the antigens have not been purified.

Molecular Identification Methods

Polymerase chain reaction (PCR) with restriction endonuclease analysis of PCR products and mass spectrometry helps in accurate identification of causative pathogens for mycetoma. For eumycetomas, the molecular techniques are based on the identification of the internal transcribed spacer (ITS). The ITS regions are amplified with panfungal primers and sequenced. The resulting sequence is identified by data in the GenBank. A PCR-restriction fragment length polymorphism has been used for identifying *M. mycetomatis*. Other techniques include restriction endonuclease analyses, random amplified polymorphic deoxyribonucleic acid, and amplification fragment length polymorphism.

Imaging Modalities

Ultrasound helps to distinguish mycetoma from other subcutaneous lesions. Eumycetomas produce single or multiple thick-walled cavities with grains causing distinct hyperreflective echoes. Actinomycetomas have similar findings except the grains are at the bottom of the cavities and produce much finer echoes.

Radiology helps in evaluating the extent of involvement. Routine X-rays may show cortical thinning, periosteal erosion, osteomyelitis, osteolysis, osteosclerosis, and disuse osteoporosis. Magnetic resonance imaging (MRI) is better than computed tomography at defining the soft tissue involvement. The characteristic finding on MRI is a "dot-in-circle sign." The tiny hypointense dots are the grains within a hyperintense spherical lesion. This is surrounded by low-intensity matrix T2-weighted image. These are the granulomas interspersed in the fibrosis areas (Figs. 24.2A to E).

■ TREATMENT

Debulking the bigger lesions is especially important in the management of eumycetomas. Establish the etiology before embarking on treatment.

Table 24.2: Differences between actinomycetoma and eumycetoma

Actinomycetoma	Eumycetoma
Caused by aerobic species of actinomycetes including *Nocardia, Actinomadura*, and *Streptomyces*	Caused by fungi
Prevalent in rainy areas	Prevalent in arid areas
More commonly involves chest, abdomen, and head	Foot involvement is more common
Rapid progression, more destruction	More circumscribed, slow progression, and less destruction
Lymph node involvement common	Lymph node involvement infrequent
Osteosclerotic and osteolytic bone lesions	Osteolytic bone lesions
Gram-positive, septate, thin branching filaments stained better by Gram stain	Gram-negative, wider, septate hyphae better stained with PAS and Gomori methenamine silver
Homogeneous eosinophilic material around the grain radiating in a star shape (Splendore-Hoeppli reaction)	Suppurative granulomas
Cultured on LJ, Columbia agar, and brain–heart infusion. Require a minimum of 10 days to grow	SDA or Kimmig's agar; requires 3–6 weeks to grow
Antibiotics for treatment	Surgery plus antifungals for treatment
LJ, Lowenstein–Jensen medium; PAS, periodic acid–Schiff; SDA, sabouraud dextrose agar.	

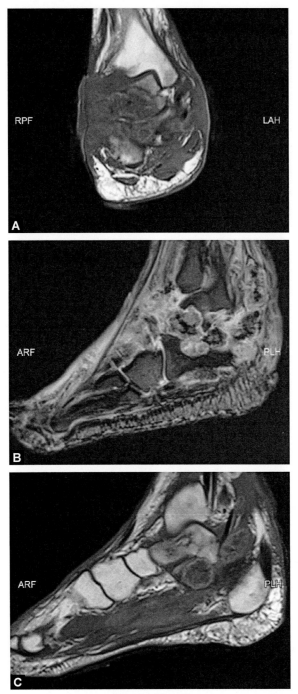

Figs. 24.2A to C

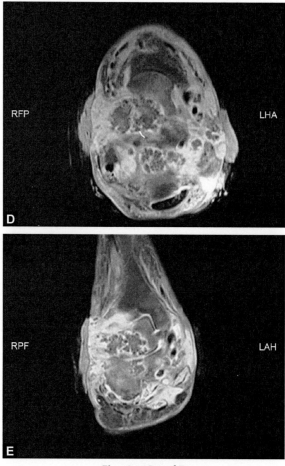

Figs. 24.2D and E

Figs. 24.2A to E: MRI foot scan. Coronal and sagittal T1-weighted PDFS and postcontrast images of ankle reveal extensive destruction of multiple bones with adjoining soft tissue thickening with contrast enhancement in a patient of eumycetoma caused by *M. mycetomatis*.

Treatment of Actinomycetoma

The various antibiotics used in the treatment of actinomycetomas include cotrimoxazole, dapsone, streptomycin, amikacin, netilmicin, trimethoprim (TMP), rifampicin, amoxycillin-clavulanic acid, ciprofloxacin, linezolid, and meropenem. Cotrimoxazole is the drug of choice. Combination therapy helps prevent resistance. Streptomycin may be used in combination with dapsone or TMP–sulfamethoxazole. The Welsh regimen uses amikacin as cyclical doses with a daily dose of cotrimoxazole. In modified Welsh regimen, rifampicin is added as the third drug. Various other combinations have been used. Amoxycillin–clavulanic acid can be used in pregnancy. Refractory cases are treated with carbapenems with amikacin.

Treatment of Eumycetoma

Eumycetomas are more difficult to treat, and a combination of surgery and medical management is required. Various azoles are used and prolonged treatment for years may be required. Itraconazole is generally used in a dose of 400 mg/day in two divided doses. Fluconazole is avoided because of intrinsic resistance. Voriconazole may be used at 400 mg/day in two divided doses. Posaconazole is highly active in vitro against *M. mycetomatis*. Liposomal amphotericin B and echinocandins lack efficacy in eumycetomas.

External beam radiotherapy has been tried successfully in a few selected cases.

Treatment is continued till the skin heals, the sinus and the mass disappear, and grains can no longer be demonstrated on FNAC. Radiological resolution of the lesions should be ascertained.

CLINICAL PEARLS

- It is important to establish etiological diagnosis of actinomycetoma or eumycetoma.
- Histopathology and culture of grains establish the diagnosis.
- Serological and molecular diagnostic tests are now available.
- Actinomycetoma should be treated with combination antibiotic therapy.
- Eumycetomas require surgical and medical management.

SUGGESTED READING

1. Al-Hatmi AM, Bonifaz A, Tirado-Sánchez A, et al. *Fusarium* species causing eumycetoma: report of two cases and comprehensive review of the literature. Mycoses. 2017;60:204.
2. Difonzo EM, Massi D, Vanzi L, et al. *Madurella mycetomatis* mycetoma treated successfully with oral posaconazole. J Chemother. 2011;23:243.
3. El Shamy ME, Fahal AH, Shakir MY, et al. New MRI grading system for the diagnosis and management of mycetoma. Trans R Soc Trop Med Hyg. 2012;106:738.
4. Hazra B, Bandyopadhyay S, Saha SK, et al. A study of mycetoma in eastern India. J Commun Dis. 1998;30:7.
5. Loulergue P, Hot A, Dannaoui E, et al. Successful treatment of black-grain mycetoma with voriconazole. Am J Trop Med Hyg. 2006;75:1106.
6. Smith EL, Kutbi S. Improvement of eumycetoma with itraconazole. J Am Acad Dermatol. 1997;36:279.
7. Troke P, Aguirrebengoa K, Arteaga C, et al. Treatment of scedosporiosis with voriconazole: clinical experience with 107 patients. Antimicrob Agents Chemother. 2008;52:1743.
8. van de Sande WW, de Kat J, Coppens J, et al. Melanin biosynthesis in *Madurella mycetomatis* and its effect on susceptibility to itraconazole and ketoconazole. Microbes Infect. 2007;9:1114.
9. van de Sande WW. Global burden of human mycetoma: a systematic review and meta-analysis. PLoS Negl Trop Dis. 2013;7:e2550.
10. Zijlstra EE, van de Sande WW, Welsh O, et al. Mycetoma: a unique neglected tropical disease. Lancet Infect Dis. 2016;16:100.

25

Penicilliosis/Talaromycosis

Monica Mahajan

INTRODUCTION

Penicillium marneffei was discovered in 1956 and is an important thermally dimorphic fungus. It has been now renamed *Talaromyces marneffei*. It causes a severe systemic fungal infection called penicilliosis or talaromycosis in human immunodeficiency virus (HIV) infected and immunocompromised individuals. The infection proves fatal if appropriate antifungals are not initiated early.

ETIOLOGY

Talaromyces marneffei belongs to the phylum *Ascomycota* and family *Trichocomaceae*. It is a dimorphic fungus that grows easily on Sabouraud dextrose agar (SDA). The growth is inhibited by cycloheximide. At 25°C, the fungus grows as a mold and produces granular colonies with greenish-yellow shades and a characteristic red pigment, which diffuses into the agar. The reverse side of the culture plate appears red. The mold form has hyaline septate hyphae and produce spherical conidia in chains. At 37°C the fungus grows as a yeast form and produces white to tan-colored colonies that lack the red pigment. These colonies may be convoluted or smooth. The yeast cells are oval to round with a central septum.

EPIDEMIOLOGY

Talaromyces marneffei was discovered in bamboo rats in Vietnam. Since the habitat of these rats is Southeast Asia, most of the cases are reported from these tropical/subtropical countries, including Thailand, Vietnam, Hong Kong, China, Taiwan, India, Indonesia, Cambodia, and Laos. However, with international travel patients may acquire infection in these locations but infection may be diagnosed anywhere in the world, including United States, Australia, and Europe. It is a common AIDS–defining illness observed in patients who have a CD4+ cell count <100 cells/mm^3. There has been a recent surge in the cases of penicilliosis in Manipur, especially in patients who are unaware of their HIV status, do not have access to antiretroviral therapy (ART), or have suboptimal response to HIV treatment. This infection is uncommon in immunocompetent individuals. The fungus may remain latent for many years or cause a subclinical infection.

Talaromyces marneffei has been isolated from the feces, liver, lungs, and spleen of these rats. It is not clear whether the rats are an asymptomatic reservoir for the fungus or are affected by the fungus. Humans may acquire the infection from eating infected rats or by inhaling aerosols from the soil containing *T. marneffei* conidia. The incidence increases in the rainy season in Thailand. Direct inoculation in the mycology laboratory can also cause a localized disease.

PATHOPHYSIOLOGY

Inhalation of microconidia results in primary disease. The spores may remain latent in the body for long periods, and there is reactivation of the disease when cellular immunity declines.

PREDISPOSING FACTORS

- Human immunodeficiency virus
- Immunological disorders
- Transplant recipients
- Use of steroids or cytotoxic drugs
- Hematological malignancies
- Diabetes
- Autoantibodies to interferon-gamma (INF-γ).

CLINICAL MANIFESTATIONS

Penicilliosis or talaromycosis occurs in immunocompromised patients with HIV, cancer, autoimmune disorders, or diabetes. The patients present with fever, anemia, weight loss, abdominal pain, diarrhea, dry cough, dyspnea, chest pain, and a skin rash. Patients with mild disease have only skin manifestations. The skin lesions are papular with a central umbilication due to necrosis and appear on the face, extremities, and genitalia. These are characteristic of the disease and need to be differentiated from molluscum contagiosum. Mucosal lesions are also noted in the oral cavity, pharynx, and gastrointestinal tract. Reticuloendothelial system involvement causes generalized lymphadenopathy and hepatosplenomegaly. Patients may have hepatomegaly with derangement of liver function test (LFT). Other organs involved due to hematogenous spread include the lungs, intestines, lymph node, bone marrow, and central nervous system (CNS). HIV-uninfected patients are more likely to have bone and joint involvement. Clinical features also include altered mental status, abdominal pain, diarrhea, arthritis and osteomyelitis, asthenia, anemia, and cachexia. Patients with severe disease may have circulatory or respiratory failure that may prove fatal.

DIFFERENTIAL DIAGNOSES

- Tuberculosis
- Melioidosis
- Histoplasmosis
- Cryptococcosis
- Aspergillosis.

DIAGNOSIS

Laboratory Diagnosis

- Wright's stain of peripheral blood smears, skin scrapings, lymph node biopsies, or bone marrow aspirates demonstrate the fungus as intracellular or extracellular basophilic, oval, elongated, or spherical yeasts with a clearly defined central septum or with hyaline, septate, and branched hyphae. The transverse central septum or crosswalls is a differentiating feature from *H. capsulatum* which lacks this. The conidiophores are located both terminally and laterally. Each conidiophore gives rise to 3–5 phialides where chains of lemon-shaped conidia are formed.
- Culture of the dimorphic fungus from blood, bone marrow, lymph nodes, urine, stool, cerebrospinal fluid, or skin biopsy provides a definitive diagnosis. The organism grows on culture media in 4–7 days. Bone marrow and lymph node biopsy cultures are more sensitive. The organism must be handled in a biosafety level-3 laboratory. The colonies on SDA are flat green with a diffusible, red pigmentation and have a filamentous reproductive morphology. Culture growth can be confirmed by mold-to-yeast conversion at 37°C, polymerase chain reaction hybridization assay, or an exoantigen test.
- Polymerase chain reaction amplification of specific nucleotide sequences is being developed.
- Anemia and deranged LFT are frequent findings with marked increase in alkaline phosphatase.
- Serologic tests including enzyme-linked immunosorbent assay and Western immunoblot are not freely available.
- Galactomannan testing for *Aspergillus* may show cross-reactivity with *T. marneffei* although the titers are lower in talaromycosis.

Imaging Studies

Chest X-ray findings include reticulonodular or alveolar infiltrates, cavitary or mass lesion. Ultrasound abdomen findings may include hepatomegaly, splenomegaly, appendicitis, peritonitis, or mesenteric lymphadenopathy.

Histopathology

The histopathology specimens are stained with Wright stain for the presence of *T. marneffei* in the bone marrow, skin, lymph node, and bronchoalveolar lavage. Methenamine silver or periodic acid-Schiff stains are better than hematoxylin and eosin in demonstrating unicellular oval, round, or elliptical yeast-like organisms within macrophages or histiocytes. Sausage-shaped or elongated cells with one or two septa are also seen extracellularly. Fine-needle aspiration cytology or biopsy from skin and lymph nodes are especially useful in establishing the diagnosis.

Liver biopsy specimens may show a diffuse infiltration with foamy macrophages containing the fungus, granulomas formation with inflammatory cell infiltration, or a mixed pattern.

TREATMENT

Delay or lack of initiation of treatment is associated with very high mortality in moderate-to-severe disease. All isolates are susceptible to 5-flucytosine, ketoconazole, itraconazole, voriconazole, and amphotericin B. Fluconazole is relatively inactive. Micafungin also shows efficacy against *Talaromyces marneffei* as part of combination therapy, but echinocandins should not be considered monotherapy. The treatment approach depends on the severity of the disease. Mild disease implies only a dermatological manifestation. Moderate disease includes multiple systems involvement. Severe disease implies circulatory collapse or respiratory failure.

Liposomal amphotericin B (LAmB) is administered at doses of 3–5 mg/kg/day intravenous (IV) for 2 weeks, followed by itraconazole 400 mg/day for 10 weeks. Subsequently the patient is put on secondary prophylaxis. Hydration of the patient prior to administering LAmB reduces nephrotoxicity. Monitor for electrolyte imbalance, infusion-related adverse reactions, and dose-dependent renal toxicity. Patients with CNS involvement should receive induction therapy with LAmB for 2 weeks, followed by itraconazole or voriconazole.

Milder disease may be treated with oral itraconazole 200 mg thrice daily for 3 days as loading dose, 400 mg/day for 8 weeks, followed by 200 mg/day as a preventive dose. Itraconazole solution is given empty stomach, whereas capsule is given with or after a meal. Serum itraconazole levels need to be monitored.

Voriconazole may be used as alternative therapy. It is used 6 mg/kg IV every 12 hours on the first day, followed by 4 mg/kg every 12 hours for 3 days. Subsequently, oral voriconazole is given 200 mg twice daily for a maximum of 12 weeks. For patients with milder disease, voriconazole is used at a dose of 400 mg 12 hourly on the first day, followed by 200 mg twice daily for 12 weeks. Therapeutic drug levels need to be monitored. Voriconazole is also used in patients with treatment failure when treated with LAmB and itraconazole.

Initiation of Antiretroviral Therapy

Antiretroviral therapy should be started as early as possible after initiation of antifungal therapy in patients with CD4+ count <50 cells/mm^3. In case the CD4+ count is more than 50 cells/mm^3, ART should be initiated 2 weeks after starting antifungal therapy for penicilliosis. Itraconazole and voriconazole can increase blood levels of protease inhibitors and nonnucleoside reverse-transcriptase inhibitors. Immune reconstitution inflammatory syndrome (IRIS) has been reported in HIV patients with penicilliosis.

Primary Prophylaxis

Primary prophylaxis is recommended in HIV-positive patients with CD4+ cell count <100 cells/mm^3 who reside in rural areas of northern Thailand, Vietnam, and southern China. Primary prophylaxis has not been recommended for residents of other areas. The drugs used for primary prophylaxis include itraconazole 200 mg/day or fluconazole 400 mg once weekly. Prophylaxis can be discontinued if the patient is on ART and has a CD4$^+$ count >100 cells/mm^3 for at least 6 months.

Secondary Prophylaxis

More than 50% patients of penicilliosis relapse within 6 months after discontinuation of antifungal therapy if they are not treated with ART. All patients who are successfully treated for penicilliosis should receive chronic maintenance therapy with itraconazole 200 mg/day and should be initiated on ART if indicated. Secondary prophylaxis can be discontinued in AIDS patients on ART who have a CD4+ cell count >100 cells/mm³ for at least 6 months. Secondary prophylaxis will need to be reintroduced if the CD4+ cell count falls to <100 cells/mm³.

Treatment during Pregnancy

Amphotericin B is the only drug found to be safe during pregnancy. All azoles are teratogenic and contraindicated.

▨ CLINICAL PEARLS

- *Penicillium marneffei* redesignated *T. marneffei* causes talaromycosis in immunocompromised patients in endemic areas in Southeast Asia.
- It is a frequent opportunistic infection in HIV patients but also occurs in diabetes, cancer, and autoimmune disorders.
- A presumptive diagnosis is made on the basis of histopathology in a patient with appropriate history and clinical features. Culture provides a definitive diagnosis.
- Treatment includes induction, followed by maintenance phase of therapy. Antifungals include amphotericin B, itraconazole, and voriconazole. Primary and secondary prophylaxis are indicated in HIV patients.

▨ SUGGESTED READING

1. Cao C, Liu W, Li R, et al. In vitro interactions of micafungin with amphotericin B, itraconazole or fluconazole against the pathogenic phase of *Penicillium marneffei*. J Antimicrob Chemother. 2009;63:340.
2. Castro-Lainez MT, Sierra-Hoffman M, LLompart-Zeno J, et al. *Talaromyces marneffei* infection in a non-HIV non-endemic population. IDCases. 2018;12:21.
3. Le T, Huu Chi N, Kim Cuc NT, et al. AIDS-associated *Penicillium marneffei* infection of the central nervous system. Clin Infect Dis. 2010;51:1458.
4. Le T, Kinh NV, Cuc NTK, et al. A trial of itraconazole or amphotericin B for HIV-associated talaromycosis. N Engl J Med. 2017;376:2329.
5. Panel on Opportunistic Infections in HIV-Infected Adults and Adolescents. Guidelines for the prevention and treatment of opportunistic infections in HIV-infected adults and adolescents: recommendations from the Centers for Disease Control and Prevention, the National Institutes of Health, and the HIV Medicine Association of the Infectious Diseases Society of America. 2018. [online] Available from <http://aidsinfo.nih.gov/contentfiles/lvguidelines/adult_oi.pdf>.
6. Ranjana KH, Priyokumar K, Singh TJ, et al. Disseminated *Penicillium marneffei* infection among HIV-infected patients in Manipur state, India. J Infect. 2002;45:268.
7. Sirisanthana V, Sirisanthana T. Disseminated *Penicillium marneffei* infection in human immunodeficiency virus-infected children. Pediatr Infect Dis J. 1995;14:935.
8. Supparatpinyo K, Khamwan C, Baosoung V, et al. Disseminated *Penicillium marneffei* infection in southeast Asia. Lancet. 1994;344:110.

26

Chromoblastomycosis

Monica Mahajan

INTRODUCTION

Chromoblastomycosis (CBM) is a chronic progressive cutaneous and subcutaneous mycoses caused by certain dematiaceous fungi including the following:

- *Fonsecaea pedrosoi*
- *Phialophora verrucosa*
- *Cladosporium carrionii*
- *Fonsecaea compacta*
- *Rhinocladiella aquaspersa*
- *Exophiala* species.

EPIDEMIOLOGY

The endemic areas for CBM are rural areas in humid tropical and subtropical countries in America, Africa, Australia, and Asia. Some sporadic cases have been reported from Russia and Finland. Cases have been reported from the sub-Himalayan belt and from western and eastern coasts of India. Maximum cases have been reported from Kerala and Karnataka.

ETIOLOGY

Max Rudolph described the first case of CBM in 1914. A year later, Lane and Medlar described the pathognomonic sclerotic cells now popularly known as "Medlar bodies," "sclerotic bodies," or "muriform cells." The International Society for Human and Animal Mycology adopted the term chromoblastomycosis in 1992.

Chromoblastomycosis is caused by melanized fungi called dematiaceous fungi of the Herpotrichiellaceae family. Infections are primarily caused by two genera—*Fonsecaea* species and *Cladophialophora* species. Other less common genera causing CBM include *Exophiala* species, *Phialophora* species, and *Rhinocladiella* species.

PATHOPHYSIOLOGY

The fungi are ubiquitous and found in soil, decaying vegetation, and rotting wood. The fungal spores/propagules from melanized fungi gain entry into the human host through traumatic inoculation, however minor, from wood splinters or thorns or through abrasions. Agricultural workers, gardeners, manual laborers who walk barefoot, and people indulging in outdoor recreational activities, such as hunting, are more likely to be exposed to contaminated material. Infection has also been associated with the habit of sitting on babacu shells in Brazil. Certain Cactaceae have the fungi on their surfaces, thorns, and medulla. CBM has been reported after natural disasters. Acupuncture has also been implicated. HLA-A29 may genetically predispose patients to CBM. There is a male predominance in countries where males are involved in outdoor activities. In countries, such as Japan and Brazil, where men and women have equal exposure to same working conditions, there is equal prevalence of the disease in both sexes. There is no human-to-human or animal-to-human transmission.

Unlike pheohyphomycosis, most patients are immunocompetent. The host defenses include the macrophages and the cell-mediated immunity. These result in granuloma formation, microabscesses, and tissue proliferation.

The fungal virulence factors include the following:
- Medlar bodies resist host immune defense mechanisms and make the fungi resistant to antifungals.
- Medlar bodies contain glycogen and lipids that permit the fungus to remain dormant in tissues for many months and years.
- Melanin in the fungi protects against proteolytic enzymes and phagocytosis.
- Fungal cells are hydrophobic which facilitates adherence to host tissues.

CLINICAL MANIFESTATIONS

The most frequent site of involvement is the lower extremities although the lesions may also involve the upper limbs, face, ears, breast, and axillae. Ear involvement due to *F. pedrosoi* has been described.

The infection starts with a minor traumatic inoculation. The inciting trauma may be forgotten or overlooked by the patient. After a gap of many years an asymptomatic solitary erythematous papule develops at the site of trauma. It gradually progresses over the years to become scaly. There are two variants of the disease:
- Nodular
- Plaque.

The surface of the lesion is verrucous, and it keeps spreading indolently to the contiguous tissues. The cicatricial plaque variety spreads peripherally with a central atrophic healed area and a raised active border of spreading vegetative lesions (Fig. 26.1). The nodular variety develops pedunculated cauliflower florets with tumor-like morphology. The surface of these lesions has small ulcerations covered by malodorous discharge having multiple black dots or a "cayenne pepper appearance" which are teeming with the fungus. Another variant may present as annular, papulosquamous, and verrucous patches. Early disease is asymptomatic, whereas pruritus and pain are late features of the disease. Fibrosis and lymphedema gradually develop leading to physical disability.

Dissemination occurs by surface spread, lymphatics, autoinoculation from scratching, and hematogenously to distant subcutaneous sites from the primary site.

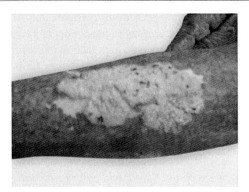

Fig. 26.1: Verrucous, plaque-like lesions in chromoblastomycosis of the lower limbs.

COMPLICATIONS

- Secondary bacterial infection with foul-smelling purulent discharge.
- Lymphatic stasis and elephantiasis.
- Osteomyelitis and osteolytic lesions.
- Flexion deformities due to fibrosis associated with mature collagen crosslinking.
- Hematogenous and lymphatic dissemination is rare, and extracutaneous spread has been documented to lymph nodes, lung, and brain. Some of these cases were of pheohyphomycosis, which were wrongly diagnosed CBM.
- Squamous cell carcinoma has been associated with CBM.

DIFFERENTIAL DIAGNOSES

- Sporotrichosis
- Blastomycosis
- Candidosis
- Rhinosporidiosis
- Tertiary syphilis
- Cutaneous leishmaniasis
- Leprosy
- Squamous cell carcinoma
- Cutaneous tuberculosis/lupus vulgaris
- Phaeohyphomycotic infections
- Conjunctival melanoma
- Cutaneous lymphoma
- Psoriasis.

DIAGNOSIS

Laboratory Studies

- About 10% potassium hydroxide (KOH) smears of skin scrapings demonstrate Medlar bodies. These are cigar-colored thick-walled sclerotic cells and are also called "copper pennies." Dematiaceous hyphae are present in the black dots on the surface of the skin lesions. Sampling is preferred from areas with black dots or cayenne pepper appearance. Calcofluor-white fluorescent stain may help in detection of the fungal elements.

- Vinyl adhesive tape collection from skin lesions may show fungal elements in the horny layer of the epidermis.
- Skin biopsy is preferred for culture instead of skin scrapings and exudative specimens. Cycloheximide containing media may be used to prevent bacterial contamination. Culture of the fungi produces darkly pigmented (black, brown, gray, or green), velvety colonies with a black obverse. They have dense aerial mycelia. *Exophiala* species is an exception that grows black colonies with a yeast morphology. The two most commonly isolated fungi for CBM are *Fonsecaea pedrosoi and Cladophialophora carrionii* (Fig. 26.2).
- A 54-kD antigen test is available for *F. pedrosoi*.
- An enzyme-linked immunosorbent assay for the diagnosis of *Cladosporium carrionii* is routinely used for diagnosis and follow-up. Asymptomatic individuals living in endemic areas may also test positive.
- Duplex polymerase chain reaction is a rapid technique for the identification of *Fonsecaea* isolates.
- Rolling circle amplification is an inexpensive and practical technique for *Fonsecaea* species.

Imaging Studies

Since this is subcutaneous mycoses, bone involvement is not a typical feature. Old, longstanding lesions may be radiographed for bony changes. Lymphoscintigraphy is not routinely available or used for the evaluation of lymphedema.

Histopathology

The skin biopsy should be an elliptical incisional biopsy over the area with black dots. It should include the epidermis, dermis, and subcutaneous tissue. Hematoxylin and eosin stain

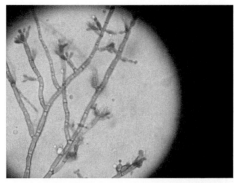

Fig. 26.2: *Fonsecaea pedrosoi* in lactophenol cotton blue mount.

Table 26.1: Staging system of chromoblastomycosis	
Feature	*Scoring*
Area of lesion	Lesions up to 25 cm²—1 point 25–100 cm²—2 points >100 cm²—3 points
Number of lesions	1 lesion—1 point 1–5 lesions—2 points >5 lesions—3 points
Complications	Lymphedema—1 point Ulceration—1 point Secondary infection—1 point
Resistance to previous treatment/unsuccessful treatment previously	1 point

demonstrates cigar-colored fungi. The epidermis shows pseudoepitheliomatous hyperplasia and hyperkeratosis, while the dermis has a lymphocytic inflammatory infiltrate. Granulomas with giant cells and intradermal microabscesses may be seen. Inside the multinucleated giant cells are muriform cells (brown colored, thick-walled fungal cells). These can be single or multiple since these multiply by septation and not by budding. There is transepithelial elimination of fungal bodies and inflammatory debris. Dermal fibrosis is prominent.

Staging System of Chromoblastomycosis (Table 26.1)

The staging system is based on the extent of diseased area, number of lesions, and complications.
- Mild disease—Up to 3 points
- Moderate disease—4-6 points
- Severe disease—7-10 points.

▓ TREATMENT

Small single localized lesions are eradicated by cryosurgery. Liquid nitrogen is applied on the affected skin, and two freeze–thaw cycles are performed in each session. CBM may be treated with cryotherapy alone or in combination with antifungals. One or multiple sessions may be required. The potential complications include pain, edema, scarring and dyspigmentation.

Surgical excision can be curative for small lesions amenable to surgery. The depth of the excision should include the subcutaneous tissue, and there should be at least 0.5 cm of healthy margin all around when excision is performed.

Severe CBM is refractory to treatment, and no single antifungal agent or regimen has demonstrated satisfactory results. Itraconazole is the drug of choice. It is used as a monotherapy or in combination with oral flucytosine (5-FC). Daily dose of itraconazole is 200–400 mg, and therapy may need to be continued for several years. Pulsed dosing of itraconazole may be attempted wherein the drug is given for 1 week every month for a long duration. A complete cure is rare even after prolonged treatment due to the fungistatic nature of the drug. Drug withdrawal may lead to relapse. Combination of itraconazole with 5-FC has a synergistic effect. Terbinafine is an expensive alternative but has suboptimal results. The usual adult dose is 250–500 mg/day. It has fewer drug–drug interactions compared to itraconazole and may have antifibrotic properties. A regimen containing itraconazole and terbinafine may be tried in severe cases. Posaconazole has been tried in the treatment of CBM refractory to conventional therapy. About 800 mg of posaconazole is used per day in divided doses. Topical imiquimod is used concurrently. Dense fibrosis reduces the penetration of antifungals.

Thermotherapy/heat therapy uses chemical pocket warmers or heating pads, which increases skin temperature and impairs fungal growth but has associated risk of skin burns. Oral and topical antibiotics are required for secondary bacterial infection. Photodynamic therapy (PTD) using 5-aminolevulinic acid irradiation may be used as adjunctive therapy for refractory CBM. Carbon dioxide laser vaporization can be useful.

Cladosporium carrionii shows better response to therapy compared to *F. pedrosoi*. Therapy is continued till there is resolution of skin lesions, and the skin scrapings, KOH mounts, and culture are negative for the fungus for 3 consecutive months. Monthly skin biopsies should be negative for fungal elements for 3 consecutive months. Follow up the patients for at least 2 years after cessation of treatment.

The best way of preventing CBM is using shoes, gloves, and appropriate clothing while working outdoors.

CLINICAL PEARLS

- Chromoblastomycosis is endemic subcutaneous mycoses. The most important etiological agents are *F. pedrosoi* and *Cladophialophora carrionii*.
- Results from traumatic inoculation in agricultural workers in tropical and subtropical regions.
- Medlar bodies or sclerotic bodies are pathognomonic.
- The polymorphic skin lesions may be nodular, papular, verrucous, or plaques. Lymphedema, elephantiasis, and secondary bacterial infection are known complications.
- Treatment includes itraconazole and terbinafine, cryotherapy, heat therapy, and PTD.

SUGGESTED READING

1. Bonifaz A, Carrasco-Gerard E, Saúl A. Chromoblastomycosis: clinical and mycologic experience of 51 cases. Mycoses. 2001;44:1.
2. de Azevedo CM, Gomes RR, Vicente VA, et al. *Fonsecaea pugnacius*, a novel agent of disseminated chromoblastomycosis. J Clin Microbiol. 2015;53:2674.
3. Hu Y, Huang X, Lu S, et al. Photodynamic therapy combined with terbinafine against chromo-blastomycosis and the effect of PDT on *Fonsecaea monophora* in vitro. Mycopathologia. 2015; 179:103.
4. Queiroz-Telles F, de Hoog S, Santos DW, et al. Chromoblastomycosis. Clin Microbiol Rev. 2017; 30(1):233-76.
5. Queiroz-Telles F, Esterre P, Perez-Blanco M, et al. Chromoblastomycosis: an overview of clinical manifestations, diagnosis and treatment. Med Mycol. 2009;47(3):233.
6. Silva-Rocha WP, Cardoso FJ, Colalto W, et al. Clinical improvement of chromoblastomycosis refractory to itraconazole successfully treated with high dose of terbinafine. J Dermatol. 2013;40:775.

27

Sporotrichosis

Monica Mahajan

INTRODUCTION

Sporotrichosis is a fungal infection involving the subcutaneous tissue. The etiological agent is the *Sporothrix schenckii* complex. Another popular name for the disease is "rose gardener's disease." It is a ubiquitous fungus found in soil and on plant matter. Cutaneous involvement is the most frequent although pulmonary sporotrichosis and disseminated sporotrichosis have been described. The credit for isolating *S. schenckii* goes to a medical student Benjamin Schenck.

ETIOLOGY

This fungus is placed in the division *Ascomycota*, class Pyrenomycetes, order Ophiostomatales; *S. schenckii* complex comprises phylogenetically different species including *S. schenckii sensu stricto*, *Sporothrix globosa*, *Sporothrix brasiliensis*, *Sporothrix mexicana*, *Sporothrix albicans*, *Sporothrix luriei*, and *Sporothrix pallida*. It is found in decomposing organic matter, sphagnum moss, rose bushes, hay, wood, and soil.

S. schenckii displays thermal dimorphism. When cultured at temperatures below the human body temperature (25°C), it produces 1–2-µm-wide hyaline, septate hyphae. The colonies are moist, glabrous, wrinkled, and vary in color from white to black. The conidiophore arises at a right angle from the hypha as a solitary structure with a tapered apex. Clusters of single-celled, hyaline or brown, ovoid or elongated, and denticulate conidia are formed. These may have a "bouquet-like" pattern of arrangement. The characteristic feature of conidia of *S. schenckii* is the dark cell wall. This is not a feature of nonpathogenic *Sporothrix* species.

At 37°C the colonies are glabrous, white to yellow, and the yeast cells are spherical or oval, 2–6 µm in diameter with cigar-shaped buds. *Sporothrix* species do not form cottony or floccose colonies.

ROUTES OF TRANSMISSION

Cutaneous inoculation occurs due to trauma while working outdoors. It is frequent in gardeners, nursery workers, landscaping, horticulture, berry picking, timber workers, carpenters, and people who carry hay bales. Zoonotic spread occurs from scratches from a cat, horse, or an armadillo. Veterinarians and cat owners are at a higher risk of acquiring the disease. Rarely, inhalation of the conidia causes pulmonary or disseminated forms of sporotrichosis. Extracutaneous manifestations including meningitis and dissemination are more frequent in immunosuppressed patients, including HIV, chronic obstructive pulmonary disease (COPD), diabetes, and alcoholics.

CLINICAL MANIFESTATIONS

Most patients have involvement of skin and subcutaneous tissues. It occurs most frequently on the hand or arm due to handling contaminated plant matter. It develops as a painless nodules, papules, pustules, or ulcerative lesions. Spread through the lymphatics results in lymphocutaneous sporotrichosis. A chain of nodules develops along the lymphatic channels. Lesions are unresponsive to oral and topical antibiotics. *S. brasiliensis* infection may result in erythema nodosum or erythema multiforme as a hypersensitivity manifestation.

Bone and joints involvement in sporotrichosis can be due to direct inoculation or through hematogenous spread. Osteoarticular sporotrichosis occurs in patients with alcoholism issues. It can be monoarticular or polyarticular. Features include tenosynovitis, joint effusion, bursitis, and limitation of joint movement. Osteomyelitis and draining sinus tracts may develop.

Pulmonary sporotrichosis due to inhalation of conidia results is frequently seen in patients with COPD and alcoholics. The disease presents as fibrocavitary lesions. Physical findings are nonspecific or predominantly related to COPD. Outcome is poor due to delay in diagnosis.

Disseminated disease occurs in immunocompromised host, including HIV, single-organ transplant recipients, corticosteroid, and chemotherapy use. These patients should be evaluated for central nervous system involvement and meningitis due to sporotrichosis. Organs involved include brain, eyes, sinuses, larynx, or prostate.

DIAGNOSTIC WORKUP

Laboratory Investigations

- Specimens are examined by making a 10% potassium hydroxide mount. It shows oval budding yeast cells 2–6 μm in size. These are scanty and detected with difficulty in human specimens. However, infected cats have a higher fungal load, and the yeast cells are easy to demonstrate in the specimens. Fluorescent-antibody staining improves chances of detection. On Gram stain, yeast cells are positively stained and may occasionally appear intracellularly within giant cells.
- Culture from skin scrapings or biopsy provides a definitive diagnosis. Other specimens which may be cultured include sputum, cerebrospinal fluid, or synovial fluid. *S. schenckii* grows as filamentous hyphae with conidia at room temperature. Confirmation is by demonstrating fungal dimorphism and growth of yeast form at 37°C. Growth may become positive within 8 days to 4 weeks.
- Sporotrichin skin test detects delayed hypersensitivity and finds utility as an epidemiological tool. The reaction will be positive not only in confirmed cases but also in the cases with previous exposure to sporotrichosis.

- Serological tests for antibody detection based on double immunodiffusion, immuno-electrophoresis, latex agglutination, and tube agglutination have been developed.

Histopathology

Skin biopsy shows granulomatous inflammation with oval or cigar-shaped yeast cells. Histopathological features include suppuration and formation of granulomas in the dermal and subcutaneous layers. Other findings include hyperkeratosis, parakeratosis, and pseudoepitheliomatous hyperplasia. Granulomas comprise cellular debris, caseous material, giant and epithelioid cells, and intracellular/extracellular *S. schenckii* yeast cells.

▓ DIFFERENTIAL DIAGNOSES

- Chromoblastomycosis
- Blastomycosis
- Cryptococcosis
- Atypical mycobacterial infections, including *Mycobacterium marinum* and *Mycobacterium fortuitum*
- Nocardiosis
- Leishmaniasis
- Cat-scratch disease
- Rheumatoid arthritis
- Sarcoidosis.

▓ TREATMENT

Treatment is recommended for all patients as spontaneous resolution of the disease is rare. Treatment of visceral and osteoarticular sporotrichosis is more challenging. Exposure at multiple sites will cause lesions on different areas of the body.

Itraconazole is the drug of choice. The formulations available are a 100-mg capsule and a solution of 100 mg/10 mL. The capsule is preferably taken after food, whereas solution is administered empty stomach. Liposomal amphotericin B (LAmB) is preferred for severe or disseminated disease and in patients with *S. schenckii* meningitis. Higher doses of terbinafine have been tried. Fluconazole has low response rates. Data on efficacy of voriconazole and posaconazole is scant (Table 27.5).

Devices using infrared waves are used to heat tissues to 42°C. Induced hyperthermia inhibits growth of *S. schenckii* and decreases the size of cutaneous lesions (Table 27.1).

The mechanism of action of saturated solution of potassium iodide (SSKI) is not clear but it is effective only in cutaneous and lymphocutaneous sporotrichosis. It is inexpensive but cumbersome to administer with a dropper. The side effects include abdominal pain, altered taste, parotid enlargement, and rash.

Itraconazole is successful in treating cutaneous sporotrichosis in 90–100% patients (Table 27.2).

Table 27.1: Disseminated sporotrichosis.

Drug	Dosage	Recommendations
LAmB	3–5 mg/kg as initial therapy	AmBd is not preferred
Itraconazole	200 mg twice daily as step-down therapy	Complete at least 12 months of therapy; monitor therapeutic drug levels. For HIV-positive, continue suppressive therapy 200 mg/day to prevent relapse

AmBd, amphotericin B deoxycholate; LAmB, liposomal amphotericin B; HIV, human immunodeficiency virus

Table 27.2: Cutaneous or lymphocutaneous sporotrichosis.

Drug	Dosage	Recommendations
Itraconazole	200 mg/day orally Nonresponders—200 mg twice daily	Continue for 3–6 months
Terbinafine	500 mg twice daily orally	Used for nonresponders to itraconazole
SSKI	Initiate with 5 drops thrice daily, increase to 40–50 drops thrice daily	For nonresponders to itraconazole
Fluconazole	400–800 mg/day	Use only for those intolerant to other agents

SSKI, saturated solution of potassium iodide

Table 27.3: Osteoarticular sporotrichosis.

Drug	Dosage	Recommendations
Itraconazole	200 mg twice daily	Continue for at least 12 months; monitor serum drug levels
AmBd LAmB	0.7–1 mg/kg daily 3–5 mg/kg daily	Use as initial therapy, followed by oral itraconazole to complete at least 12 months of therapy

AmBd, amphotericin B deoxycholate; LAmB, liposomal amphotericin B

Amphotericin B is recommended if the disease is unresponsive to itraconazole therapy or is more severe. Intra-articular amphotericin B is not recommended. Other therapies including fluconazole, SSKI, and terbinafine are ineffective.

Surgical debridement alone is not effective and needs to be combined with antifungal therapy. Aspiration of involved joint or removal of sequestrum improves recovery (Table 27.2).

Surgery is recommended for localized pulmonary involvement in combination with amphotericin B. Fluconazole is ineffective (Table 27.3).

Amphotericin B is the drug of choice for meningeal sporotrichosis. LAmB is preferred. Combination therapy of amphotericin B with azoles does not offer a survival benefit. For AIDS patients, lifelong immunosuppressive therapy is recommended to prevent relapse. Fluconazole and voriconazole have no role in treatment of meningeal sporotrichosis. Posaconazole may have some efficacy but lacks sufficient data (Table 27.4).

Table 27.4: Pulmonary sporotrichosis.

Disease severity	Treatment	Duration
Severe/life-threatening disease	LAmB 3–5 mg/kg or AmBd 0.7–1 mg/kg as initial therapy. Maintenance therapy with itraconazole 200 mg twice daily	Continue therapy for at least 12 months, monitor therapeutic drug levels of itraconazole
Mild disease	Itraconazole 200 mg twice daily	Continue therapy for at least 12 months

AmBd, amphotericin B deoxycholate; LAmB, liposomal amphotericin B

Table 27.5: Meningeal sporotrichosis.

Drug	Dosage	Recommendations
LAmB	5 mg/kg as initial therapy	Continued for 4–6 weeks; AmBd is not preferred
Itraconazole	200 mg twice daily as step-down therapy	Complete at least 12 months of therapy; monitor therapeutic drug levels. For HIV-positive, continue suppressive therapy 200 mg/day to prevent relapse

AmBd, amphotericin B deoxycholate; LAmB, liposomal amphotericin B; HIV, human immunodeficiency virus

Amphotericin B is preferred as initial therapy. LAmB is preferred due to lesser nephrotoxicity. Itraconazole is used as suppressive therapy in AIDS. Therapy may be discontinued once the cluster of differentiation 4 count is 200 cells/μL for ≥1 year.

Sporotrichosis in Pregnancy

Treatment onset may be delayed in cutaneous sporotrichosis as it does not worsen during pregnancy and does not disseminate to the fetus.

Liposomal amphotericin B 3–5 mg/kg daily or amphotericin B deoxycholate (AmBd) 0.7–1 mg/kg daily is recommended. All azoles are contraindicated. Local hyperthermia may be offered as treatment for cutaneous sporotrichosis. Terbinafine is a pregnancy category B drug, and it is not expected to harm the fetus. It passes into breast milk.

Sporotrichosis in Children

Itraconazole 6–10 mg/kg or SSKI at the dose of one drop per kg body weight using an eye dropper is used for cutaneous or lymphocutaneous sporotrichosis. AmBd 0.7 mg/kg daily is used as initial therapy in disseminated sporotrichosis.

Prevention of Sporotrichosis

Personal protection measures include use of gloves and long-sleeve clothes and high boots while gardening, landscaping, or baling of hay.

CLINICAL PEARLS

- Sporotrichosis is caused by the thermally dimorphic fungus *S. schenckii* following traumatic inoculation from contaminated plant matter.
- Zoonotic transmission from cats may result in minor outbreaks.
- In humans, it causes subcutaneous mycosis with involvement of adjacent lymphatics.
- Culture is diagnostic, and itraconazole is the preferred antifungal for both humans and cats.

SUGGESTED READING

1. Aung AK, Teh BM, McGrath C, et al. Pulmonary sporotrichosis: case series and systematic analysis of literature on clinico-radiological patterns and management outcomes. Med Mycol. 2013;51:534.
2. Barros MB, de Almeida Paes R, Schubach AO. *Sporothrix schenckii* and sporotrichosis. Clin Microbiol Rev. 2011;24:633.
3. Freitas DF, de Siqueira Hoagland B, do Valle AC, et al. Sporotrichosis in HIV-infected patients: report of 21 cases of endemic sporotrichosis in Rio de Janeiro, Brazil. Med Mycol. 2012;50:170.
4. Kauffman CA, Pappas PG, McKinsey DS, et al. Treatment of lymphocutaneous and visceral sporotrichosis with fluconazole. Clin Infect Dis. 1996;22:46.
5. López-Romero E, Reyes-Montes Mdel R, Pérez-Torres A, et al. *Sporothrix schenckii* complex and sporotrichosis, an emerging health problem. Future Microbiol. 2011;6:85.
6. Tiwari A, Malani AN. Primary pulmonary sporotrichosis: case report and review of the literature. Infect Dis Clin Pract. 2012;20:25.

28

Lobomycosis

Monica Mahajan

INTRODUCTION

Lobomycosis is a subcutaneous mycosis caused by *Lacazia loboi*. It is endemic in the Amazon basin with cases being reported in both humans and dolphins. The most common clinical presentation is keloid-like lesions. Since dolphins are found in every coastal region, there is a need for clinicians to be aware of this disease entity.

ETIOLOGY

Lobomycosis was described by Brazilian dermatologist Jorge Lobo in 1931. It has also been called by several other names, including keloid blastomycosis, Jorge Lobo mycosis, Amazonic pseudolepromatous blastomycosis, and lacaziosis.

The taxonomy of this fungus has changed numerous times. Based on genotyping, it is now designated *L. loboi*. It belongs to the order Onygenales and family Ajellomycetaceae. Although it has similarities regarding cellular structure with *Paracoccidioides brasiliensis*, the two differ phylogenetically.

L. loboi is visible in tissues as a round yeast with a birefringent membrane and a thick wall and melanin pigmentation. Formation of blastoconidia leads to a rosary bead appearance. It is predominantly an intracellular fungus.

PATHOGENESIS

L. loboi produces a cutaneous mycosis in humans and dolphins by skin inoculation. The fungus exists as a saprophyte in soil and water. Transmission is suspected to be through insect or animal inoculation, including after insect bite, snake bite, or stingray trauma.

Interleukin-10 and transforming growth factor β1 levels increase and inhibit the cellular immune response and the phagocytic activity of macrophages. This allows the fungus to proliferate in the dermis. Inflammatory response with histiocytes and multinucleated giant cells develops. Cluster of differentiation 8 T-lymphocyte proliferation causes increase in production of immunoglobulin A antibodies by plasma cells which, in turn, results in fibrosis and keloid-like lesions. Melanin within the fungus helps to evade the immune attack. An immunodominant antigen with an approximate 193-kDa molecular weight is recognized by the host to produce an antibody response.

There can be lymphatic dissemination and regional lymphadenopathy. Autoinoculation and contiguous spread have been documented. Human-to-human transmission does not occur.

EPIDEMIOLOGY

Lobomycosis has been described in forest areas with large rivers, high temperatures, and humidity. Most cases have been reported from the Amazon basin. Countries with lobomycosis include Brazil, Columbia, Venezuela, Peru, and Bolivia. Imported cases have been detected in the United States, France, Canada, Germany, and Greece.

The fungus has been detected in bottlenose dolphins in the Gulf of Mexico, Guyana dolphin in Suriname River, dolphins in the Indian Ocean, Japanese coast, African coast, and the European coast.

Lobomycosis can be an occupational hazard for people dealing with dolphins, including veterinarians, marine biologists, and those who undertake rescue and rehabilitation of injured dolphins. Certain recreational activities, such as swimming with dolphins in recreational parks, deep-sea diving, and swimming in the sea, may make humans more prone to lobomycosis.

CLINICAL FEATURES

The exact incubation period is not known and can be a few months to years. Lesions involve the exposed areas, including the ear pinna, upper and lower limbs. A superficial or a deep papule develops at the site of trauma. It is covered by shiny erythematous skin with or without telangiectasia. It resembles a scar or a keloid. Gradually the lesion may acquire a more polymorphic appearance. There are varying degrees of hyperpigmentation to hypopigmentation and achromia. During the rainy season, there can be maceration of skin and ulceration. Further growth leads to exophytic or wart-like lesions. Verrucous lobomycosis needs to be distinguished from chromoblastomycosis. New lesions developing around the index lesion may indicate autoinoculation or lymphatic dissemination. Confluence of these lesions forms a plaque.

Lobomycosis is generally asymptomatic. Extensive lesions cause pruritus, ulceration, cosmetic disfigurement, and secondary bacterial infection. Two cases of squamous cell carcinoma have been described in association with lobomycosis. The disease may be classified as:
- Localized
- Multifocal—restricted to one anatomical area
- Disseminated—involvement of more than one anatomical area

DIFFERENTIAL DIAGNOSES
- Leprosy
- Chromoblastomycosis
- Squamous cell carcinoma

- Sporotrichosis
- Keloid and hypertrophic scars
- Leishmaniasis
- Paracoccidioidomycosis

DIAGNOSTIC WORKUP

Diagnosis is made on the basis of the following clinical features:

- Direct examination of skin scrapings is used to visualize the fungus. Round-to-oval yeast cells which are 6–12 μm in diameter and have a birefringent membrane are found in the dermis. The fungal structures can be in isolation or in a rosary beads distribution.
- Vinyl adhesive tape or exfoliative cytology are other techniques for obtaining samples that may be used.
- Skin biopsy shows a dense diffuse histolytic infiltrate in the dermis and a number of fungal elements. There are epithelioid, multinucleate, and Langerhans cells with or without granuloma formation. "Pseudo-Gaucher cells" are large xanthomatous histiocytes with clear or finely granular cytoplasm and no intracellular organisms. Fibrosis is a dominant feature, and asteroid bodies may be seen.

TREATMENT

The ideal treatment is surgical excision. Itraconazole is the only antifungal that works as an adjuvant to surgery. It is sometimes used in combination with clofazimine. Patients with lobomycosis and concurrent leprosy show improvement in both when treatment for multibacillary treatment is administered. Posaconazole may have variable efficacy.

CLINICAL PEARLS

- Lobomycosis/lacaziosis is a self-limited, chronic fungal infection endemic in South and Central America.
- It leads to keloid-like lesions.
- Surgical excision is recommended.

SUGGESTED READING

1. Fonseca JJ. Lobomycosis. Int J Surg Pathol. 2007;15:62.
2. Paniz-Mondolfi A, Talhari C, Sander Hoffmann L, et al. Lobomycosis: an emerging disease in humans and delphinidae. Mycoses. 2012;55:298.
3. Reif JS, Schaefer AM, Bossart GD. Lobomycosis: risk of zoonotic transmission from dolphins to humans. Vector-borne Zoonotic Dis. 2013;13:689.
4. Talhari S, Talhari C. Lobomycosis. Clin Dermatol. 2012;30:420.

29

Phaeohyphomycosis

Monica Mahajan

INTRODUCTION

The term phaeohyphomycosis was coined by Ajello in 1974 to describe dematiaceous or melanized fungi. It means a disease condition caused by fungi with dark hyphae. Apart from phaeohyphomycosis, other conditions caused by dematiaceous fungi include mycetoma and chromoblastomycosis (CBM). Mycetoma is characterized by production of mycotic granules while hallmark of CBM is sclerotic bodies in tissues. There has been an increase in the number of case reports of disseminated phaeohyphomycosis. The most serious infection caused by these pathogens is infection of the central nervous system (CNS).

ETIOLOGY

There is conflicting nomenclature for the fungi that cause phaeohyphomycosis. These are fungi that contain melanin in their cell wall and spores. There are more than 100 species classified in approximately 60 different genera. Molecular methods are being applied for identifying these dematiaceous fungi.

The neurotropic fungi include *Cladophialophora bantiana*, *Bipolaris* species, *Exophiala* species, and *Rhinocladiella mackenziei* (Box 29.1).

EPIDEMIOLOGY

The fungi are ubiquitous and found in the soil, polluted water, and decaying vegetation. Cases have been reported worldwide, but some species, such as *R. mackenziei*, are more frequent in the tropical and subtropical countries, including India, Pakistan, Saudi Arabia, Kuwait, and Afghanistan.

PATHOGENESIS

The spores are inhaled from the soil and reach the paranasal sinuses. There can be contiguous or hematogenous spread. The fungi may also gain access to human host through penetrating trauma, contaminated wounds, or even abrasions from thorns or wood splinters. The incubation period is unknown.

Box 29.1: Dematiaceous fungi causing phaeohyphomycosis

- *Cladophialophora bantiana* (previously known as *Cladosporium trichoides, Xylohypha bantiana, Cladosporium bantianum*)
- *Wangiella dermatitidis* (also known as *Exophiala dermatitidis*)
- *Dactylaria gallopava* (also known as *Ochroconis gallopava*)
- *Fonsecaea pedrosoi*
- *Bipolaris spicifera* (also known as *Drechslera spicifera*)
- *Rhinocladiella mackenziei* (also known as *Ramichloridium mackenziei* and *Ramichloridium ovoideum*)
- *Aureobasidium* species
- *Alternaria* species
- *Curvularia* species (Figs. 29.1A and B)
- *Exserohilum* species
- *Phialophora* species
- *Scedosporium prolificans*

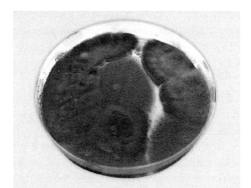

Fig. 29.1A: Black, hairy colonies of *Curvularia* species on SDA. (SDA, Sabourad dextrose agar)

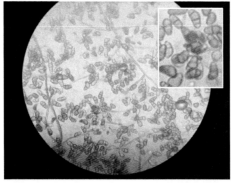

Fig. 29.1B: *Curvularia geniculata* in *LPCB mount*: Erect, unbranched conidiophore. Smooth walled, dark brown, 4-septate, central cell largest, conidia unilaterally flattened to distinctly curved. (LPCB, Lactophenol cotton blue)

An outbreak of fungal meningitis and septic arthritis occurred in the United States in 2012 when several patients received epidural injection or intra-articular injections of methyl-prednisolone from a single compounding center. The pathogens isolated from these patients included *Exserohilum* species, *Aspergillus fumigatus*, and *Cladosporium* species.

PREDISPOSING FACTORS

- Malignancy
- Bone marrow and solid-organ transplant (SOT) recipients
- Chemotherapy-induced neutropenia
- Acquired immune deficiency syndrome
- Intravenous (IV) drug abuse
- Traumatic inoculation
- Inoculation during surgery
- Allergic fungal sinusitis
- Prematurity
- Cardiac surgery and valve replacement, especially bioprosthetic (porcine) valves.

Bipolaris spicifera has been diagnosed as the cause of invasive fungal infection in a cardiac transplant patient. Infections due to phaeohyphomycosis are also known to occur in immuno-competent patients.

Melanin as a Virulence Factor

Melanin in the cell wall of these fungi imparts a dark color to their hyphae and conidia. It plays an important role in the pathogenesis of the disease. Mechanisms by which melanin is an important virulence factor, include:

- Melanin scavenges free radicals produced by oxidative burst in phagocytic cells. These free radicals would have killed the pathogens in the absence of melanin.
- Melanin binds with hydrolytic enzymes and prevents disruption of plasma membrane.
- Melanin plays a role in the formation of a structure called fungal appressorium that helps in penetrating host cells. An appressorium is a specialized cell that is used to infect host plants. It is a flattened hyphal pressing organ that helps enter the host cells by using turgor pressure.

Melanin is also a virulence factor in *Cryptococcus neoformans*.

CLINICAL FEATURES

Subcutaneous phaeohyphomycosis presents as an asymptomatic nodule at the site of trauma. The most common sites include the feet, legs, hands, arms, and head. In immunocompetent hosts, lesion is solitary and does not ulcerate. Immunocompromised patients may have a varied presentation, including nodules, papules, pustules, eschars, or ulcers. They may develop draining sinuses.

Invasive rhinosinusitis due to phaeohyphomycosis in immunocompetent patients involves the ethmoid and sphenoid sinus more frequently compared with the other sinuses. Patients present with gradually progressive symptoms of unilateral blockage, mucopurulent discharge, anosmia, and persistent headache. Complications include spread to the orbit, resulting in proptosis, restricted extraocular movements, and visual impairment. Cavernous sinus thrombosis is a dreaded complication. Immunocompromised hosts have higher propensity for maxillary and ethmoid involvement, eschar formation, and brain abscess.

Allergic rhinosinusitis occurs more frequently in individuals who have had previous sinus surgeries. Presenting complaints include nasal polyposis and thick yellow mucus discharge. Nasal polyps may cause bony erosion. Complications include invasion of orbit by allergic mucin and deviation of nasal septum to contralateral side due to pressure effects. The resected tissue contains eosinophilic mucin with noninvasive fungal elements in the mucin.

Pulmonary phaeohyphomycosis resembles invasive aspergillosis with features including pulmonary infiltrates, nodules, cavities, and a halo sign on computed tomography (CT) scan. *Curvularia* species cause allergic symptoms resembling allergic bronchopulmonary aspergillosis, and investigations reveal eosinophilia and high immunoglobulin E levels.

The most common manifestation is fungemia with positive blood cultures. *Scedosporium prolificans* is most frequently implicated, and infection may result in septic shock. Other organs frequently involved in disseminated phaeohyphomycosis are the lungs, heart, brain, kidney, and skin. There can be multiorgan involvement. Organs, such as liver, spleen, lymph nodes, bones, and joints, are less frequently involved. *S. prolificans* can cause bone and joint involvement in immunocompetent patients. Presenting complaints include fever, rash, ulcers, respiratory, CNS, and gastrointestinal symptoms.

Brain abscess is the most common manifestation due to cerebral phaeohyphomycosis and presents as focal neurologic deficit, altered mental status with or without seizures. Fever and headache may be absent. Frontal lobes are most frequently involved. Abscess is mostly solitary, but multiple abscesses have been reported in immunocompromised hosts. Meningitis, encephalitis, and arachnoiditis have been described. The most common cause of CNS phaeohyphomycosis is *C. bantiana* (Figs. 29.2A and B).

Other manifestations include endocarditis, peritonitis, osteomyelitis, and pericarditis.

▩ DIFFERENTIAL DIAGNOSES

- *For cutaneous phaeohyphomycosis:*
  - ♦ Chromoblastomycosis
  - ♦ Cutaneous leishmaniasis
  - ♦ Sporotrichosis
  - ♦ Blastomycosis
  - ♦ Coccidioidomycosis
  - ♦ Paracoccidioidomycosis.
- *For rhinosinusitis:*
  - ♦ Aspergillosis
- *For cerebral phaeohyphomycosis:*
  - ♦ Bacterial cerebral abscess
  - ♦ Nocardiosis
  - ♦ Toxoplasmosis
  - ♦ Cryptococcosis
  - ♦ Histoplasmosis
  - ♦ Coccidioidomycosis
  - ♦ Listeriosis.

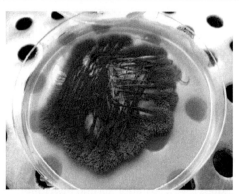

Fig. 29.2A: Spreading, velvety, olive-grey to black colonies of *Cladophialophora bantiana*.

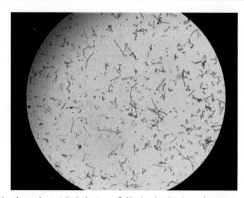

Fig. 29.2B: Sparsely branched, oval conidial chains of *Cladophialophora bantiana*.

DIAGNOSIS

These dematiaceous fungi are found in the soil and may grow as contaminants during fungal culture. Isolation of these fungi from sputum or bronchoalveolar lavage may represent contamination, colonization, or a true infection.

- Microscopic examination of skin scrapings, pus, or aspirate from cerebral abscess shows brown-pigmented, thin, septate hyphae, and irregular swelling with septae showing constrictions. There is occasional branching. Terminal or intercalated vesicular swellings with thick walls may be confused with chlamydoconidia. Pigmented yeast cells with budding and separation can be occasionally detected. The Masson–Fontana stain is melanin-specific and used to detect the dematiaceous fungi in the tissue. Other fungi that may stain positive include *A. fumigatus* and *Zygomycetes* species. The distinguishing feature from CBM and mycetoma is the absence of sclerotic cells and grains, respectively. Silver stains may obscure the fungi, and the brown color may not be visible.
- Blood cultures are positive in more than 50% cases of fungemia. *S. prolificans* is positive in majority of the patients. These fungi are frequent contaminants in the laboratory, but growth is considered significant if isolated from a normally sterile site.

- Fungal culture demonstrates irregularly swollen hyphae with yeast-like structures. It is the only definitive technique to confirm diagnosis. Growth occurs on Sabouraud dextrose agar at 25–30°C in 1–2 weeks. Dark-brown or black mold is seen. Growth may be delayed up to 4 weeks. Molecular techniques play an important role in species identification. Sequencing of the internal transcribed spacer regions of ribosomal deoxyribonucleic acid gene complex is used for genotyping the species (*See* Figs. 29.1 and 29.2).
- Eosinophilia can be a feature with *Curvularia* and *Bipolaris* species since these are also associated with allergic fungal sinusitis.
- Cerebrospinal fluid (CSF) examination findings include raised opening pressure, increased proteins, reduced glucose, and pleocytosis. CSF culture is negative, and resection of the abscess is the only method for confirming the diagnosis.
- Imaging studies, including CT scan and magnetic resonance imaging, of the brain reveal single or multiple enhancing lesions in the frontal or parietal lobe. Meningeal enhancement is infrequent. CT scan in the cases of invasive rhinosinusitis reveals a hyperdense mass within one sinus with erosion of the sinus walls. Allergic rhinosinusitis is seen as a serpiginous sinus opacification of multiple sinuses with mucosal thickening and bony erosion.

TREATMENT

Itraconazole is the preferred antifungal. Terbinafine also demonstrates efficacy against dematiaceous fungi, including pathogens causing phaeohyphomycosis. Combination therapy with itraconazole and terbinafine may have a synergistic effect against *S. prolificans*. Both drugs work at different levels of the ergosterol synthetic pathway and can be a useful combination. Some of these fungi can be resistant to amphotericin B and echinocandins. The newer azoles, including voriconazole and posaconazole, show activity against these fungi.

Scedosporium prolificans is generally resistant to all available antifungal agents, whereas *Scedosporium apiospermum* is susceptible to miconazole, voriconazole, and posaconazole.

Management of *subcutaneous phaeohyphomycosis* requires complete surgical resection of the lesion. Partial resection or incision and drainage will result in recurrence. There is no role of antifungals subsequent to surgery. Unresectable lesions are managed with azoles or terbinafine. A combination of both may be used. The duration of treatment is not defined.

Patients with *invasive fungal rhinosinusitis* should undergo extensive debridement with the removal of necrotic material. Recurrent debridements may be needed. Various antifungals, including itraconazole, voriconazole, posaconazole, terbinafine, and amphotericin B, have been tried in these patients with varying success.

Allergic fungal rhinosinusitis treatment includes nasal polypectomy and debridement of eosinophilic fungal debris. Antifungals are used along with postoperative corticosteroids to reduce recurrence of the disease. Since the underlying cause is thought to be an immune response to the fungus, the role of itraconazole or other antifungals is controversial. Two-thirds of patients tend to relapse.

Solitary pulmonary nodules are resected. Immunocompromised hosts with pulmonary phaeohyphomycosis are managed with azoles (itraconazole, voriconazole, or posaconazole) or amphotericin B.

Cerebral abscess due to phaeohyphomycosis requires complete resection of the lesion rather than CT-guided aspiration of the abscess. Partial resection is associated with high mortality. Surgery alone is not sufficient. However, treatment protocols have not been standardized as susceptibility testing for dematiaceous fungi is not available. Various antifungals, including azoles, terbinafine, echinocandins, and amphotericin B, have been tried. A reasonable option is a combination therapy with liposomal amphotericin B (3–5 mg/kg IV daily) and IV voriconaozle (4–6 mg/kg IV twice daily) or itraconazole (200 mg orally twice daily) or posaconazole delayed release tablets (300 mg twice daily on day 1, followed by 300 mg once daily). Voriconazole may be preferred since it is available as an IV formulation and has good CNS penetration. Therapy is continued from 6 months to 2 years. Despite recent advances in antifungal therapy, the mortality associated with cerebral phaeohyphomycosis is more than 50%. Patients with *C. bantiana* or *R. mackenziei* infection are refractory to antifungals and have poor outcomes.

Granulocyte colony-stimulating factors may be used in neutropenic patients. Surgery may be required in fungal endocarditis or osteomyelitis.

Disseminated phaeohyphomycosis is associated with very high mortality rates, especially in immunodeficient patients. Persistent neutropenia is associated with worst outcomes.

PROPHYLAXIS

Due to rarity of this infection, role of chemoprophylaxis has not been adequately studied. Bone marrow transplant and SOT recipients may already be on itraconazole prophylaxis for aspergillosis, and the same may reduce probability of developing phaeohyphomycosis. Other measures, including positive-pressure ventilation and high-efficiency particulate matter filters, can be beneficial.

CLINICAL PEARLS

- Phaeohyphomycosis is caused by dematiaceous fungi with melanin in their cell walls. These fungi are ubiquitous.
- Brain abscess is the most severe manifestation.
- Infection is common both in immunocompetent and immunocompromised patients.
- Surgical resection and antifungals are required as combined approach to treatment.

SUGGESTED READING

1. Centres for Disease Control and Prevention (CDC). Multistate outbreak of fungal infection associated with injection of methylprednisolone acetate solution from a single compounding pharmacy—United States, 2012. MMWR Morb Mortal Wkly Rep. 2012;61:839.
2. Deng S, Pan W, Liao W, et al. Combination of amphotericin B and flucytosine against neurotropic species of melanized fungi causing primary cerebral phaeohyphomycosis. Antimicrob Agents Chemother. 2016;60:2346.
3. Kantarcioglu AS, Guarro J, De Hoog S, et al. An updated comprehensive systematic review of *Cladophialophora bantiana* and analysis of epidemiology, clinical characteristics, and outcome of cerebral cases. Med Mycol. 2017;55:579.
4. Li DM, de Hoog S. Cerebral phaeohyphomycosis—a cure at what lengths? Lancet Infectious Dis. 2009;9:376-83.
5. Proia LA, Trenholme GM. Chronic refractory phaeohyphomycosis: successful treatment with posaconazole. Mycoses. 2006;49:519.

30

Hyalohyphomycosis

Monica Mahajan

INTRODUCTION

Hyalohyphomycosis is an infection caused by molds that have hyaline, light-colored hyphal elements that can be branched or unbranched but lack pigment in their cell wall. These can produce localized or disseminated infections. These nondematiaceous molds are the counterpart of phaeohyphomycosis, which collectively refers to brown-walled septate hyphae. Hyalohyphomycosis does not refer to one disease entity; instead, it is a spectrum of diseases caused by hyaline molds. Histopathologically, these may be misidentified as *Aspergillus*.

ETIOLOGY

The organisms causing hyalohyphomycosis include various species of *Fusarium, Penicillium, Scedosporium, Acremonium, Paecilomyces, Scopulariopsis, Basidiomycota, Schizophyllum, Beauveria, Trichoderma, Chaetoconidium, Chrysosporium*, and *Microascus*.

PATHOGENESIS

Infection is more common in immunocompromised host. The fungi produce various myco-toxins that suppress cellular and humoral immunity. Proteases and collagenases cause tissue breakdown and invasion. Adhesion molecules facilitate adhesion to catheters, prosthetic valves, or contact lenses.

FUSARIOSIS

Fusarium are ubiquitous soil saprophytes and plant pathogens. A few species are a frequent cause of both superficial and invasive infections in humans. The spectrum of disease includes onychomycosis, keratitis, pneumonia, fungemia, or disseminated disease depending on the immune status of the host.

Etiology

Genus *Fusarium* comprises at least 300 phylogenetically different species.

The *Fusarium* species most frequently implicated for disseminated infection include *F. solani* complex, *F. oxysporum* complex, *F. verticillioides* (includes *Fusarium moniliforme*), *F. proliferatum*, *F. chlamydosporum*, *F. subglutinans*, *F. sacchari*, and *F. anthophilum*. *F. verticillioides* and *F. proliferatum* are part of *Fusarium fujikuroi* complex. Most pathogenic species are found in the *F. solani* complex and include *Fusarium falciforme* and *Fusarium lichenicola*.

Colonies are pale or bright colored depending on the species (Fig. 30.1). These may or may not have an aerial mycelium. The thallus varies in color from white to yellow, red, purple, or pink. The macroconidia are hyaline, two or multicelled, and are sickle/crescent shaped, banana shaped, or fusiform (Fig. 30.2). They have an elongated apical cell and a pedicellate basal cell. Microconidia are one to two celled, hyaline, fusiform, pyriform or ovoid, straight or curved, and are smaller in size than macroconidia. Macroconidia can be occasionally absent on subculture. Chlamydospores can be present or absent. Culture growth on potato dextrose agar requires daily exposure to light for 10–14 days for pigmentation to develop. Cycloheximide in culture media inhibits growth. Database for molecular identification of species on the basis of multilocus sequence data is available on the Internet. Fusarium MLST or FUSARIUM-ID are the preferred databases rather than GenBank. Matrix-assisted laser desorption/ionization–time-of-flight (MALDI–TOF) assists in species identification.

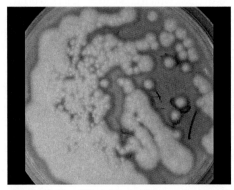

Fig. 30.1: White to cream-colored colonies of *Fusarium* species on sabourad dextrose agar (SDA).

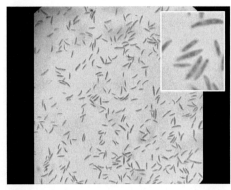

Fig. 30.2: *Fusarium* species with bean-shaped macroconidia on lactophenol cotton blue (LPCB) mount.

Epidemiology

These fungi are found in soil, polluted waters, and decaying vegetation. They are important plant pathogens. In humans, the routes of infection include entry of spores through traumatized skin in burns, cellulitis, insect bite, onychomycosis, patients with indwelling catheters, and central lines and through inhalation of airborne spores. Direct inoculation of the pathogen may occur into the skin, bone, or joint. Other portals of entry are the paranasal sinuses and the lungs. Consumption of food contaminated with *Fusarium* mycotoxin may result in *Fusarium* mycotoxicosis. Although it is a ubiquitous fungus, the incidence of infection may show geographical variations. In Brazil, it is the leading invasive fungal infections, followed by aspergillosis and candidiasis.

Predisposing Factors

- Prolonged (>14 days) or severe (<100 cells/mm^3) neutropenia
- Hematologic malignancy, especially during induction phase of chemotherapy for acute myeloid leukemia
- Hematopoietic stem cell transplant (HSCT) recipients
- Graft-versus-host disease (GVHD)
- Corticosteroid therapy
- Solid-organ transplant (SOT) recipients
- T-cell immunodeficiency
- Smoking.

Clinical Manifestations of Fusariosis

Immunocompetent hosts have milder superficial disease, whereas immunosuppressed hosts have invasive/disseminated disease.

Clinical Manifestations in Immunocompetent Host (Table 30.1)

- *Onychomycosis and superficial cutaneous infections:* There is whitish, brownish, or yellowish discoloration of the nail, which is indistinguishable from onychomycosis produced by other fungi. Features favoring *Fusarium* as a causative pathogen include:

Table 30.1: Clinical manifestations of fusariosis.

Immunocompetent host	Immunocompromised host
- Onychomycosis - Keratitis - Mycotoxicosis - Allergic bronchopulmonary fusariosis - Cutaneous, sinusitis, thrombophlebitis, peritonitis, endocarditis, endophthalmitis (uncommon)	- Cellulitis - Sinusitis - Pneumonia - Disseminated fusariosis - Fungemia - Cerebritis - Endophthalmitis - Septic arthritis

- ◆ Predominantly toe-nail involvement rather than fingernail
- ◆ Acute/subacute paronychia
- ◆ Proximal subungual involvement
- ◆ *Tinea pedis*
- ◆ Intertrigo.

■ *Keratitis*: *Fusarium* is a common cause of fungal keratitis (Fig. 30.3). It can be due to poor ocular hygiene in contact lens users or due to traumatic inoculation. It was the causative pathogen for an outbreak amongst contact lens users due to a contaminated contact lens solution. The clinical features include pain, photophobia, and conjunctival injection. The eye is less inflamed compared with bacterial keratitis. Development of hypopyon is a late feature. Corneal perforation is a dreaded complication (Fig. 30.4).

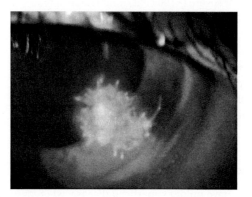

Fig. 30.3: Fungal keratitis.

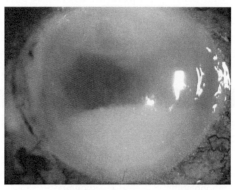

Fig. 30.4: Fungal hypopyon.

- Subcutaneous/deep infections: Patients with skin burns or pre-existing onychomycosis may develop subcutaneous involvement with abscess formation or cellulitis.
- *Fusarium* also causes localized infection, including endophthalmitis, cellulitis, arthritis, osteomyelitis, cystitis, and peritonitis in immunocompetent patients. Infection is caused by direct inoculation following trauma or instrumentation.

Clinical Manifestations in Immunocompromised Host (Table 30.1)

Disseminated infection is common in immunocompromised patients with underlying malignancy, burns, or neutropenia. It presents as fever that is unresponsive to antibiotics, multiple cutaneous lesions, rhinocerebral infection, pneumonitis, endophthalmitis, or pyomyositis.

- Cutaneous lesions due to disseminated fusariosis are present in 60–80% of hosts. These may present as:
  - Multiple erythematous subcutaneous nodules
  - Ecthyma gangrenosum, such as lesions with painful, erythematous macules, and papules with central necrosis
  - Red or gray macule with a central ulceration or black eschar that appears as a target lesion with a thin rim of erythema surrounding a papule or nodule
  - Extensive cellulitis of the extremities or the face.

  Lymphatic spread and dissemination are known. Metastatic skin lesions develop especially on the extremities. Lesions are multiple and can be in different stages of evolution. Bullae are very rare. Aspergillosis and mucormycosis can produce similar lesions.
- Sinusitis can be in isolation or as part of disseminated disease. It resembles aspergillosis or mucormycosis. Patient presents with nasal discharge, periorbital cellulitis, and destruction of nasal mucosa due to angioinvasive nature of the fungus.
- Pneumonia can be a primary presentation or secondary to disseminated disease. In the latter case, it tends to be bilateral. Lung involvement is seen in half of the patients with fusariosis. Presenting complaints include dry cough, dyspnea, and pleuritic chest pain.
- Fungemia is associated with high blood culture positivity as the fungus tends to sporulate in vivo and then spreads hematogenously. Central venous catheter infections may have fungemia without any organ involvement.
- Disseminated disease is frequent in the setting of severe/prolonged neutropenia. There can be cutaneous involvement with cellulitis, sinusitis, and pneumonitis. Fever is refractory to antibiotics, and blood culture is positive for *Fusarium*.

Similarities between Fusariosis and Aspergillosis

- Skin manifestations with necrosis and erythema
- Sinusitis with black eschar formation
- Vascular invasion and thrombosis, resulting in tissue infarction
- Hyaline septate hyphae with acute angle branching
- Spores present in air and soil.

Differences between Fusariosis and Aspergillosis

- Skin lesions are more frequent in patients with disseminated *Fusarium* infection rather than in disseminated aspergillosis.
- Lesions caused by *Fusarium* are smaller, numerous, widespread, and in various stages of evolution. *Aspergillus* lesions are larger, fewer, coalescing, and generally have a black eschar.
- Blood culture is positive frequently for *Fusarium* species, whereas culture positivity in aspergillosis is very low. *F. solani* is the most virulent and most frequently isolated species.

Differential Diagnoses

Keratitis

- Bacterial keratitis—*Staphylococcus*, *Streptococcus*, gram-negative bacilli, mycobacteria, *Nocardia* species
- Viral keratitis—herpes simplex virus, varicella zoster, adenovirus
- Fungal keratitis—*Candida, Aspergillus*
- Parasitic keratitis—*Acanthamoeba*
- Keratitis secondary to hypersensitivity reaction, autoimmune disorders, trauma.

Onychomycosis

- *Trichophyton rubrum*
- *Scopulariopsis brevicaulis*
- *Candida* species
- *Aspergillus* species.

Disseminated Fusariosis

- Aspergillosis
- *Paecilomyces* infection
- *Scedosporium* infection
- *Acremonium* species infection.

Laboratory Diagnosis

- Fungal culture is the gold standard for definitive diagnosis. The specimens that may be cultured include blood, nail scrapings, skin scrapings, corneal scrapings, skin biopsy, sputum, bronchoalveolar lavage, sinus aspirate, and cerebrospinal fluid (CSF). *Fusarium* grows much more easily on blood culture compared with *Aspergillus* and other opportunistic molds. Blood culture can be positive in 40–60% of patients since the fungus sporulates in vivo. Growth becomes positive on incubation of aerobic culture bottles for 3 days. It is important to use special stains, including Fontana–Masson stain for melanized fungi causing phaeohyphomycosis to avoid confusion. Culture is also important to rule out aspergillosis. Culture on potato dextrose agar produces white, pink, lavender, salmon, or gray-colored colonies that can be cottony or velvety.

- Histopathology examination of biopsy specimens shows hyaline septate hyphae with acute angle branching and adventitious sporulation (ability to sporulate in vivo in blood and tissues). Multicellular macroconidia are hyaline, banana or crescent shaped. Since the hyphae resemble those of aspergillosis and scedosporiosis, in situ hybridization and real-time polymerase chain reaction (PCR) help in species identification. Skin lesions are the most accessible tissue for biopsy.
- β-1,3,-D-glucan test is positive in fusariosis but does not aid in distinguishing it from other fungi, including *Candida* and *Aspergillus.*
- Radiological findings on chest radiography are nonspecific. Computed tomography (CT) findings include nodules or masses with absence of halo sign. CT scan is better imaging modality compared with X-rays in immunocompromised host and is preferred.
- Molecular-based techniques, including multiplex PCRs, panfungal PCR assays, and in situ hybridization techniques, have varying specificities and sensitivities and need further validation.

Treatment

Antifungal susceptibility testing may not necessarily help in guiding treatment as the clinical breakpoints are not well defined, and there is poor *in vitro* to *in vivo* correlation. Interpreting the minimum inhibitory concentrations data of antifungal agents for molds is inconclusive with no established breakpoints.

F. solani complex is frequently resistant to all azoles. Other species show variable response to azoles and amphotericin B. In immunocompromised host, therapy is initiated with voriconazole and liposomal amphotericin B (LAmB). Lipid formulations of amphotericin B have been successful in the treatment of some patients with invasive fusariosis. It is used at a dose of 3–5 mg/kg intravenous (IV) daily. Voriconazole is fungicidal against filamentous fungi. Posaconazole is recommended as salvage therapy. Voriconazole has been tried in combination with terbinafine in some patients. Therapeutic drug monitoring is required for voriconazole. There is intrinsic resistance to echinocandins. Isavuconazole is being evaluated for treatment of fusariosis.

Management of Onychomycosis

Treatment includes prolonged use of systemic antifungals or topical therapy along with nail avulsion in selected cases. Immunocompetent patients respond to itraconazole or terbinafine. Voriconazole and posaconazole have greater efficacy than itraconazole and terbinafine and are preferred in immunocompromised host. Topical amphotericin B may be used in unresponsive patients.

Management of Keratitis

The challenge with treating fusarial keratitis includes limited susceptibility of *Fusarium* to various antifungals, poor tissue penetration of topical antifungals, and potential complications, including corneal perforation and endophthalmitis. *F. solani* keratitis is associated with poor prognosis. Topical natamycin (5 mg/mL) has been traditionally used for keratitis. Amphotericin B (1.5 mg/mL) or topical voriconazole are used as alternatives. The eye drops are used hourly with subsequent dose modification based on response to therapy. Systemic therapy in hospitalized patients comprises IV voriconazole. The loading dose of voriconazole is 6 mg/kg IV every 12 h for two doses, followed by 4 mg/kg IV every 12 h. Oral voriconazole is used as a loading dose of 400 mg every 12 h, followed by 200 mg orally twice daily. Intracorneal injections are used in patients who are not responding to a combination of topical and systemic antifungals. Oral posaconazole may be used as salvage therapy. Therapy is continued till there is resolution of infiltrate and complete epithelial healing. The duration of therapy may vary from few weeks to months. Patients who are unresponsive may require keratoplasty.

Adjuvant Therapy

Other important measures in management of fusariosis include:
- Reversal of immunosuppression
- Removal of venous catheters associated with infection
- Extensive surgical debridement of affected tissues
- Granulocyte colony-stimulating factor or granulocyte-macrophage colony-stimulating factor to shorten the period of neutropenia
- Postponing further cytotoxic therapy if possible
- Evaluation and treatment of skin lesions, including treatment of onychomycosis.

Secondary Prophylaxis

Patients who have had a prior episode of fusariosis should receive secondary prophylaxis during periods of immunosuppression, including further chemotherapy, HSCT, or GVHD. Evaluate for residual disease by blood cultures and CT scan before starting immunosuppressive therapy. Drugs used for secondary prophylaxis include voriconazole, posaconazole, or LAmB.

Prevention of Fusariosis

- Fusariosis is an airborne and waterborne infection. The fungus is also isolated from tap water, wash basins, showers, and saunas. Identification of source is important for infection control in the hospitals. Avoid exposure of patients to contaminated tap water.
- Air quality in hospitals should be monitored. Use of high-efficiency particulate air filters and positive pressure ventilation should be encouraged.
- A thorough examination of the skin should be conducted on admission to the hospital. Onychomycosis and skin infections should be treated before starting immunosuppressive therapy.

Prognosis

The outcome of *Fusarium* infection is either resolution with recovery of neutropenia or death secondary to fulminant infection. Severe immunosuppression and neutropenia are associated with mortality rates up to 50–70%.

SCEDOSPORIOSIS

Scedosporium species cause disseminated infection in immunocompromised hosts.

Etiology

The species include:

- *Scedosporium boydii* (teleomorphic state—*Pseudallescheria boydii*)
- *Scedosporium apiospermum* (teleomorphic state—*Pseudallescheria apiosperma*)
- *Scedosporium prolificans*
- *Scedosporium aurantiacum*

These are ubiquitous fungi. *S. prolificans* grows as greyish-white to olive-gray colonies and cannot be truly a part of hyalohyphomycosis.

Pathophysiology

Scedosporium species are present in soil, polluted waters, manure, and compost. It is a saprophytic fungus with predilection for central nervous system (CNS) and infects the immunocompromised host.

Clinical Features

In immunocompetent host, *Scedosporium* infection causes eumycotic mycetoma, keratitis, otitis, sinusitis, soft-tissue infection, and bone involvement. Pneumonia has been reported following near-drowning in polluted water in an immunocompetent patient. CNS involvement follows trauma or contiguous spread from sinusitis.

However, in immunocompromised patients, infection is more severe and disseminated. Manifestations include endophthalmitis, sinusitis, pneumonitis, or meningitis. Meningitis is secondary to hematogeneous dissemination. Brain abscess formation is associated with high mortality.

Diagnosis

- Direct microscopy, culture, and histopathology reveal irregular branching, septate, hyaline hyphae resembling *Aspergillus*. Annelloconidia developing from the extruded end of the conidiophore may be present in the tissue. Use of selective media supplemented with cycloheximide allows growth of *Scedosporium* over other filamentous fungi (Fig. 30.5).
- Blood culture can be positive in half the patients.
- Chest radiography shows bilateral patchy nodular opacities, alveolar infiltrates, or consolidation. Cavitation or crescent sign are absent.
- Panfungal PCR and multiplex PCR may be used in combination with conventional laboratory tests. Species identification by MALDI-TOF and PCR needs further validation.

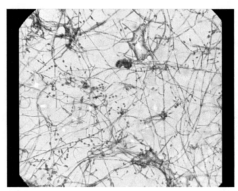

Fig. 30.5: *Scedosporium* species on LPCB mount with conidia arise alongside the hyphae.

Treatment

Voriconazole shows activity against *S. aurantiacum*. *P. apiosperma* shows variable susceptibility to itraconazole, voriconazole, posaconazole, and micafungin. *S. prolificans* is resistant to azoles, amphotericin B, and caspofungin.

Voriconazole is the first-line agent for therapy. It may be used alone or in combination with terbinafine. Some patients have been treated with voriconazole in combination with caspofungin. Therapeutic drug monitoring is recommended for voriconazole.

Surgical resection can be curative for a localized lesion. Amphotericin B may be used as intra-articular or intravitreal injections for arthritis and endophthalmitis, respectively.

Scedosporium prolificans has the worst outcome since it is pan-resistant to antifungals. Surgical debridement and early reversal of immunosuppression are recommended.

■ *PAECILOMYCES* SPECIES

The two important species responsible for infection in humans are *Paecilomyces lilacinus* and *Paecilomyces variotii*. These are rarely isolated as human pathogens. These cause infections including endophthalmitis, keratitis, and peritonitis in continuous ambulatory peritoneal dialysis patients.

Pathogenesis

Paecilomyces is an opportunistic saprophytic fungus also called the "bottle imp" since it resists sterilization and frequently contaminates sterile solutions, laboratory solutions, or moisturizing body lotions. It is found in soil and in contaminated medical supplies. It can be airborne. It causes iatrogenic infections during surgery or use of implants. Cases involving cataract surgery with intraocular lens implantation have been reported due to contamination of solution used during the surgery. The fungus may enter through a break in the skin in the cases with tinea pedis, onychomycosis, or indwelling catheters. *Paecilomyces* has also been isolated from air conditioning systems.

Paecilomyces infection is frequent in immunocompromised patients with SOT or bone marrow transplant, chronic granulomatous disease (CGD), lymphoma, corticosteroid use, or immunosuppressive therapy. A major outbreak of *P. lilacinus* was reported in a bone marrow transplant center, resulting in fatalities.

Clinical Features

Lower limbs are involved more frequently than the upper limbs due to the fungus remaining hidden in the toenails. Clinical features include macules, pustules, vesicles, or nodules. These can be confused with bacterial cellulitis or furunculosis. Satellite lesions may develop.

Immunocompromised patients may present with disseminated infection, fungemia, pneumonitis, or pyelonephritis.

Diagnosis

Confirmatory diagnosis of *Paecilomyces* infection is based on fungal culture and histopathology findings of the lesions. *P. lilacinus* produces reproductive structures, including phialides and conidia in infected tissues. This type of sporulation in infected tissue is known as adventitious sporulation. It is seen with *Paecilomyces*, *Fusarium*, and *Acremonium*. Species identification is essential because antifungal susceptibilities vary. *P. lilacinus* and *P. variotii* are the two species most frequently isolated, but other species causing infection include *Paecilomyces marquandii*, *Pipistrellus javanicus*, and *Psychotria viridis* (Figs. 30.6 and 30.7).

Treatment

Treatment includes removal of implant, vigorous debridement, and antifungal therapy for a successful outcome. *P. lilacinus* is intrinsically resistant to fluconazole, flucytosine, and amphotericin B but is susceptible to voriconazole and posaconazole. On the other hand, *P. variotii* is susceptible to amphotericin B.

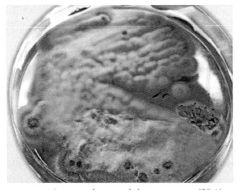

Fig. 30.6: Colony of *Paecilomyces* species on sabouraud dextrose agar (SDA).

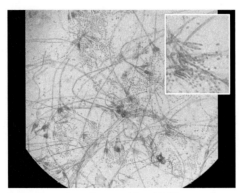

Fig. 30.7: *Paecilomyces* species on lactophenol cotton blue (LPCB) mount.

◾ *ACREMONIUM* SPECIES/*CEPHALOSPORIUM* SPECIES

These fungi cause nail infection, mycetoma, keratitis, osteomyelitis, peritonitis in dialysis patients, endocarditis in prosthetic valves, meningitis following CSF tap, and cerebritis in IV drug users. Disseminated *Acremonium* infections with features of peritonitis, cerebritis, and pneumonia have been reported in immunosuppressed patients.

Etiology

Species responsible for infection in humans are *Acremonium falciforme*, *Acremonium kiliense*, *Acremonium recifei*, *Acremonium strictum*, *Acremonium potronii*, *Acremonium murorum*, *Acremonium alabamense*, and *Acremonium roseogriseum*. More than 80% of human infections are caused by the first three. *Acremonium* growth on culture is slow, and cultures must be kept for at least 2 weeks to ensure the detection of the growth of the fungus.

Pathogenesis

Acremonium (Cephalosporium) species are environmental fungal contaminants and soil saprophytes but rarely cause disease in humans. They are most often considered laboratory contaminants. The fungus is angioinvasive and releases large volume of spores in the blood stream due to adventitious sporulation.

Clinical Features

Immunocompetent hosts suffer from mycetomas or fungal keratitis following skin or ocular trauma, respectively. Other manifestations include peritonitis and dialysis fistula infection, osteomyelitis, or meningitis following a spinal tap.

Immunocompromised patients suffering from hematological malignancies, CGD or SOT recipients may have pneumonia, CNS involvement, endocarditis or fungemia due to *Acremonium* species. Skin involvement includes cutaneous and subcutaneous nodules, painful violaceous papules with necrotic centers or skin/muscle abscesses.

Diagnosis

Definitive diagnosis requires isolation of the fungus by blood or tissue culture.

Treatment

Mycetoma requires surgical management. Voriconazole, posaconazole, and amphotericin B are recommended for use. Catheters implicated for infection should be removed.

■ *SCOPULARIOPSIS*

Scopulariopsis bears phylogenetic resemblance to *Scedosporium*.

Etiology

Scopulariopsis is a ubiquitous soil saprophyte. It has also been isolated from food, paper, beaches in California, caves in Mexico, and saunas in Germany. Eight species of *Scopulariopsis* have been reported as causing infection in humans (*Scopulariopsis acremonium*, *Scopulariopsis asperula*, *Scopulariopsis flava*, *Scopulariopsis fusca*, *Scopulariopsis koningii*, *Scopulariopsis brevicaulis*, *Scopulariopsis brumptii*, and *Scopulariopsis candida*). Some species of *Scopulariopsis* have either *Microascus* or *Kernia* teleomorphs (sexual states, perfect form) and have been reported under these names as human pathogens. The majority of cases of *Scopulariopsis* species infections in humans are due to *S. brevicaulis*.

Pathogenesis

The infection may result from inoculation and hematogenous spread. Lesions can be multifocal suggesting angioinvasion.

Clinical Features

Scopulariopsis species have an affinity for keratin and are associated with onychomycosis particularly involving large toenails. It differs from other dermatophytes as other toenails are not affected, and there is absence of tinea pedis. It also causes keratitis, otomycosis, sinusitis, and prosthetic valve endocarditis in healthy individuals.

In immunocompromised hosts, it has myriad presentations, including an eschar, exophytic ulcerative subcutaneous nodules, necrotic ulcers, cellulitis, or otomycosis. There can be lung involvement. Infection is severe and can be fatal.

Treatment

Scopulariopsis can be resistant to itraconazole, 5-fluorouracil, and fluconazole. It can be variably susceptible to amphotericin B, miconazole, and ketoconazole. Management includes surgical debridement and use of newer antifungals. Oral itraconazole, terbinafine, and topical natamycin are used for treating onychomycosis.

▚ *TRICHODERMA*

Although *Trichoderma* are ubiquitous soil saprophytes, they are being increasingly isolated in immunocompromised patients. The fungus is found in waterlogged soil, decaying vegetation, and damp buildings. The fungus is also present in food grains.

Etiology

Six species resulting in infections in immunocompromised hosts are *Trichoderma harzianum*, *Trichoderma koningii*, *Trichoderma longibrachiatum*, *Trichoderma pseudokoningii*, *Trichoderma citrinoviride*, and *Trichoderma viride*.

Pathogenesis

The fungus may be acquired by inhalation, inoculation, or ingestion of contaminated food grains.

Clinical Features

Risk factors for invasive *Trichoderma* include prolonged and severe neutropenia, prolonged use of broad-spectrum antimicrobial agents, corticosteroids, mucosal barrier damage, and transplantation. Skin lesions include ulcerated plaques especially at the site of IV line insertion. Disseminated *T. pseudokoningii* infection with skin, lung, and brain involvement

Table 30.2: Management of fungal endophthalmitis.	
Definition	Infection within the eye involving the vitreous and/or aqueous
Endogenous endophthalmitis	Fungal or bacterial seeding of the eye via the bloodstream. The posterior segment or choroid is involved first, followed by the anterior segment
Exogenous endophthalmitis	Infection enters the eye from outside following eye surgery, trauma, or keratitis. The aqueous is involved first, and the vitreous/posterior segment may or may not get involved
Etiology	Bacterial Fungal—*Candida, Fusarium, Aspergillus, Cryptococcus, Paecilomyces lilacinus, Scedosporium apiospermum, Lecythophora mutabilis, Sporothrix, Coccidioides*
Epidemiology	Common in tropical countries, including India
Symptoms	Red eye, pain, photophobia, floaters, scotomas, visual loss
Signs	Chorioretinal lesions, hemorrhage and choroidal neovascular membranes, retinal detachment, retinal necrosis, iridocyclitis, hypopyon
General principles of treatment	▪ Vitrectomy ▪ Intravitreal and/or intracameral injections ▪ Removal of foreign material ▪ Antifungal treatment

Contd...

Contd...

Vitrectomy	▪ Surgical removal of part of vitreous is done under LA and sedation using a vitrector to cut and aspirate. Balanced salt solution is infused into the vitreous cavity to maintain IOP. Vitreous washings are sent for microbiology studies. Intravitreal antibiotics are injected. In case retina is not visualized or patient is too sick, needle aspirate of vitreous sent for tests ▪ Important for reducing the fungal burden in the eye ▪ In case aqueous alone is involved, aqueous is aspirated and samples sent. Apart from intracameral injections, intravitreal injections are given to prevent spread to vitreous
Keratoplasty	May be required in the case of extensive mold involvement of cornea, corneal melting, and impending perforation
Removal of foreign material	Intraocular lens introduced during cataract surgery or any foreign body causing trauma should be removed to avoid persistent infection or relapse
Intravitreal antifungals	Intravitreal AmBd—5–10 µg in 0.1-mL sterile water, may be repeated a few days later up to a maximum cumulative dose of 30 µg to avoid retinal toxicity Intravitreal voriconazole—100 µg in 0.1-mL sterile water
Intracameral antifungals	In the cases with severe aqueous involvement, AmBd 5 µg in 0.1-mL sterile water or voriconazole 50–100 µg in 0.1-mL sterile water used as multiple injections. It may cause transient pain, inflammation, or hypopyon formation
Topical antifungals	Voriconazole 1% or AmBd 0.15% solution is not commercially available and has to be prepared for use. Penetrate through the debrided cornea and are used as adjunctive therapy
Antifungal therapy	▪ Voriconazole is the drug of choice and achieves vitreous concentration 40% of plasma levels. Active against *Aspergillus*, *Fusarium*, and other molds. Systemic amphotericin B has little role in treatment of exogenous endophthalmitis. ▪ LAmB achieves higher vitreous concentration than AmBd. Measure voriconazole levels 1 week after initiating therapy. IV caspofungin has been used in *Aspergillus* endophthalmitis, but echinocandins have no role in *Fusarium* infection. ▪ Fluconazole not recommended due to poor activity against molds. Intraconazole has low vitreous levels. Posaconazole is used as salvage therapy.

AmBd, amphotericin B deoxycholate; IOP, intraocular pressure; IV, intravenous; LA, local anesthesia; LAmB, liposomal amphotericin B

has been reported in a bone marrow transplant recipient. The fungus can disseminate after mucosal damage in the oral cavity or intestine. The fungus may involve the lung, liver, bowel, bone, or brain.

■ *BLASTOSCHIZOMYCES CAPITATUS*

Blastoschizomyces capitatus was earlier known as *Geotrichum capitatum* and *Trichosporon capitatum*. *Blastoschizomyces capitatus* is found in soil and in feces of pigeons. It is present as normal human skin flora and also in the respiratory and digestive tract mucosa.

In immunocompetent host, *B. capitatus* causes onychomycosis. Leukemic patients receiving intensive chemotherapy causing neutropenia develop invasive disease. It resembles invasive candidiasis. From the gastrointestinal and respiratory tract the fungus spreads by hematogenous route and localizes in the skin and lungs. Patients may develop pruritic rash, papules, nodules, gingival ulcers, or nodular pneumonia.

Patients may have hepatosplenomegaly with microabscesses, deranged liver function test, and bull's-eye lesions on ultrasound similar to those in hepatosplenic candidiasis.

Chest scans reveal pulmonary nodular infiltrates with a crescent sign.

CONCLUSION

Treatment for hyalohyphomycosis can be curative in normal hosts but difficult to treat in immunosuppressed. It can be refractory to conventional antifungals. The choice of antifungals and the duration of therapy have not been well defined. Therapy should be continued till there is complete resolution of clinical and laboratory findings, discontinuation of immuno-suppression, recovery from neutropenia, and resolution of significant GVHD.

CLINICAL PEARLS

- Organisms causing hyalohyphomycosis include various species of *Fusarium, Penicillium, Scedosporium, Acremonium, Paecilomyces, Scopulariopsis, Basidiomycota, Schizophyllum, Beauveria, Trichoderma, Chaetoconidium, Chrysosporium*, and *Microascus*.
- The fungi can be resistant to conventional antifungals and management, including combined medical and surgical approach (Table 30.2).

SUGGESTED READING

1. Lingappan A, Wykoff CC, Albini TA, et al. Endogenous fungal endophthalmitis: causative organisms, management strategies, and visual acuity outcomes. Am J Ophthalmol. 2012;153:162-6.
2. Tortorano AM, Richardson M, Roilides E, et. al. ESCMID and ECMM joint guidelines on diagnosis and management of hyalohyphomycosis: *Fusarium* species, *Scedosporium* species and others. Clin Microbiol Infect. 2014;20:27-46.

Section **5**

INVASIVE FUNGAL INFECTIONS

31

Invasive Fungal Infections: Definitions
(Based on EORTC/MSG Consensus Group Recommendations)

Monica Mahajan

▨ INVASIVE FUNGAL DISEASE

Invasive fungal disease (IFD) is classified as a disease process caused by a fungal infection when adequate diagnostic evaluation of the infectious disease process rules out an alternative etiology.

Revised definitions of IFD have been provided by the *European Organization for Research and Treatment of Cancer/Invasive Fungal Infections Cooperative Group* and the *National Institute of Allergy and Infectious Diseases Mycoses Study Group* (EORTC/MSG) consensus group.

Definitions for "proven" and "probable" IFD have been revised to include recent advances in indirect tests if they have been standardized and validated.

"Possible" IFD includes those cases that are highly likely to be caused by a fungal etiology but lack mycological evidence.

The criteria for "probable" and "possible" IFD are based on:
- The host factors
- Clinical manifestations
- Mycological evidence.

These definitions do not apply to *Pneumocystis jiroveci* infections.

Host Factors

Host factors imply characteristics that predispose an individual to acquire IFD. Host factors include:
- Recent neutropenia temporally related to the onset of invasive fungal infection
- Allogenic stem cell transplant recipient
- Prolonged corticosteroids use (excluding among patients with allergic bronchopulmonary aspergillosis) at a mean minimum dose of 0.3 mg/kg/day of prednisone equivalent for >3 weeks
- Human immunodeficiency virus
- Solid organ transplant
- Connective tissue disorders

- Hereditary immunodeficiencies, such as chronic granulomatous disease or severe combined immunodeficiency
- Use of immunosuppressive agents, including chemotherapeutic drugs, calcineurin inhibitors, antilymphocyte antibodies, anti–tumor necrosis factor-α drugs, monoclonal antibodies, such as alemtuzumab or nucleoside analogs, in the past 90 days.

Fever has been excluded from the new definitions as a host factor since it is a clinical feature and not a host factor.

Clinical Criteria

The clinical criteria are no longer divided into major and minor criteria but are now based on objectively verifiable evidence including medical imaging that indicate that the disease is consistent with IFD (Table 31.1).

For example, patients with computed tomography or ultrasound lesions typical of chronic disseminated candidiasis were earlier labeled "probable," hepatosplenic candidiasis without

Table 31.1: Clinical Criteria for IFD	
Clinical criteria	*Signs*
Lower respiratory fungal disease	The presence of one of the three following signs on CT: 1. Dense, well-circumscribed lesions with or without a halo sign 2. Air crescent sign 3. Cavity
Tracheobronchitis	Tracheobronchial ulceration, nodule, pseudomembrane, plaque, or eschar seen on bronchoscopic analysis
Sinonasal infection	Imaging showing sinusitis plus at least 1 out of 3 signs: 1. Acute localized pain, including pain radiating to eye 2. Nasal ulcer with black eschar 3. Extension from the paranasal sinus across bony barriers including into the orbit
CNS infection	One of the following two signs: 1. Focal lesions on imaging 2. Meningeal enhancement on MRI or CT
Disseminated candidiasis	At least 1 of the following 2 entities after an episode of candidemia within the previous 2 weeks: 1. Small, target-like abscesses or bull's-eye lesions in liver or spleen 2. Progressive retinal exudates on ophthalmologic examination
CNS, central nervous system; CT, computed tomography; MRI, Magnetic resonance imaging.	

any need for mycological support. Now they are reclassified as "possible" IFD. Patients with invasive pulmonary aspergillosis have focal pulmonary infiltrates with at least one macronodule with or without a halo sign. This may be used as clinical criteria to support the diagnosis of IFD.

Mycological Criteria

Mycological criteria include direct tests including cytology, direct microscopy or culture, including mold in sputum, bronchoalveolar lavage (BAL), bronchial brush, or sinus aspirate samples indicated by the following:

- Presence of fungal elements indicating a mold
- Recovery by culture of a mold-like *Aspergillus, Fusarium, Zygomycetes,* or *Scedosporium* species

A case may be classified as "probable" pulmonary IFD, if the BAL fluid yields *Aspergillus, Zygomycetes, Fusarium,* or *Scedosporium* species or other pathogenic molds as mycological support in the presence of appropriate clinical evidence and host factors.

Indirect tests are included if they are validated and standardized. The thresholds recommended by the manufacturer are being relied on for interpretation of results. Since it has been standardized, the *Platelia Aspergillus galactomannan* enzyme immunoassay has been approved for plasma, serum cerebrospinal fluid (CSF), and BAL. β-D-Glucan detected in serum is present in fungal disease other than cryptococcosis and zygomycosis.

On the other hand, polymerase chain reaction-based tests and molecular techniques for detecting fungi are not included as they have not been standardized and validated.

▨ PROVEN INVASIVE FUNGAL DISEASE

Proven IFD requires demonstration of fungal elements in diseased tissue. It does not rely on the host factors or clinical features. The revised definition includes indirect assays that are highly specific for a fungal infection being detected. In the case of culture positivity the results include both the genus as well as the species.

Proven aspergillosis requires both culture and identification; otherwise, it is labeled "proven mold IFD."

Molds

- Microscopic examination of specimen from a sterile site: Histopathologic, cytopathologic, or direct microscopic examination of a specimen obtained by needle aspiration or biopsy demonstrates hyphae or melanized yeast-like forms accompanied with the evidence of tissue damage. Grocott-Gomori methenamine silver or periodic acid–Schiff (PAS) stain are useful in delineating the fungal structures. Wet mounts from sites of infection should be stained with fluorescent dyes, including calcofluor or blankophor, whenever possible.
- Culture of a specimen for a mold obtained by a sterile procedure from a normally sterile and clinically or radiologically abnormal site consistent with an infectious disease process excluding culture from BAL fluid, a cranial cavity sinus specimen or urine.

- Blood culture that yields a mold-like *Fusarium* spp. in the context of a compatible infectious disease process. Recovery of *Aspergillus* from blood culture invariably represents contamination.
- Serologic analysis of CSF is not applicable for molds.

Yeasts

- Microscopic examination of specimen from a sterile site: Histopathologic, cytopathologic, or direct examination of a specimen obtained by needle aspiration or biopsy from a normally sterile site other than mucous membranes shows yeast cells, e.g. encapsulated budding yeasts in the case of *Cryptococcus* species and *Candida* species showing pseudohyphae or true hyphae. *Candida*, *Trichosporon*, and yeast-like *Geotrichum* species and *Blastoschizomyces capitatus* may also form pseudohyphae or true hyphae. Grocott-Gomori methenamine silver or PAS assist in identifying the fungus. Wet mounts are stained with fluorescent dyes, including calcofluor and blankophor, whenever possible.
- Growth of yeast by culture of a sample obtained by a sterile procedure, including a freshly placed drain, placed less than 24 h ago, from a normally sterile site showing a clinical or radiological abnormality consistent with an infectious disease process.
- Blood culture that yields yeast, e.g. *Candida* spp. or *Cryptococcus* or a yeast-like fungus, e.g. *Trichosporon* spp.
- Serologic analysis of CSF for cryptococcal antigen indicates disseminated cryptococcosis.

PROVEN IFD: ENDEMIC DIMORPHIC FUNGI

For endemic dimorphic fungi the histological appearance is characteristic for each fungus to form a definitive diagnosis (Table 31.2).

HISTOPATHOLGY

Histoplasma capsulatum needs to be distinguished from *Candida glabrata* or *Leishmania* by histopathology demonstrating characteristic granulomatous inflammation in histoplasmosis with silver staining demonstrating the presence of this fungus.

The presence of coccidioidal antibody in CSF is sufficient criteria for "proven" coccidioidomycosis.

Table 31.2: Proven IFD for endemic dimorphic fungi.

Endemic dimorphic fungus	Histological appearance
Histoplasma capsulatum	Small intracellular budding yeasts
Coccidioides spp.	Spherules
Paracoccidioides brasiliensis	Large yeasts with multiple daughter yeasts in a 'pilot-wheel' configuration
Blastomyces dermatitidis	Thick-walled, broad-based budding yeasts

The demonstration of capsular antigen in CSF is sufficient for the diagnosis of proven disseminated cryptococcosis.

Urinary *Histoplasma* antigen is present not only in the cases with histoplasmosis but also in patients with coccidioidomycosis and blastomycosis and is considered insufficient evidence for diagnosing proven histoplasmosis.

PROBABLE INVASIVE FUNGAL DISEASE

Probable IFD cases require the presence of:
- A host factor
- Clinical features
- Mycological evidence.

POSSIBLE INVASIVE FUNGAL DISEASE

Possible IFD includes those cases that have:
- Appropriate host factor
- Sufficient clinical evidence of IFD
- *Lack* mycological evidence.

This category has limited value for inclusion in clinical trials, evaluation of diagnostic tests, or collection of epidemiological data. Every effort should be made to upgrade these patients to a category of probable or proven IFD.

LIMITATIONS OF REVISED INVASIVE FUNGAL DISEASE DEFINITIONS

- These definitions are more applicable for immunocompromised hosts but may not apply to the other categories of patients admitted in the intensive care unit since the appropriate host factors can be different.
- The definitions cannot replace the clinical, histopathological, and radiological descriptions and criteria for classifying IFDs.
- In case there is inadequate evidence to meet the criteria of IFD, it does not altogether exclude the diagnosis. There can be more evidence available later on in the course of the disease to support the diagnosis. This limits the practical use of these definitions in daily clinical practice and cannot be used as a guide for clinical practice. These definitions are more useful for studying the epidemiology of IFD and for testing efficacy of therapeutic regimens and strategies.

CLINICAL PEARLS

- Invasive fungal disease may be proven, probable, or possible.
- These definitions help in testing efficacy of therapeutic regimens and strategies and also in collecting epidemiological data of IFD.

■ SUGGESTED READING

1. Badiee P, Hashemizadeh Z. Opportunistic invasive fungal infections: diagnosis & clinical management. Indian J Med Res. 2014;139(2):195-204.
2. De Pauw B, Walsh TJ, Donnelly JP, et al. Revised definitions of invasive fungal disease from the European Organization for Research and Treatment of Cancer/Invasive Fungal Infections Cooperative Group and the National Institute of Allergy and Infectious Diseases Mycoses Study Group (EORTC/MSG) consensus group. Clin Infect Dis. 2008;46:1813-21.
3. Tsitsikas D, Morin A, Araf S, et al. EORTC/MSG definitions for invasive fungal disease on the rates of diagnosis of invasive aspergillosis. Med Mycol. 2011;50:538-42.

32

Invasive Cutaneous Fungal Infections

Sunil Choudhary, Soumya Khanna, Raghav Mantri,
Prateek Arora, Rohit Jain, Shaunak Dutta

INTRODUCTION

Invasive fungal infections of the skin and soft tissue are increasingly being seen with the rising incidence of diabetes and growing use of immunosuppressive drugs for many conditions, including organ transplants. The common organisms are *Candida*, *Aspergillus*, and zygomycetes (mucormycosis). Infections due to mucormycosis can present as pulmonary, rhinocerebral, cutaneous, gastrointestinal, and disseminated forms.

The objective of this chapter is to highlight mainly cutaneous mucormycosis and its management because it happens to be the most common form of invasive cutaneous infections and carries high morbidity and mortality. Mucormycotina is found universally all over the world in farmlands, forests, garden soils, and decaying organic materials. Common species of cutaneous mucormycosis are *Mucor*, *Rhizomucor*, *Rhizopus*, and *Lichtheimia* (previously called *Absidia*).

Predisposing factors for invasive skin and soft-tissue fungal infections are patients with hematological malignancies, diabetes, cirrhosis, and renal failure, which all cause immunocompromised status in the host body. Patient on anti-tumor necrosis factor-α therapy are also at risk of developing invasive cutaneous infections. Patients with primary immunodeficiency disorders are vulnerable to invasive fungal diseases. Patients with dyserythropoietic iron overload are another unique group with high risk of invasive fungal infections.[1,2] The presence of invasive fungal infection in any patient should prompt further investigations to rule out any immunodeficiency disorder.

Even patients with normal immune status can fall prey to invasive cutaneous fungal infections, especially after burns and trauma. Many such cases have been reported in significant numbers after natural calamities, such as tsunami.

EPIDEMIOLOGY

Mucormycosis is a rare condition, and its incidence is difficult to calculate accurately but seems to be rising in recent years.[3,4] An estimated 500 cases occur in the Unites States annually.[5] The incidence is appearing to be rising due to increased immunocompromised state and excessive use of antifungal drugs prophylactically.[6,7] An audit of all the soft tissue

Flowchart 32.1: Enumerates the common fungal subphylum and species of pathogenic cutaneous mucormycosis.

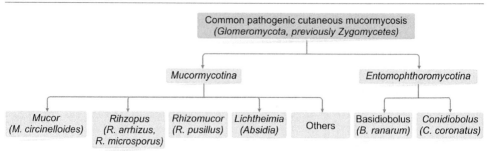

infections reported by our microbiology laboratory over 2 consecutive years showed that fungal infections constituted less than 4% of all isolates and consisted only mucormycosis and aspergillosis (Flowchart 32.1).

An Indian study of 38 patients done by Bala et al.[8] claimed that the frequency of cutaneous mucormycosis was 31% and rhino-orbital mucormycosis was 61.5%, which was comparable to a larger study of 178 patients done by Chakrabarti et al.[9] who found that rhino-orbito-cerebral type (54.5%) was the most common presentation, followed by cutaneous (14.6%).

In a study by Lanternier et al.,[10] the mortality rate with invasive cutaneous fungal infections was found to be very high at 22% but still lower than the other forms, such as rhinocerebral and pulmonary fungal infections.

In a review of 929 patients by Roden et al.,[4] 24% of cutaneous infections were deep involving muscle, tendon, or bone. About 20% of patients with primary cutaneous fungal infection developed hematogenous spread, resulting in a mortality of 94%. In a reverse scenario, cutaneous involvement from primary disseminated fungal infection was found to be very low (6 patients out of 220 cases).

PATHOGENESIS

Cutaneous mucormycosis generally occurs after direct inoculation of spores from the environment following a *trauma* or *burns*. Many reports of wounds with invasive fungal infection came in highlight after *natural calamities*, such as tsunami, as they are present in decaying matter, wood, soil, cotton, bread, fruits, vegetables, and animal excreta. Gardening is also a common source of fungal spore inoculation. Other unusual sources of infection reported were adhesive tape, wooden tongue depressors, ostomy bags, building construction contamination, vascular devices, and nitroglycerine patches.[7]

Patients with *end-stage renal disease* have high iron overload, and desferrioxamine is routinely given in them, which acts like a siderophore for mucorales causing its proliferation because iron is an essential element for fungal cell growth and development.

Patients with *hematological malignancies* have low count of mononuclear polymorphonuclear phagocytes that are responsible for inhibiting germination of spores. The *Mucor* species have high affinity for vessels and which is its hallmark.

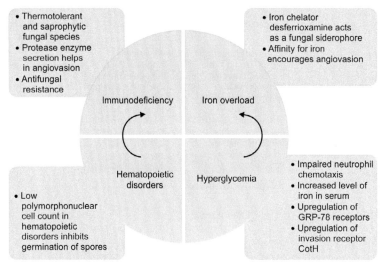

Fig. 32.1: Host and pathogen factors responsible for mucormycosis.

In patients with *diabetic ketoacidosis*, there are multiple mechanisms that facilitate invasive fungal infection:

- Acidic pH dissociates iron from protein, leading to free iron delivery to fungus.
- Hyperglycation of iron-sequestering proteins, which results in free iron in blood.
- Hyperglycemia upregulates glucose-regulated protein 78 epithelial receptor that binds to fungus and facilitates tissue penetration.
- Activation of coat protein H, a fungal protein which binds to mammalian receptor to initiate invasion in host cells.
- Hyperglycemia induces poorly characterized defects in phagocytosis.[11,12]

The invasive fungal infections are associated with high mortality. The cause for this mortality is multifactorial that is environmental, host, and virulence of the fungus (Fig. 32.1). Figure 32.2 depicts the natural progression of the disease in patients with poor immunity. The pathogen is usually acquired from the immediate environment. The *Mucor* is thermotolerant saprophytic organisms that thrive well in body temperature. Many of these fungi acquire virulent genes aiding angioinvasion by secreting protease enzyme. The antifungal resistance in patients receiving prophylactic antifungals makes them more susceptible to more virulent and resistant variety of invasive fungus. Poor polymorphonuclear cell functions in hyperglycemia and hematological malignancies further enhance the spread of fungus in the host. Angioinvasion eventually causes tissue infarction, necrosis, and then death (Fig. 32.2).[4]

CLINICAL PRESENTATION

The common sites affected by cutaneous mucormycosis are arms and legs as these are easily accessible. However the other sites reported are face scalp, back, thorax, abdomen, perineum, breast, and neck. The mechanism is mostly due to the direct inoculation from surrounding environment.

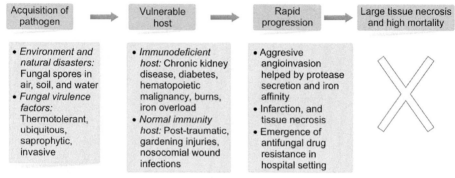

Fig. 32.2: Natural history of progressive invasive mucormycosis.

Clinical manifestations are classified as follows:

- Primary mucormycosis
- Secondary mucormycosis.

Primary Mucormycosis

In a primary disease, there is a direct inoculation in skin; whereas in secondary disease, there is local spread or dissemination from other sites, such as in rhinocerebral mucormycosis. Primary mucormycosis can present as localized, deep, or disseminated form. Most of these cases remained localized to the total depth of the skin, with 24% showing extension to bone or muscle, and 20% developing hematogenous dissemination to other noncontiguous organs.[4,13]

It usually starts as cellulitis and progresses to necrosis and eschar formation. The eschar is progressive, which is indicative of vascular invasion. Other presentations include targetoid lesions, tender nodules, ulcers, purpuric lesions, and swollen and scaly plaques. The onset may be gradual or fulminant and may take days to years.

Secondary Mucormycosis

Secondary mucormycosis develops following rhinocerebral or disseminated mucormycosis. It begins as sinusitis and extends intraorally as eschar or in the orbit as orbital cellulitis, proptosis, and loss of vision. Here they present as necrotic eschars with blackish ulcers and foul odor from the mouth. It has a cute onset and is associated with high mortality. The final stage can involve intracranial extension. The disease has three stages:[13]

1. *Stage I*: Disease restricted to sinonasal area
2. *Stage II*: Sino-orbital infections
3. *Stage III*: Disease with intracranial infiltration

Stage III is associated with mortality of 62%.[4]

◼ DIFFERENTIAL DIAGNOSES

Aspergillosis versus Mucormycosis

Aspergillosis and mucormycosis are both cutaneous fungal infections; thus, it is important to determine the species for correct antifungal management. Aspergillus infection mainly affects lung and cutaneous manifestations are a secondary phenomenon after severe dissemination. These infections are common in immunodeficient hosts. They can be hospital acquired from intravenous cannula or injection sites, bandages, or even adhesive tapes. Primary cutaneous invasive aspergillus infections are seen in patients with burns. They usually present as deterioration in burn wound with eschar formation and local cellulitis. Microscopic examination and *polymerase chain reaction (PCR)* can differentiate it from mucormycosis. *Voriconazole* is usually the first line of treatment. It is also important to differentiate mucormycosis from aspergillosis since mucormycosis usually show in vitro resistance to some of the new antifungal drugs and voriconazole and capsofungin.[13]

Systemic Nonfungal Conditions versus Mucormycosis

The other conditions that need to be differentiated from mucormycosis are autoimmune disorders, drug reactions, and bacterial synergistic infections—anthrax, tuberculosis, neoplasms, and infiltrative diseases, such as Wegener's granulomatosis. The history and biopsy from the ulcer will help distinguish from mucormycosis.[12]

Secondary mucormycosis with rhinocerebral extension mimics lymphomas, rhinoscleromas, and sinusitis. These may be differentiated from biopsy and microscopic examination. Table 32.1 summarizes the differential diagnosis.

Mycetoma versus Mucormycosis

Mycetoma is another differential diagnosis. It is a localized long-standing granulomatous infection of soft tissue with extension into bones. It is endemic in tropics and subtropics. The infection is acquired from the soil, after a penetrating injury, in those who walk barefoot. Mycetoma can be caused by fungus or actinomycetes bacteria. However, the presentation and clinical course is different from *Mucor* infections. It starts as a cutaneous or subcutaneous swelling with multiple nodules. These nodules may suppurate and drain through sinuses discharging grains during its

Table 32.1: Differential diagnosis of mucormycosis.		
Disorder	*Clinical presentation*	*Treatment strategy*
Cutaneous aspergillosis	▪ Most commonly cutaneous lesions present secondary to disseminated aspergillosis ▪ Hospital acquired in immunodeficient hosts ▪ Predilection for IV catheter sites, surgical wounds, and burns ▪ Microscopy and histopathology can differentiate	▪ Azole derivatives, such as voriconazole and itraconazole ▪ Amphotericin B in nonresponders
Autoimmune disorders, vasculitis	▪ History of nonhealing chronic painful ulcer ▪ Biopsy from the ulcer can differentiate	Appropriate immunotherapies
Drug reactions	▪ History of drug intake ▪ Acute onset ▪ Biopsy from the lesion can differentiate	▪ Cessation of drug ▪ Wound dressings ▪ Supportive therapies
Bacterial infections, such as anthrax, tuberculosis	Microscopic examination and tissue culture	Antibiotics with or without surgical debridement
IV, Intravenous		

Table 32.2: Differences between mucormycosis and mycetoma (Madura foot).

Fungal factors	Invasive cutaneous mucormycosis	Mycetoma or Madura foot
Organisms and species	Glomeromycota	Eumycetoma (Fungal), Actinomycetoma (Bacteria)
Host factors	Commonly seen in patients with poor immunity	Seen in farmers in tropical climate who walk barefoot
Clinical manifestation	Mostly acute presentation with rapid progression. With cellulitis and eschar formation. The spread is horizontal with angioinvasion. No colored granules seen in the wound	Mostly chronic presentation with osteomyelitis and discharging spores from the sinuses extruding colored spores. The infection is localized and mostly spread in vertical direction involving bone. Wound shows colored granules (spores) which can differentiate fungal or bacterial species. *Eumycetomas* ▪ *Black grains: Madurella mycetomatis* ▪ *Pale grains: Petriellidium boydii, Aspergillus nidulans, Aspergillus flavus* *Actinomycetomas* ▪ *Red grains: Actinomadura pelletieri* ▪ *Yellow grains: Streptomyces somaliensis* ▪ *Pale grains: Nocardia brasiliensis, Nocardia cavae, Nocardia asteroides, Actinomadura madurae*
Patient outcome	High mortality	Low mortality but risk of loss of limb
Treatment	Surgery with antifungals, such as amphotericin and voriconazole	Fungal infection mandates antifungal drugs, such as ketoconazole, iatraconazole with local wound debridement or amputation in severe cases. Bacterial infections settle with cotrimoxazole and streptomycin.

active phase. The characteristic feature of mycetoma is extrusion of colored granules from the sinus tract, which are organism specific. Between the abscesses/nodules, there are extensive granulation tissues, resulting in deformity that mimics neoplasm. Infections often involve bone, resulting in osteomyelitis. The diagnosis is made clinically, and culture from granules identifies the agent correctly. Imaging of the limb is also required to rule out osteomyelitis. Cytology, histology, and immunodiagnostics are organism specific to guide appropriate treatment. Table 32.2 enlists the differentiating features of mycetoma and mucormycosis.

■ LABORATORY DIAGNOSIS

Quick Direct Microscopy with Potassium Hydroxide Mount

Tissue impression smear from the wound edges or biopsy from the center of the lesion may be taken for direct microscopy with 10% potassium hydroxide mount. *Mucor* species are characterized by aseptate, hyaline, hyphae with irregular branching at right angles, mainly at the periphery of the lesion (Fig. 32.3). Microscopic features are nonspecific, and differential diagnosis with other filamentous fungi must be considered.

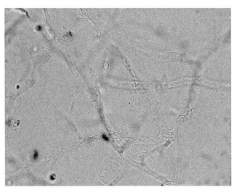

Fig. 32.3: Direct microscopy image of *Mucor* species with potassium hydroxide (KOH) mount. Note the broad aseptate hyphae with right angle branching.

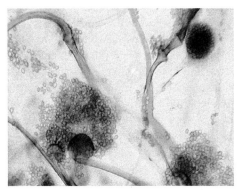

Fig. 32.4: *Rhizopus* fungal culture growth wooly texture, dark grayish brown colonies. Sporangiophores are produced singly or in group of four measuring around 8 µm. The sporangia are spherical bluish black in color, columella is pyriform. Rhizoids are present.

Histopathology

Biopsy is taken from the center of the lesion with subcutaneous fat. One part is sent in saline to microbiology, and another part is sent to the pathology laboratory in formalin solution. Histopathology typically reveals fungal hyphae, tissue edema, thrombosis, infarction, and necrosis with fungal hyphae. The interstitial infiltrate is flooded with polymorphonuclear cells, plasma cells, and eosinophils.

Fungal Culture

Sabouraud and potato dextrose agar media without antibiotics are preferable culture media for fungal growth. Culture can take a long incubation time of up to 6 weeks and hence is often not helpful in treating acute cases. (Fig. 32.4)

Quantitative Polymerase Chain Reaction Assay

The positive yield of fungal cultures even for cases where histopathology shows fungal elements, has been very low. *PCR assays can help in accurate diagnosis by detecting fungal DNA in biopsy specimens even when cultures are negative.* It makes very early diagnosis possible and can be used as a screening tool in very high-risk patients. As PCR is highly specific and hence can accurately differentiate between the various fungal species, which is extremely helpful in deciding the class of antifungals for the treatment.[12]

■ MANAGEMENT

The treatment of invasive cutaneous mucormycosis involves multimodality approach. It includes aggressive antifungal regime for an adequate duration, radical debridement, and treatment of predisposing underlying disease. ***In spite of aggressive management, the results may be dismal with high mortality.*** The medical management must be initiated after proper identification of species. The duration of drug dosages is protocol based generally lasting 6–8 weeks.

Liposomal amphotericin B is the most common and effective drug in mucormycosis, which is also the first-line treatment. Minimum recommended dosage is 5 mg/kg/day (range 3–10 mg/kg/day). High dose of 10 mg/kg/day can cause nephrotoxicity (Table 32.3).[14]

Use of deoxycholate amphotericin B is usually discouraged; however, it is still used where resources are limited. Posaconazole is recommended in patients with refractory diseases or in the cases in intolerance to amphotericin or previous therapy (Table 32.3).

Caspofungin with amphotericin B formulation may be combined in a limited number of patients with rhinocerebral mucormycosis who are diabetic.

The recommendations in children are similar to adults. There is no substantial data or trials specific for pediatric population.

In the patients with hematological malignancy, deferasirox 20 mg/kg/day is the recommended iron chelator, for enhancing the efficacy of liposomal amphotericin. These patients also require granuloctye colony-stimulating factor to cure infection due to neutropenia.

Table 32.3: Recommended antifungals in mucormycosis.	
Antifungal drug	*Dosage and route*
Amphotericin B deoxycholate	*Intravenous* Standard dose 0.25–0.75 mg/kg/day Severe cases 1.0–1.5 mg/kg/day
Liposomal amphotericin B	*Intravenous* 5–10 mg/kg/day
Amphotericin B lipid complex	*Intravenous* 5–7.5 mg/kg/day
Posaconazole	*Per oral* 400 mg bid
Isavuconazole	*Per oral, intravenous* 200 mg tid for 6 doses, then 200 mg qd
bid, bis in die (twice daily); tid, ter in die (thrice daily); qd, quaque die (once daily)	

Glucocorticosteroid treatment is a risk factor for infection, and it should be avoided. If it is not possible, then dose should be reduced to minimum.

Role of hyperbaric oxygen therapy—This can be used as an adjunctive treatment along with aggressive debridement and antifungal therapy. The quality of evidence is limited on its benefits and recommended optimal duration to make it a standard of care. The value of this therapy should be considered on individual basis.[14]

Based on the need for differential medical and surgical management, the patients may be grouped into three distinctive types (Flowchart 32.2):

1. *Group I*: Patients with locally aggressive infections that can be acquired after trauma or local inoculation from the environment—in primary type, or the spread from contiguous structures, such as rhino-cerebro-orbital mucormycosis like in secondary type. These patients must be treated with radical debridement and systemic antifungals. The debridement may mandate multiple revisions.
2. *Group II*: Patients usually have localized indolent or chronic infection which starts like a nodule and slowly increases in size. Such lesions may be managed by wide excision may suffice with a cover of azoles.
3. *Group III*: Patients with multiple wounds due to systemic fungal infections fall in Group III wherein systemic antifungals and aggressive treatment of underlying cause suffice. The prognosis is generally poor in such patients.[15]

The wound due to invasive fungal infections may require multiple debridements as the fungal elements infiltrate the vessels at the microscopic level and may be difficult to eliminate with naked eye. The wound must be assessed during and after debridement for fungal growth with fungal culture

Flowchart 32.2: Surgical management plan of invasive fungal cutaneous infections based on groups.

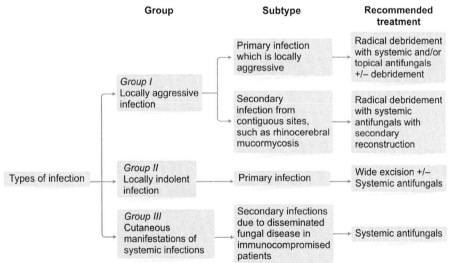

and biopsy. The negative margins must be confirmed on biopsy from the edge of the wound prior to definitive reconstruction of the defect. The wound bed may be prepared with negative pressure wound therapy once the biopsy is negative. Wound once covered with healthy granulation tissue can be covered with skin grafting of local flaps. Wounds where critical structures, such as bone, vessels, or tendons, are exposed, covering the defect with flap may be required. Large cavities will also require cover with muscle or fasciocutaneous flap. Abdominal full thickness defects will require reconstruction with component separation and mesh repair (Flowchart 32.3).

Florid infection of the limb may result in amputation of the part, depending on the extent of involvement and condition of the patient (Figs. 32.5A and B).

Complex facial defects will require free microvascular flap reconstruction with anterolateral thigh flap, free fibula flap, or radial forearm flap (Figs. 32.6A to F).

Flowchart 32.3: MIRACLES *algorithm* for surgical management of invasive cutaneous fungal infection.

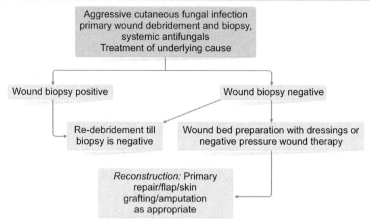

Aggressive cutaneous fungal infection primary wound debridement and biopsy, systemic antifungals Treatment of underlying cause

Wound biopsy positive

Wound biopsy negative

Re-debridement till biopsy is negative

Wound bed preparation with dressings or negative pressure wound therapy

Reconstruction: Primary repair/flap/skin grafting/amputation as appropriate

Courtesy: Max Institute of Reconstructive, Aesthetic, Cleft & Craniofacial Surgery (MIRACLES), New Delhi, India.

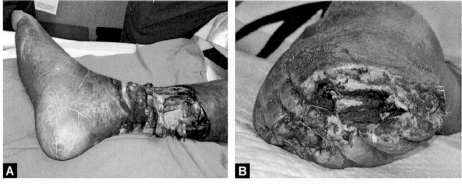

Figs. 32.5A and B: (A) Primary invasive mucormycosis in a patient with chronic kidney disease. Note all the compartments of the leg were involved with necrotic bone; (B) Post-below-the-knee amputation showing regrowth of fungus in the stump after 48 hours. The patient then underwent above knee amputation. The patient expired due to systemic spread of fungus and multiorgan failure.

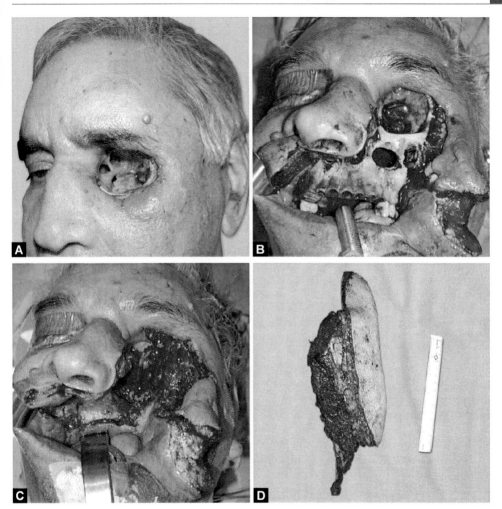

Figs. 32.6A to D: (A) Case of diabetes with rhino-orbital mucormycosis (treated) post-exenteration with maxillary bone osteomyelitis; (B) Note the necrotic maxilla and orbit. There was granulation tissue over the orbital roof; (C) Residual defect after extensive debridement; (D) A free microsurgical anterolateral thigh musculocutaneous flap measuring 20 cm × 7 cm elevated to fill the defect and reconstruct the maxilla and orbit.

CONCLUSION

Invasive fungal cutaneous infections are a challenging problem to treat with high mortality rates. Poor local host factors and virulence of the fungus are the factors responsible for its recalcitrant nature. They cause severe local destruction, leading to secondary deformities that may be difficult to correct. It is important to differentiate the fungal species to start appropriate

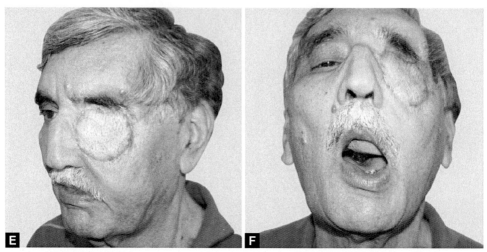

Figs. 32.6E and F: Post-reconstruction pictures of the same patient with free double paddle anterolateral thigh musculocutaneous flap. Reconstruction of both palate and orbital defect was achieved at the same sitting.

antifungal, which play a synergistic role in treatment along with wound debridement. Classification of the wounds into locally aggressive, indolent, and cutaneous manifestation of systemic infections also aids in management. The successful treatment encompasses multispecialty team approach comprising a physician, microbiologist, and reconstructive team working in synchronization aggressively (Figs. 32.4 to 34.6).

■ CLINICAL PEARLS

- Mucormycosis is the most common fungal cutaneous infection. Affinity for iron and release of protease enzyme encourages angioinvasion that is responsible for high mortality and morbidity.
- Predisposing factors are patients with hematological malignancies, diabetes, cirrhosis, and renal failure on desferrioxamine therapy.
- Microscopy with potassium hydroxide mount and fungal culture is a quick aid for diagnosis; however, PCR assays help in accurate diagnosis by detecting fungal deoxyribonucleic acid in biopsy specimens even when cultures are negative.
- Based on the need for differential medical and surgical management, the patients may be grouped into three distinctive types:
  Group I: Aggressive local infections,
  Group II: Indolent infections, and
  Group III: Systemic manifestations of local infection. These groups can be subclassified into primary and secondary types.
- Medical management with liposomal amphotericin B is the first-line treatment with optimization of underlying medical disorders.

- Surgical management of the wound usually requires multiple debridement followed by staged reconstruction of the defect depends on the wound bed and loss of tissue.

REFERENCES

1. Lanternier F, Cypowyj S, Picard C, et al. Primary immunodeficiencies underlying fungal infections. Curr Opin Pediatr. 2013;25(6):736-47.
2. Camargo JF, Yakoub D, Cho-Vega JH. Successful treatment of primary cutaneous mucormycosis complicating anti-TNF therapy with a combination of surgical debridement and oral posaconazole. Mycopathologia. 2015;180(3-4):187-92.
3. Guinea J, Escribano P, Vena A, et al. Increasing incidence of mucormycosis in a large Spanish hospital from 2007 to 2015: epidemiology and microbiological characterization of the isolates. PLoS One. 2017;12(6):e0179136.
4. Roden MM, Zaoutis TE, Buchanan WL, et al. Epidemiology and outcome of zygomycosis: a review of 929 reported cases. Clin Infect Dis. 2005;41:634-53.
5. Holzheimer RG, Dralle H. Management of mycosis in surgical patients—review of literature. Eur J Med Res. 2002;7(5):200-26.
6. Kontoyiannis DP, Lewis RE. Agents of mucormycosis and entomophthoromycosis. Mandell, Douglas and Bennett's Principles and Practice of Infectious Diseases, 7th edition. Philadelphia, PA: Churchill Livingstone; 2010. pp. 3257-69.
7. Petrikkos G, Skiada A, Drogari-Apriranthitou M. Epidemiology of mucormycosis in Europe. Clin Microbiol Infect. 2014;20(Suppl 6):67-73.
8. Bala K, Chander J, Handa U, et al. A prospective study of mucormycosis in North India: experience from a tertiary care hospital. Med Mycol. 2015;53(3):248-57.
9. Chakrabarti A, Das A, Mandal J, et al. The rising trend of invasive zygomycosis in patients with uncontrolled diabetes mellitus. Med Mycol. 2006;44(4):335-34.
10. Lanternier F, Dannaoui E, Morizot G et al. A global analysis of mucormycosis in France: the RetroZygo Study (2005–2007). Clin Infect Dis. 2012;54(Suppl 1):S35-43.
11. Binder U, Maurer EC, Lass-Florl C. Mucormycosis—from the pathogens to the disease. Clin Microbiol Infect. 2014;20(Suppl 6):60-6.
12. Spellberg B. Mucormycosis pathogenesis: beyond *Rhizopus*. Virulence. 2017;8(8):1481-2.
13. Castrejón-Pérez AD, Welsh EC, Miranda I, et al. Cutaneous mucormycosis. An Bras Dermatol. 2017;92(3):304-11.
14. Cornley OA, Arikan-Akdagli S, Dannaoui E, et al. ESCMID and ECMM joint clinical guidelines for the diagnosis and management of mucormycosis 2013. Clin Microbiol Infect. 2014;20(Suppl 3):5-26.
15. Heinz T, Perfect J, Schell W, et al. Soft tissue fungal infections: surgical management of 12 immuno-compromised patients. Plast Reconst Surg. 1996;97(7):1391-98.

33

Invasive Fungal Infections in Neutropenic Cancer Patients

Pramod Kumar Julka , Shaik Maheboob Hussain, Tarun Mohindra

INTRODUCTION

Prolonged or profound neutropenia in cancer patients, myelodysplasia, and aplastic anemia, is associated with a high rate of invasive fungal infection (IFI) that adds to the morbidity and mortality in this group of patients. The mortality rate may increase by 50–100%. This is especially true in cases with hematological malignances, hematopoietic stem cell transplantation (HSCT), dose-intensive chemotherapy regimens, and corticosteroid use. There is a recent trend toward non-*albicans Candida, Aspergillus*, and rare fungi being responsible for IFI in this group. Increasing drug resistance amongst these pathogens is a major challenge. On the other hand, diagnostic techniques and imaging have made significant advances in the past two decades facilitating the diagnosis of these infections. The armamentarium of available antifungals has expanded to help prevent and treat these IFIs. Echinocandins for managing invasive candidiasis and voriconazole for invasive aspergillosis (IA) have improved survival rates.

EPIDEMIOLOGY

Invasive fungal diseases (IFDs) in cancer patients remain an important complication causing considerable mortality and morbidity. The risk of IFI depends on the primary diagnosis of neoplasm as well as the degree of immunosuppression of the host. Fungal infections evolve while treatment of underlying malignancies with newer chemotherapies, and new biological agents negatively impact the protective immune system. Outcome for patients with IFDs depends on the type of cancer and its treatment. It is essential that clinicians assess both the general risks of IFDs in a particular patient and the specific local risks within the context of hospital practices, patient populations, and local infection control effectiveness. There are subgroups within cancer risk groups that have even higher or lower risks for IFDs.

The overall frequency of IFIs in patients with acute leukemia and following allogeneic HSCT (the patient populations at highest risk) is between 10% and 25%; the overall case fatality rate exceeds 50% and is close to 100% in disseminated infections or persistent neutropenia. Neutropenic enterocolitis and pneumonia are associated with poor prognosis.

PATHOGENESIS

Neutropenia can be consequent to:
- Chemotherapeutic agents
- Radiotherapy
- Bone marrow failure in myelodysplasia and aplastic anemia
- Infiltration of bone marrow with malignant cells

Neutropenia is associated with an increase in incidence of IA and other IFIs. Profound neutropenia with absolute neutrophil count <100 increases risk of IFIs manifold. Neutropenia is also associated with lymphopenia and impaired cell-mediated immunity. Agents, including fludarabine, are cytotoxic for cluster of differentiation 4+ lymphocytes. Corticosteroids impact cytokine and chemokine expression, oxidative function thereby affecting the capacity of neutrophils to cause hyphal damage for filamentous fungi. Steroids also impair phagocytic activity of macrophages.

Use of broad-spectrum antibiotics in neutropenic patients may change the intestinal flora and promote fungal invasion.

Fever can be the only clinical manifestation of IFI in some neutropenic patients, whereas 30% neutropenic patients with IFI may remain afebrile.

RISK FACTORS AND FREQUENCY OF INFECTIONS

Multiple risk factors account for the increased frequency of IFDs.

The most important risk factor for the development of fungal infection includes patients with:
- Hematologic malignancies [with or without bone marrow transplant (BMT)], severe and prolonged neutropenia
- Chronic graft-versus-host (GVHD) disease
- Immunosuppressive therapy, including steroid use. Prednisone use equivalent to 0.5 mg/kg for longer than 1 month duration significantly increases risk of IFI
- Multiple courses of broad-spectrum antibiotic therapy
- The presence of vascular access catheters
- Parenteral nutrition
- Colonization at multiple sites
- Prolonged intensive care unit stay
- Environmental exposure (hospital construction sites, contaminated cooling/heating systems) can also be a significant contributory factor.

Candida and *Aspergillus* species have accounted for most of yeast and mold infections reported in immunocompromised cancer patients. However, in the last decade, there has been a perceptible emergence of non-*Candida* yeast, non-*fumigatus Aspergillus* species, yeast-like organisms (*Trichosporon beigelii* and *Blastoschizomyces capitatus*), hyaline molds (including *Fusarium* species, *Pseudallescheria boydii*, *Paecilomyces* species, and *Scedosporium* species), zygomycetes, and the phaeohyphomycoses from various cancer centers around the world.

Histoplasma capsulatum, Blastomyces dermatitidis, and *Coccidioides immitis* cause more severe and disseminated disease in the neutropenic cancer host.

Yeast-like organisms resemble *Candida* in their clinical spectrum and dissemination. The filamentous fungi cause embolic skin lesions and fungemia. The hyaline molds disseminate through the bloodstream.

Increased awareness, improved blood culture techniques, and the advent of high-resolution imaging techniques have had considerable impact on improving the clinical diagnosis of IFDs. In spite of these advances, however, IFDs remain difficult to diagnose and to manage, and there is a continuing and urgent need for improved diagnosis, treatment, and prevention.

OPTIONS FOR PREVENTING INVASIVE FUNGAL INFECTION IN CANCER PATIENTS

The approaches include the following:
- Implementation of a strict handwashing policy to prevent nosocomial fungal infections
- High-efficiency particulate air filters and positive air pressure
- Avoid construction activities in vicinity of the patient care areas.
- Chemoprophylaxis—Use of fluconazole as chemoprophylaxis at a dose of 400 mg/day has been shown to be effective in allogeinic BMT recipients in decreasing frequency and severity of invasive candidiasis and gut-related GVHD, thereby providing a survival benefit. Fluconazole (400 mg/day) and itraconazole (2.5 mg/kg administered orally twice daily) are effective in preventing IFI and break through candidemia despite colonization by *Candida* species in patients undergoing remission induction chemotherapy for hematological malignancies. The main disadvantage and concern with use of chemoprophylaxis is the selection of drug-resistant non-*albicans Candida* species, such as *Candida glabrata* and *Candida krusei,* and a nosocomial spread of these pathogens. Efficacy of antifungal agents as chemoprophylaxis for aspergillosis is less well established. Use of voriconazole chemoprophylaxis has caused increased incidence of fungal pathogens belonging to the *Mucorales, Fusarium,* and *Scedosporium* species.
- Empiric antifungal therapy may be considered in high-risk neutropenic patients with allogeneic HSCT or hematologic malignancies who present with persistent/recurrent fever in spite of being treated with appropriate broad-spectrum antibiotics. Liposomal amphotericin B (LAmB) has been approved for this indication. Voriconazole has shown comparative efficacy with lesser nephrotoxicity. Fluconazole is not active against molds and cannot be a good option. Trials are being conducted on empiric use of echinocandins and newer triazoles. The Infectious Diseases Society of America recommends empirical antifungal therapy if a neutropenic patient remains febrile for >5 days despite use of broad-spectrum antibiotics.

TREATMENT OF FUNGAL INFECTIONS IN NEUTROPENIC CANCER PATIENTS

Yeast-like Fungi

Trichosporon Species

Trichosporon is an extremely rare but one of the important emerging pathogens in immunocompromised cancer patients causing IFDs. Most common species associated with disseminated trichosporonosis is *T. beigelii* of which *T. asahii* is the most important.

These species are normal commensals of the human respiratory and gastrointestinal tract as well.

Risk factors:
- Hematological malignancy
- Hematopoietic stem cell transplantation
- Hemochromatosis or other iron overload conditions.

Clinical features: *Trichosporon* often coexists with other opportunistic fungi and has been frequently associated with fungemia and skin lesions; pneumonia, catheter-related infections, and funguria; prosthetic valve infections, peritoneal dialysis catheter-associated peritonitis, brain abscess; and ventriculo-meningeal infections, prosthetic joint infections, renal failure, and disseminated infections (Figs. 33.1A and B).

Diagnosis:
- Bronchoalveolar lavage (BAL) and tissue cultures are frequently negative.
- Blood cultures occasionally are positive for yeast-like forms, and hence, diagnosis relies on histopathological examination of tissue specimens (hyphae and pseudohyphae with characteristic arthroconidia).
- Serum galactomannan antigen or 1,3-β-D-glucan testing
- Molecular diagnosis using panfungal polymerase chain reaction (PCR) assay
- Matrix-assisted laser desorption ionization–time-of-flight (MALDI-TOF) mass spectrometry appear promising.
- It may result in false-positive cryptococcal antigen test due to cross-reactivity.

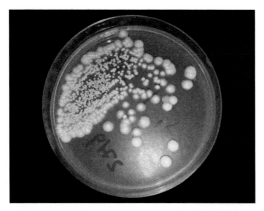

Fig. 33.1A: Colony of *Trichosporon* species on sabouraud dextrose agar (SDA).

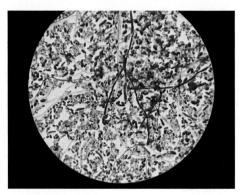

Fig. 33.1B: *Trichosporon* species on Gram stain.

Management strategies for disseminated trichosporonosis:

- Poorly defined due to paucity of clinical data
- Amphotericin B, fluconazole, miconazole, and ketoconazole have been used in the past with variable success rates.
- Voriconazole has been used with limited success.
- Resistant to triazoles and polyenes due to biofilm produced by the species
- Treatment with a combination of LAmB and caspofungin with a successful outcome in a patient who had breakthrough infection on voriconazole.
- Data with posaconazole is insufficient except for a liver transplant patient with disseminated *Trichosporon mucoides* who responded well to posaconazole therapy.
- Several antifungal combinations of polyene with azoles (ketoconazole, miconazole, and fluconazole) or 5-flucytosine (5-FC) have been reported in literature with variable success rates.
- It has low virulence with an associated mortality rate of approximately 12%.

Rhodotorula Species

Rhodotorula rubra and *Rhodotorula mucilaginosa* are red yeasts that were long considered to be nonpathogenic saprophytic organisms but have now been identified as pathogens in immunocompromised patients.

Risk factors:

- Indwelling central venous catheter
- Hematological or solid organ cancers
- Corticosteroid or cytotoxic chemotherapy
- Prolonged hospitalization for >1 month and exposure to broad-spectrum antibiotics for more than 1-month duration.

The most common presentation is catheter-related fungemia.

Diagnosis:
- Standard culture methods
- Panfungal PCR.

Management:
- Good response to amphotericin therapy with or without catheter removal
- Reduction in immunosuppressive therapy plays a crucial role in management.
- Successful treatment with catheter removal alone without antifungal therapy has also been reported.
- These fungi are capable of producing biofilms that make more resistant to antifungal therapy.
- Polyenes are the drug of choice with amphotericin B exhibiting the lowest minimum inhibitory concentration (MIC) of ≤1 µg/mL, compared with azoles and echinocandins that have poor activity against these yeasts (voriconazole MIC90 4 µg/mL; caspofungin MIC ≥ 64 µg/mL; fluconazole >4 µg/mL).
- Breakthrough infections with *Rhodotorula* species have occurred in patients receiving azole or echinocandin prophylaxis that is partly attributed to its intrinsic resistance to these antifungal agents.
- Posaconazole (MIC50 0.25 mg/L) and flucytosine (MIC50 0.12 mg/L) have demonstrated good in vitro activity but data on clinical efficacy is lacking.

Malassezia Furfur

The classical presentation is pityriasis versicolor and folliculitis.

Risk factors: Increased incidence of infection is reported in neonates, children, and immuno-compromised cancer patients; particularly those requiring lipid-containing parenteral nutrition. This is likely related to the lipophilic nature of the yeast with lipids presumably providing growth factors required for replication.

Clinical features: In cancer patients, it causes invasive infections, including catheter-related fungemia. The fungus causes colonization of intravenous catheters with subsequent dissemination.

Diagnosis: Standard microbiological culture: The yield is improved by adding olive oil to the culture plates.

Management:
- Imidazoles and triazoles have a variable in vitro susceptibility pattern with MIC in the range of 0.03–16 mg/L and cannot be used in serious infections.
- *Malassezia* breakthrough pachydermatitis has been reported on posaconazole prophylaxis in a patient with acute myeloid leukemia. The antifungal drug of choice with the most available clinical data is amphotericin B although the fungus has been shown to be resistant to the same in some studies. Catheter removal is in general associated with the best outcome.

Geotrichum Capitatum (Formerly Blastoschizomyces Capitatus)

G. capitatum is a yeast ubiquitous in nature and like *Candida* species is a normal flora of the human respiratory and gastrointestinal tracts and has been isolated from sputum and feces of healthy humans. Mode of infection is inhalation or ingestion.

Risk factors:
- Profound, prolonged neutropenia in hematological malignancies
- Disseminated infections in immunocompromised patients, particularly those with hematological cancers
- Broad-spectrum antibiotic exposure.

Diagnosis:
- Standard microbiological identification, culture on SDA (Figs. 33.2A and B)
- MALDI–TOF
- Galactomannan assays
- Molecular diagnosis based on PCR analysis is under evaluation.

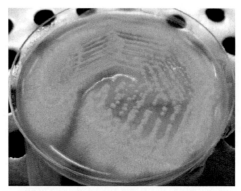

Fig. 33.2A: Dry, creamy, hairy colonies of *Geotrichum* species on SDA.

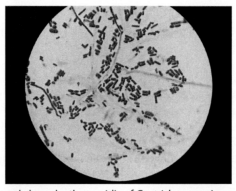

Fig. 33.2B: Rectangular or barrel-shaped arthroconidia of *Geotrichum* species on Gram stain.

Management:

- Polyenes and voriconazole have demonstrated good in vitro antifungal activity.
- Amphotericin B has been the drug of choice.
- Clinical success with voriconazole alone or in combination with amphotericin B has been reported in literature.
- Breakthrough infections in patients on caspofungin prophylaxis have occurred due to its intrinsic resistance to echinocandins.
- A combination of voriconazole and caspofungin was successfully tried in a case of probable geotrichosis in a leukemic patient.
- Despite appropriate therapy, geotrichosis has an extremely poor prognosis with a mortality rate approaching 60–75%.

Candida Species

Risk factors:

- Approximately half of the patients with hematological malignancy or those undergoing HSCT have *Candida* colonization at baseline. About 15% of these will develop candidemia or acute disseminated candidiasis in the absence of chemoprophylaxis. The mortality rate may range from 50% to 100%.
- Degree of neutropenia
- High Acute Physiology and Chronic Health Evaluation II score
- Indwelling/central venous catheters
- Hypogammaglobulinemia.

There is a recent surge of cases with non-*albicans Candida* infections. A multicenter study in patients with hematological malignancies conclude that 87.5% infections were caused by non-*albicans Candida* species; of which, *Candida parapsilosis* was the most frequent. Fluconazole chemoprophylaxis has resulted in an overall decrease in incidence of invasive candidiasis.

Since *Candida* is present as a part of endogenous microbiome, any disruption of alimentary tract mucosa and mucositis will permit *Candida* to invade the bloodstream. This is especially true in leukemia patients.

Clinical features:

- Oropharyngeal and esophageal candidiasis
- Acute disseminated candidiasis with deep tissue involvement
- Fungemia/candidemia
- Hepatosplenic/chronic disseminated candidiasis.

Diagnosis:

- Blood culture, including BacT/Alert
- Detection of $1,3$-β-D-glucan
- Imaging, including ultrasonography, computed tomography (CT) scan, and magnetic resonance imaging (MRI) for invasive disease
- Nucleic acid amplification-based techniques for diagnosis and detection of resistance.

Treatment:

- *C. glabrata* can be resistant to all triazoles. *C. krusei* is resistant to fluconazole. Patients of allogeneic HSCT who are on fluconazole chemoprophylaxis are treated with LAmB as the breakthrough infection is more likely to be due to fluconazole-resistant *Candida*, including *C. glabrata* and *C. krusei*. *C. parapsilosis* is associated with infection of central venous catheters. *Candida tropicalis* is frequently responsible for disseminated disease with cutaneous lesions, circulatory collapse, and renal failure. Choice of antifungal depends on the susceptibility testing. Since most patients have been exposed to fluconazole, voriconazole, or posaconazole as part of chemoprophylaxis, the echinocandins are the drugs of choice for initial therapy. *Candida albicans* can be treated with echinocandin followed by fluconazole.
- Removing indwelling catheters whenever feasible may or may not improve outcomes since the most common portal of entry remains the gastrointestinal tract. In patients with a multilumen catheter, the antifungal drug should ideally be administered through all the lumens if the catheter is not being removed.
- On recovery of neutropenia, the patient needs to undergo an ophthalmological examination and abdominal imaging for potential complications including, visual loss and chronic disseminated candidiasis, respectively. Liver and spleen develop multiple target lesions. The patient may present with new-onset fever after neutropenia has already recovered. Chronic disseminated candidiasis is not a contraindication for further chemotherapy.
- Patients with hemodynamic instability, persistent fungemia, and disseminated disease may benefit from a combination therapy with LAmB and 5-FC.
- Echinocandins and newer triazoles show efficacy against invasive candidiasis.
- Management of oropharyngeal candidiasis includes clotrimazole troches and fluconazole.
- Esophageal candidiasis is treated with fluconazole, whereas refractory cases require an echinocandin. Patients with *C. glabrata* and *C. krusei* may have persistent odynophagia if the strains are fluconazole resistant.

Mold/Filamentous Fungi

Aspergillus Species

Most common cause of IA include:
- *Aspergillus fumigatus*
- *Aspergillus terreus*
- *Aspergillus flavus*
- *Aspergillus niger*
- *Aspergillus lentulus*
- *Aspergillus ustus.*

Several cancer centers around the world have reported the emergence of *A. niger*, *A. flavus*, and *A. terreus* over the last several years, which is thought to be a consequence of the widespread use of voriconazole prophylaxis in cancer patients.

Non-*fumigatus Aspergillus* species have a variable susceptibility pattern to the available antifungal agents. *A. flavus*, *A. ustus*, and *A. lentulus* are known to have higher MIC to voriconazole.

Risk factors:

- Clinical syndromes associated with aspergillosis in patients with preexisting lung disease include allergic pulmonary aspergillosis, chronic necrotizing aspergillosis, and aspergilloma.
- Prolonged neutropenic phase in the early post-HSCT period (13% of mismatched allograft recipients. Profound or recurrent neutropenia increases risk.

However, recent observations have noted a shift in the time of occurrence of IA with late-onset disease being increasingly reported in the following groups:

- Unrelated HSCT with GVHD requiring intense immunosuppression with corticosteroid
- Lymphopenia/T-cell-depleted patients
- Respiratory viral infections, including cytomegalovirus disease.

Clinical features:

Invasive aspergillosis mainly involves the lungs and paranasal sinuses and can be the most common cause of pneumonia-related mortality in allogeneic HSCT recipients. Patients present with fever, sinus congestion, cough, hemoptysis, or pleuritic chest pain.

Diagnosis (Fig. 33.3):

- Demonstration of the acute-angle septate hyphae from histopathological examination of tissue from tissue biopsy specimens.
- Bronchoscopy, followed by culture of the BAL, has a poor sensitivity of 30–50%.
- Noninvasive techniques, such as galactomannan antigen by double-sandwich enzyme-linked immunosorbent assay and β-D-glucan. Serial monitoring of galactomannan levels in neutropenic patients monitors response to therapy.
- Polymerase chain reaction analysis for identification of fungal DNA directly from blood and BAL can be a valuable diagnostic tool for IA.

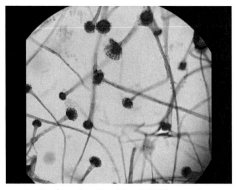

Fig. 33.3: *Aspergillus* species on Lactophenol cotton blue (LPCB) mount.

- In patients with invasive pulmonary aspergillosis, a combination of high-resolution CT scan of the thorax with galactomannan antigen testing of bronchoalveolar fluid after fiberoptic bronchoscopy (more sensitive than serum) and serum may aid in earlier diagnosis and better outcome.
- The CT scan findings include pulmonary nodules or infiltrates with halo sign in neutropenic phase and the air crescent sign in the neutrophil recovery phase although these are not entirely specific for aspergillosis and may be seen with other molds as well. Early phase scans may be nonspecific and may only demonstrate air-space consolidation. The pneumonia may be lobar or segmental and may result in cavitation.
- Computed tomography scan/MRI of sinuses shows opacification of sinuses, bony, and septal version and involvement of hard palate, orbit or central nervous system (CNS).

Treatment: The drugs at present approved for the treatment of IA include polyenes, voriconazole, and the latest addition isavuconazole. Voriconazole is the drug of choice. It is useful not only for management of IA but also shows efficacy against hyaline and dematiaceous filamentous fungi.

Amphotericin B (conventional or its lipid formulations) may be preferred in certain clinical situations as follows:
- Previous use of a mold-active agent for prophylaxis or empiric therapy
- Concomitant use of drugs with major interactions with voriconazole (cytochrome 450 interaction), such as tacrolimus, sirolimus, rifampin, or warfarin
- Hepatic impairment
- Adverse effects to voriconazole
- High suspicion for concomitant infection with zygomycosis or other mold that may not be susceptible to voriconazole. About 10–15% patients with proven IA may have a coinfection with another mold.
- Presence of cardiac risk factors, such as prolonged QT interval or cardiomyopathy.

Posaconazole has been approved for prophylaxis of IA in acute leukemia and HSCT. It is used as salvage therapy for refractory IA.

Isavuconazole is the novel addition to the antifungal armamentarium with several advantages over voriconazole, such as (1) fewer drug interactions, (2) fewer adverse effects, (3) availability of water-soluble parenteral formulation, (4) excellent oral bioavailability, and (5) excellent pharmacokinetic parameters.

All echinocandins show efficacy against *Aspergillus* infection. Echinocandins, although approved exclusively for salvage therapy, have also been evaluated for primary therapy against IA. The overall response rate to caspofungin or micafungin monotherapy for IA ranges from 50% to 56% and has been dismal. Combination of voriconazole with echinocandins improves response and outcomes.

Non-*fumigatus Aspergillus* species, including *A. terreus*, can be resistant to treatment with amphotericin B.

Surgery is lifesaving in clinical manifestations involving progressive sinusitis, endophthalmitis, endocarditis, CNS lesions, and skin/soft tissue infections. It prevents extension to contiguous tissues as well as hematogenous dissemination. Surgery may be performed even while neutropenia is present.

Secondary prophylaxis is indicated if the patient needs to undergo HSCT or further cycles of chemotherapy.

Scedosporium Species

Scedosporium apiospermum (the asexual form of *P. boydii*) and *Scedosporium prolificans* are two of the most common species associated with infections in cancer patient, which are found in soil and decaying organic matter.

Risk factors:
- Neutropenia
- Immunosuppression in post-transplant period.

Clinical features: Spectrum of infection in immunocompromised hosts includes:
- Pneumonia
- Cutaneous infections
- Invasive fungal sinusitis
- Brain abscess
- Osteomyelitis
- Endophthalmitis
- Disseminated scedosporiosis with septic shock.

Diagnosis:
- Conventional culture
- Morphological characterization of isolates from histopathological examination of tissue
- MALDI–TOF mass spectrometry has aided in the rapid diagnosis of these infections.
- Antigen-based diagnostic tests and molecular tools for microbiological detection are under investigation.

Management:
- All species of *Scedosporium* are resistant to polyenes.
- Triazoles have good efficacy against *S. apiospermum*. Cross-resistance has been reported among all triazoles except posaconazole.
- Echinocandins have demonstrated good in vitro antifungal activity against *S. apiospermum*, although clinical data is insufficient.
- The combination of voriconazole and terbinafine was efficacious with successful outcome in an orthopedic infection.
- Most published reports are on the successful use of voriconazole, data on posaconazole use is scarce, but it has been used with favorable outcome.
- A reduction in immune-suppressive therapy and surgical resection of localized lesions, if feasible, must be an integral part of management of these difficult-to treat-fatal infections.
- *S. prolificans* is resistant to all systemic antifungals.

Fusarium Species

Among the 50+ species reported so far, only the ones which are pathogenic include the following:

- *Fusarium oxysporum* species complex
- *Fusarium solani* species complex (*most common*)
- *Fusarium verticillioides*
- *Fusarium moniliforme*
- *Fusarium dimerum*
- *Fusarium proliferatum*

Risk factors:

- High-dose corticosteroid therapy
- Severe T-cell dysfunction
- Prolonged neutropenia.

Clinical features:

- Cutaneous infections, including onychomycosis and cellulitis
- Brain abscess
- Invasive fungal sinusitis
- Fungemia or disseminated infections with hepatic, ophthalmic, or joint involvement.
- *F. solani* is considered to be the most virulent of all fungal pathogens reported.
- The fungus may gain entry into the host through the periungual/soft tissue infection or through sinopulmonary tract.

Diagnosis:

- Histopathological examination of tissue specimens where the presence of acute dichotomously branching septate hyphae along with yeast-like structures in tissue (adventitious sporulation) is strongly suggestive of fusariosis.
- A positive $1,3$-β-D-glucan test with a negative galactomannan antigen test in the appropriate clinical context is highly suggestive of fusariosis.
- MALDI–TOF mass spectrometry has good sensitivity and specificity.
- Molecular testing using PCR is still in development and not standardized.

Treatment:

- *F. solani* and *F. verticillioides* are usually resistant to triazoles.
- *F. oxysporum* and *F. moniliforme* can be susceptible to voriconazole and posaconazole. Most species are resistant to polyenes. Posaconazole (minimal data) has demonstrated modest success rates.
- Combination of amphotericin B with caspofungin, voriconazole or terbinafine, and voriconazole plus terbinafine has been tried with variable success rates.
- Granulocyte transfusions, granulocyte-colony stimulating factor (G-CSF), and granulocyte-macrophage colony-stimulating factor (GM-CSF) have also been employed as adjuncts in combination with antifungal agents and can be lifesaving.

Zygomycetes

- Zygomycosis is an aggressive and often lethal infection, which occurs most commonly in immunocompromised patients representing 5-20% of all IFIs in this population.
- Etiological agents reported in order of frequency are *Rhizopus* species and *Mucor* species, followed by *Lichtheimia* and *Rhizomucor*.
- Illness is rapidly progressive with angioinvasion and tissue infarction (hallmark features of this disease).
- Mortality despite appropriate therapy remains high.

Risk factors:
- Underlying myelodysplastic syndrome associated with repeated blood transfusions resulting in an iron overload condition
- Prolonged neutropenia
- Diabetes mellitus
- Chronic GVHD on corticosteroids
- Recipients of antithymocyte globulin.

Spectrum of infection: The manifestations include:
- Rhinocerebral
- Sino-orbital
- pulmonary
- Cutaneous
- Gastrointestinal
- Disseminated zygomycosis.

The symptoms may include facial pain, sinus congestion, extraocular muscles involvement, proptosis, cavernous sinus thrombosis, cough, hemoptysis, chest pain, headache, or fever depending on the site of involvement. An eschar may be present over the nasal turbinates, palate, or skin.

Diagnosis:
- Histopathological examination of tissue that demonstrates broad aseptate hyaline hyphae on Gomori methenamine silver staining.
- Frozen sections of tissue at the time of surgical intervention.

Management:
- Management not been well defined owing to the lack of controlled prospective trials involving this relatively uncommon opportunistic mycosis.
- Polyenes have been the only agents available for treatment of infections due to zygomycetes. LAmB or amphotericin B deoxycholate is used as therapy.
- The novel extended spectrum of triazole, posaconazole has demonstrated good efficacy in vivo against zygomycetes and is currently being used as salvage therapy for zygomycosis.

- The role of echinocandins against zygomycetes has not been well established.
- It is important to debride the necrotic tissue.
- Correct neutropenia, immunosuppression, hyperglycemia.
- Withdraw corticosteroids if plausible.

Phaeohyphomycetes

Dematiaceous or black molds are a heterogeneous group of organisms that obtained their nomenclature from the presence of a brown–black pigment (melanin) incorporated in their cell wall. The genera include *Bipolaris, Alternaria, Curvularia, Exophiala, Exserohilum*, and *Wangiella* species.

Bipolaris spicifera is the etiological agent frequently reported from immunocompromised cancer patients. It is also known to cause serious disseminated infections in cancer patients.

Being distributed widely in soil, wood, and decomposing plant debris, infections are airborne, involve the skin or the sinuses and are commonly reported from tropical countries and usually affect immunocompetent individuals.

Clinical spectrum:
- Fatal meningitis
- Localized epidural or paraspinal infection
- Peripheral joint infections.

Diagnosis:
- Observation of yeast-like cells, hyphae, and pseudohyphae alone or in combination and the dark wall seen on special staining procedures.
- Blood and tissue cultures have poor sensitivity and there are no antigen-based or standardized PCR tests currently available.
- Immunohistochemistry and PCR from infected tissue.

Management:
Antifungal agents known to be efficacious include:
- Amphotericin B deoxycholate
- Itraconazole
- Fluconazole and echinocandins have no activity against any of the species. The azole, UR 9825, in development has good in vitro activity against *Exophiala spinifera*.
- Surgical resection of localized lesions with a reduction in immunosuppression is recommended in all cancer patients if feasible.

Cryptococcus Species

Cryptococcus neoformans and *Cryptococcus gattii* are the two major species associated with cryptococcal infections.

Risk factors: *Cryptococcus* meningitis and meningoencephalitis are frequently seen in human immunodeficiency virus infections and relatively less common in immunocompromised cancer patients and hematopoietic stem cell recipients.

Spectrum of infection: Cryptococcal meningitis and meningoencephalitis are frequent manifestations.

Diagnosis: A positive serum cryptococcal antigen titer and has been documented in 33–90% of transplant recipients with pulmonary cryptococcosis. A negative serum cryptococcal antigen test does not exclude pulmonary cryptococcosis. Patients with CNS disease or disseminated cryptococcosis have been shown to have a positive serum cryptococcal antigen test (95% and 97%, respectively). Therefore, an organ transplant recipient with a positive serum cryptococcal antigen test needs to be worked up for cryptococcal meningitis or dissemination infection.

Management:
- For CNS disease, LAmB [3–4 mg/kg/day intravenous (IV)] or amphotericin B lipid complex (5 mg/kg/day IV) plus flucytosine (100 mg/kg/day in four divided doses) for at least 2 weeks.
- If induction therapy does not include flu cytosine, LAmB is indicated for at least 4–6 weeks as induction therapy.
- A dosage of 6 mg/kg/day of LAmB may be considered in high fungal burden disease or relapse.
- Fluconazole 400 mg (6 mg/kg/day) for 6–12 months is indicated for mild-to-moderate non-CNS disease.
- Fluconazole maintenance therapy should be continued for at least 6–12 months.
- Decreasing the dosage of steroids and a reduction in immunosuppressive therapy if feasible.

▓ RECONSTITUTING IMMUNE DEFENSE MECHANISMS

Patients with profound neutropenia may be offered the following management options:
- Reduce or stop corticosteroids if feasible use of recombinant hematopoietic cytokines, such as G-CSF and GM-CSF, reduce risk of IFIs by reducing the intensity and duration of neutropenia. These have a synergistic response with antifungals to suppress fungal growth.
- Cytokine-elicited granulocyte transfusions involve administering G-CSF to a healthy donor, leukapheresis, cytokine exposure of harvested and irradiated granulocytes. This improves the function of transfused granulocytes.
- T-helper 1-dependent immune response is crucial in host defenses against IFIs, including candidiasis and aspergillosis. Mechanisms to improve this response include interleukin (IL)-12 and anti-IL-4.
- Improvement in cellular immunotherapy during HSCT include cotransplantation of granulocytes and monocyte progenitor cells and adoptive transfer of immunocompetent T cells.
- Research on T-cell vaccines.

■ SUGGESTED READING

1. Bow EJ. Considerations in the approach to invasive fungal infection in patients with haematological malignancies. Br J Haematol. 2008;140:133-52.
2. Bow EJ. Neutropenic fever syndromes in patients undergoing cytotoxic therapy for acute leukemia and myelodysplastic syndromes. Semin Hematol. 2009;46:259-68.
3. Gamaletsou MN, Sipsas NV, Kontoyiannis DP. Invasive candidiasis in the neutropenic host. Curr Fungal Infect Rep. 2011;5:34-41.
4. Lionakis MS, Bodey GP, Tarrand JJ, et al. The significance of blood cultures positive for emerging saprophytic moulds in cancer patients. Clin Microbiol Infect. 2004;10:922-5.
5. Mermel LA, Allon M, Bouza E, et al. Clinical practice guidelines for the diagnosis and management of intravascular catheter-related infection: 2009 update by the Infectious Diseases Society of America. Clin Infect Dis. 2009;49:1-45.
6. Otto C, Buonocore D, Cohen N, et al. Comparison of fungal culture to surgical pathology exam in the detection of dimorphic fungi and the impact on treatment and outcomes: a 25-year retrospective review at a tertiary cancer center. Am J Clin Pathol. 2017;147(Suppl 2):S176.
7. Sipsas NV, Bodey GP, Kontoyiannis DP. Perspectives for the management of febrile neutropenic patients with cancer in the 21st century. Cancer. 2005;103:1103-13.
8. Ullmann AJ, Akova M, Herbrecht R, et al. ESCMID guideline for the diagnosis and management of *Candida* diseases 2012: adults with haematological malignancies and after haematopoietic stem cell transplantation (HCT). Clin Microbiol Infect. 2012;18(Suppl S7):53-67.

34

Postrenal Transplant Fungal Infections

Dinesh Khullar, Sahil Bagai

INTRODUCTION

Renal transplantation offers the best cure for chronic kidney disease end-stage renal disease patients. It ensures a better quality and quantity of life as compared to patients on waiting list for transplant. The improvement in immunosuppressive agents, graft preservation, and surgical methods have all contributed to better graft survival; however, this has been accompanied by high incidence of opportunistic infections.[1] There has been a surge in post-transplant invasive fungal infections (IFIs) of late, and the angioinvasive fungal infections are associated with high morbidity across the globe; and in India, the outcomes are more dismal. Calcineurin inhibitor, namely cyclosporine and tacrolimus, affects calcineurin-induced upregulation of interleukin-2 expression, affecting T-lymphocyte functions resulting in increased susceptibility to invasive fungal diseases (IFI).[2] The hot and humid climate, overcrowding, nonaffordability, malnutrition, and inaccessible healthcare facilities have made the developing nations more susceptible to these infections and have huge bearing on countries' economy. As per one study, post-transplant infections rank second as the cause of death in patients with allograft.[3] The state of net immunosuppression (IS) seals the final fate of the transplant recipient. However, there is scarcity of data on the etiology and course of post-transplant infections in tropical countries.[4] An Indian study by Jha et al. estimated that infections complicate the course in 50–70% of transplant recipients in tropical countries; with mortality ranging from 20% to 60%.[4] However, in spite of new antimicrobials, infection rates following transplantation have not come down.[5] About 5% of all post-transplant infections are fungal in origin.[6] As per Rubin's timeline of infections post-renal transplantation, fungal infections can dominate right from immediate post-transplant period to any time after that. This is consistent with the study by Sharma where fungal infections contributed to 55% of total opportunistic infections.[7] However, most of the fungal infections occur within first 6 months of transplantation.[8] Mortality rates due to IFIs range between 25% and 80% in transplant recipients.[1]

Fungal conidia are being constantly inhaled eliminated by innate mechanisms in healthy individuals. These then can lead to invasive mycosis in immunosuppressed individuals.

PRESENTATION

Kidney transplant recipients usually have nonspecific complaints, and early laboratory results may appear normal, hence a high index of suspicion is necessary for correct diagnosis.

Unexplained fever despite broad-spectrum antibiotics, recurrent episodes of fever, or the presence of pulmonary infiltrates or ground glassing on radiological imaging or nonresolving pneumonias or hemoptysis with cough and fever can be indirect pointers toward fungal infection.

RISK FACTORS

Fungal infections in renal transplant recipients occur as: disseminated primary or reactivation infection of "geographically restricted" mycoses (histoplasmosis, coccidioidomycosis, blastomycosis, and paracoccidioidomycosis).[9] The probability of the patient getting invasive mycosis depends upon the epidemiological exposures and the net state of IS.

Epidemiological Exposures

These can be stratified into four types based on the source of the infection. It includes donor derived, recipient derived, community acquired, and nosocomial.

Donor-derived infections: Infections acquired from donor's tissues get activated in the immunosuppressed host following transplantation. Blood-transmitted viral infections and parasitic infections have been reported in literature. Cytomegalovirus, Epstein–Barr virus, and varicella zoster virus are important viruses that get transmitted to host and pose a significant threat in the case of recipient serology being negative for them. Active infection in donor at the time of transplantation is a contraindication to transplantation.

Recipient-derived infections: These are latent infections that get activated in the setting of IS. *Herpes simplex, varicella zoster, hepatitis B, hepatitis C, HIV,* and *Mycobacterium tuberculosis* are some common pathogens encountered.

Community-acquired pathogens: Water-borne, food-borne, respiratory viral, fungal, and parasitic organism exposure in community can lead to infection. These infections are usually seen 1 year post-transplant and present in a similar way as to normal community inhabitant.

Nosocomial infections: These are hospital-acquired infections and are of significance as are mostly antimicrobial resistant. Methicillin-resistant *Staphylococcus*, vancomycin-resistant *enterococci*, and fluconazole-resistant *Candida* are common pathogens encountered.[10] They occur within the first month of transplantation.

Net State of Immunosuppression[11]

- Immunosuppressive therapy including dose, duration, and sequence of agents—certain immunosuppressive drugs, such as antithymocyte globulin, alemtuzumab, OKT3, rituximab, antiproliferative agents, steroids, and calcineurin inhibitors, are potent drugs used in transplantation that can lead to variable degree of IS, hence predispose patients to infections.
- Underlying or comorbid diseases—underlying liver and renal dysfunction, uremia, diabetes, and malnutrition have seen to have independent effect on patient's outcome post-renal transplant.

- Prolonged use of broad-spectrum antibiotics.
- Prolonged use of indwelling catheters, invasive lines.

TIMING OF INFECTIONS: POST-TRANSPLANT

Post-transplant infections follow a timeline usually as suggested by Rubin.[12] Early infections (within the first month) are mostly due to acquired pathogens or some donor-derived infections. Opportunistic pathogens often occur during the subsequent months, reflecting the greater impact of immunosuppressive therapies. Late infections (more than 6 months) usually are secondary to opportunistic pathogens or community-acquired pathogens. Fungal infections can occur during any period post-transplant. *Aspergillus* dominates in the first month, endemic fungi rule till the next 5 months and *Aspergillus* and atypical molds commonly seen thereafter.[3]

INCIDENCE OF FUNGAL INFECTION

Invasive fungal infection incidence has been on the rise in the past. Incidence varies with type of transplant organ such that highest numbers are for small bowel (11.6%) and lowest for kidney transplant recipients (1.3%).[10] The incidence varies ranging from 5% to 42% following solid-organ transplantation (SOT).[13] Higher incidence of IFI has been reported from the developing countries as compared with the West. In one study from Chandigarh, India, incidence of IFI was 6.1% with a mortality of 63%.[14] In another study from South India, IFI incidence was 3.8–6.1% with an overall mortality of 70%.[15] *Candida* and *Aspergillus* dominated amongst the fungal infections in the past.[16]

However, Gupta et al. reported a recent rise in angioinvasive infections, such as aspergillosis and mucormycosis, which are associated with high mortality.[17]

INVASIVE MYCOSES

Mucormycosis

It is fungal infection caused by fungi of the order Mucorales and genera *Rhizopus*, *Absidia*, and *Mucor*.[18] These ubiquitous fungi occur in decaying vegetative and organic matter. They release large numbers of spores; hence, inhalation seems to be major portal of entry for them. However, ingestion, contamination of skin wounds, and ascending infection from bladder or intravenous drips have also been postulated to be other modes of entry in the host. They have minimal intrinsic pathogenicity but in compromised host infection, can be fatal. Diabetes, viral hepatitis, and chronic renal failure are independent risk factors for acquiring mucormycosis.[19] The presentation may range from rhinocerebral, pulmonary, gastrointestinal (GI), and disseminated to involving isolated organs including bone, heart, and kidneys.[18] The incidence reported is variable, ranging from 0.2% to 1.2% as reported by Nampoory et al. to 11% as reported by Chugh et al. in their study.[20]

The hallmark of mucormycosis is vascular invasion with thrombosis of large and small arteries, resulting in infarction and necrosis. Demonstration of broad aseptate hyphae histo-logically is the gold standard (Fig 34.1).[17] KOH mount of the biopsy material shows broad, aseptate, ribbon-like hyphae with wide angle branching (Fig 34.2). On fungal culture, the

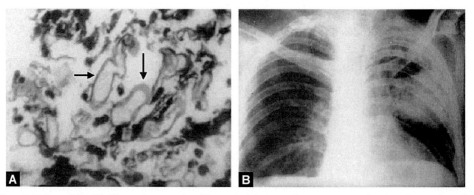

Figs. 34.1A and B: (A) Photomicrograph of bronchial biopsy showing mucor hyphae (arrows) in the inflamed necrotic tissue (H&E × 880); (B) Chest X-ray showing cavitation pneumonia left upper lobe. H&E, Hematoxylin and eosin
Reproduced after permission from Gupta KL, Khullar DK, Behera D, et al. Pulmonary mucormycosis presenting as fatal massive haemoptysis in a renal transplant recipient. Nephrol Dial Transplant. 1998; 13:3258-60.

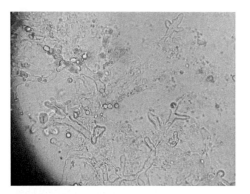

Fig. 34.2: Broad aseptate hyphae on potassium hydroxide (KOH) mount.

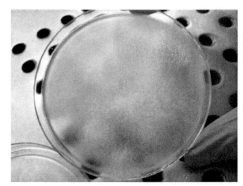

Fig. 34.3: *Rhizopus* colony on Sabouraud dextrose agar (SDA).

colonies grow rapidly as cottony growth (Fig 34.3). LPCB mount of the colonies shows ribbon-like hyphae with sporangiospore and rhizoids (Fig 34.4) Timely initiation of treatment is crucial and associated with better survival. The optimal management of mucormycosis is based upon early recognition and initiation of treatment, surgical resection of necrotic tissue if possible, and reversal of predisposing factors, such as uncontrolled glycemia, IS, and neutropenia. Amphotericin B (AmB), conventional or liposomal, and posaconazole are the only antifungals approved for Mucorales. AmB is considered the drug of choice. Lipid formulations of AmB are thought to have better activity and safety profile compared with conventional AmB deoxycholate. In the absence of surgical intervention, response to medical therapy is poor as

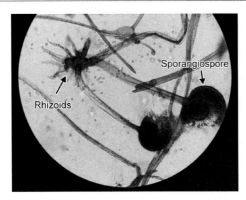

Fig. 34.4: *Rhizopus* spp. on lactophenol cotton blue (LPCB) mount.

antifungals are not able to reach necrotic tissue. The overall mortality ranges from 38% to 56.5% with marked increase in mortality reaching up to 100% in disseminated disease.[21]

Aspergillosis

Aspergillosis is a very common opportunistic infection in renal transplant recipients with a prevalence of 0.5–4%.[22] It usually presents as angioinvasive, chronic necrotizing, and tracheobronchial aspergillosis in compromised hosts making other forms of presentation rare in kidney transplant recipients.[23]

Invasive Pulmonary Aspergillosis

Neutropenia (absolute neutrophil count $<500 \times 10^6$ L^{-1}) and prolonged high-dose steroids with poor host immune response leads to the maturation of inhaled spores into hyphae that invade the pulmonary structures, particularly blood vessels leading to pulmonary arterial thrombosis, hemorrhage, lung necrosis, and systemic dissemination.[24] Mortality rates from infections can be high (50–70%).[24]

On radiographs, one can see multiple ill-defined 1- to 2-cm nodules that gradually coalesce into larger masses or areas of consolidation. Gold standard for diagnosis is made by the demonstration of septate hyphae branching at acute angles.

Ulcerative *Aspergillus* tracheobronchitis has mostly been seen in lung transplant patients as described by Kramer et al.[25]

Chronic necrotizing or semi-invasive aspergillosis typically occurs in patients with mild IS, such as respiratory airway disease or malignancy. It is slowly progressing. Treatment is usually medical. Voriconazole is superior to AmB in terms of efficacy for primary treatment (Figs. 34.5 to 34.8).[2]

Candidiasis

Candida species occur normally in the human GI tract, female gynecological tract, and skin. It becomes pathogenic in immunocompromised host. It has mortality rate of around 1.5%.[26]

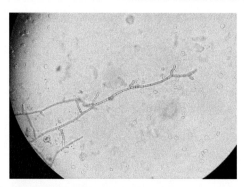

Fig. 34.5: Septate fungal hyphae with branching at acute angle.

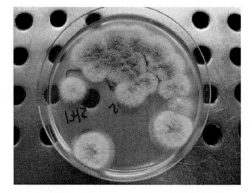

Fig. 34.6: Colony of *Aspergillus* spp. on Sabouraud dextrose agar (SDA) agar.

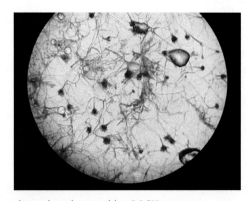

Fig. 34.7: *Aspergillus* spp. on lactophenol cotton blue (LPCB) mount.

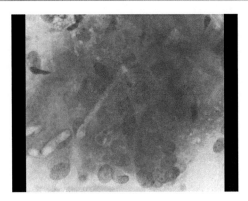

Fig. 34.8: Giant cells engulfing septate hyphae.

Fig. 34.9: Budding yeast cell on potassium hydroxide (KOH) mount.

Bloodstream, intra-abdominal, and urinary tract are the common sites of infection. In a study from North India, 2.8% patients had candidiasis post-renal transplantation.[17] A study from Iran evaluated fungal colonization by mouth, vagina, urine, and rectal swabs. Fifty-four kidney recipients (45%) had *Candida* colonization in different sites of their bodies. Fungal infections presented in 13 of 120 recipients (10.8%). This showed that patients with previous colonization had increased predisposition to have candidiasis post-renal transplantation.

Treatment: Azoles and echinocandins are the preferred agents. *Candida glabrata* and *Candida krusei* are resistant to azoles so echinocandins are preferred therapy. AmB is an alternative but usually not preferred because of relatively higher toxicities with the agent (Fig. 34.9).

Pneumocystis Jiroveci

Pneumocystis jiroveci is a quintessential opportunistic infection in immunocompromised patients. Its incidence was high before cotrimoxazole introduction.[27] Incidence of infection varies from 5% to 15%.[28] Amongst all SOTs, the incidence is lowest in renal transplantion.[29]

Fever, cough, shortness of breath, and hypoxia out of proportion to physical and radiologic findings is a typical presentation. Diagnosis relies on identification of the organism in induced sputum, bronchoalveolar lavage, or transbronchial biopsy samples. The identification of the organism, either by tinctorial (dye-based) staining, fluorescent antibody staining, or polymerase chain reaction-based assays of respiratory specimens, is essential for correct diagnosis. Elevated beta-D-glucan assay and lactate dehydrogenase enzymes are the indirect indicators of *P. jiroveci* pneumonia. High-dose trimethoprim–sulfamethoxazole (15–20 mg/kg/day) in divided doses or intravenous pentamidine (4 mg/kg/day) for 14–21 days is the treatment of choice. Atovaquone or the combination of clindamycin and pyrimethamine act as alternatives in the cases one has sulfa allergy. In patients with hypoxia (partial pressure of oxygen in the alveoli <70 mm Hg on room air), high-dose corticosteroids are coadministered with antimicrobial agents. The current recommendations are to give 80–120-mg steroids in two divided doses for 5–7 days, followed by tapering over the next 7–14 days.[30]

Cryptococcus

Cryptococcosis is caused by *Cryptococcus neoformans* or *Cryptococcus gattii*. They are basidiomycetous, encapsulated yeasts. Risk factors acquiring cryptococcal infection are HIV, prolonged therapy with steroids, organ transplantation, and liver disease. Incidence of cryptococcal infection in post-transplant period is around 2.8% as per one study and median time to acquire infection is 21 months post-transplant period. Central nervous system (CNS) and lungs are the two most common organs affected and almost one quarter of transplant recipients has fungemia.[31]

Although cryptococcal infection begins in the lungs, brain is the most frequently affected organ of cryptococcosis in compromised host. Brain parenchyma is almost always seen affected in patients presenting with meningitis-like symptoms on histological examinations.[32] Clinically, symptoms typically begin indolently over a period of 1–2 weeks. Fever, malaise, and headache are the most common presentations. Stiff neck, photophobia, and vomiting occur in a quarter to one-third of patients. In transplant patients, subacute presentation is more common. Definitive diagnosis is by identification of the cryptococcal antigen in lumbar puncture (LP), Indian ink positivity in cerebrospinal fluid, or by isolating organism on culture when CNS is not involved. LP must be done in all post-transplant patients if non-CNS cryptococococcal infection is isolated. CNS infection, disseminated infection, or pulmonary infection is treated in a similar way. Skin and soft tissue involvement is relatively rare (10% a 20%) but is almost always considered a marker for disseminated disease, and can sometimes precede the diagnosis of systemic infection (Fig 34.10). Treatment is done in two phases—induction and maintenance. AmB and flucytosine are given in induction phase. Duration of induction is 2 weeks, followed by repeat LP in the absence of neurological involvement but is 6 weeks in patients with neurological involvement.[33] Consolidation or maintenance phase constitutes of fluconazole 400–800 mg for 8 weeks, followed by 200 mg/day for 1 year.

Histoplasmosis

Histoplasmosis, caused by *Histoplasma capsulatum*, is a common endemic fungus in America, Asia, and Africa. It is acquired by inhalation. Microconidia, mold form transforms to the yeast form in tissues. Most infections are not clinically recognized but incidentally detected on imaging.

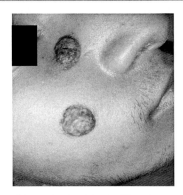

Fig. 34.10: Photograph of post-renal transplant recipient with cutaneous cryptococcal skin nodules.

Lung is the most common site of localization but brain, GI tract, or disseminated disease may occur in immunocompromised patients. Approximately, 90% of these infections result in mild and clinically significant respiratory infections. The other 10% of the patients suffer serious pulmonary or disseminated infection.[17]

Dematiaceous Fungi (Phaeohyphomycosis)

Phaeohyphomycosis is caused by a large, heterogeneous group of darkly pigmented fungi. The presence of melanin in their cell walls is characteristic and is likely an important virulence factor. They normally are seen on soil and organic vegetable material. Some common agents of phaeohyphomycosis are the genus *Alternaria*, *Exophiala*, *Cladosporium*, and *Bipolaris*. Brain abscess and pneumonia can occur with these infections and is associated with high mortality of about 25–40% of patients. These fungi can also cause subcutaneous phaeohyphomycosis, including mycotic cysts. Itraconazole for at least 6 months plus surgical excision offers best cure.

To conclude, there are array of fungal infections one can acquire in post-transplant period. One should always have a high index of suspicion and aggressively investigate to find the correct diagnosis.

CLINICAL PEARLS

- Invasive mycosis is common in renal transplant recipients in developing world and depends upon the epidemiological exposures and net state of IS.
- Nonresolving fever, use of broad-spectrum antibiotics, ground glassing/cavitation on Chest X-rays are soft pointers toward fungal infection.
- Classical signs and symptoms of the infection cannot be seen in transplant recipients, and high index of suspicion is required for diagnosis.
- Endemic fungi, aspergillosis, mucormycosis, and candidiasis are common infections encountered and are associated with high mortality, in spite of appropriate therapy.

■ REFERENCES

1. Munksgaard B. Fungal infections. Am J Transplant. 2004;4:110–34.
2. Khan A, El-Charabaty E, El-Sayegh S. Fungal infections in renal transplant patients. J Clin Med Res. 2015;7(6):371–8.
3. Karuthu S, Blumberg EA. Common infections in kidney transplant recipients. Transplant Proc. 1994;26:2072–4.
4. Jha V, Chugh S, Chugh KS. Infections in dialysis and transplant patients in tropical countries. Kidney Int. 2000;57(74):S85–93.
5. Snyder JJ, Israni AK, Peng Y, et al. Rates of first infection following kidney transplant in the United States. Kidney Int. 2009;75:317–26.
6. Patel R, Paya CV. Infections in solid-organ transplant recipients. Clin Microbiol Rev. 1997;10:86–124.
7. Gupta RK. Opportunistic infections in renal allograft recipients. Transplant Proc. 2007;39:731–73.
8. Venkataramanan R, Zang S, Gayowski T, et al. Voriconazole inhibition of the metabolism of tacrolimus in a liver transplant recipient and in human liver microsomes. Antimicrob Agents Chemother. 2002;46:3091–3.
9. Moradi M, Abbasi M, Moradi A, et al. Effect of antibiotic therapy on asymptomatic bacteriuria in kidney transplant recipients. Urol J. 2005;2:32–5.
10. Pappas PG, Alexander BD, Andes DR, et al. Invasive fungal infections among organ transplant recipients: results of the Transplant-associated Infection Surveillance Network (TRANSNET). Clin Infect Dis. 2010;50:1101–11.
11. Fishman, J. Infection in kidney transplant recipients. In: Morris PJ, Knechtle SJ (Eds). Kidney transplantation: principles and practice. China: Elsevier Saunders; 2014. pp. 491–510.
12. Fishman JA. Infection in solid-organ transplant recipients. N Engl J Med. 2007;357:2601–14.
13. Patel MH, Patel RD, Vanikar AV, et al. Invasive fungal infections in renal transplant patients: a single center study. Ren Fail. 2017;39:294–8.
14. Chugh KS, Sakhuja V, Jain S, et al. High mortality in systemic fungal infections following renal transplantation in third-world countries. Nephrol Dial Transplant. 1993;8:168–72.
15. John GT. Infections after renal transplantation in India. Transplant Rev. 1999;13:183–91.
16. Paya CV. Fungal infections in solid-organ transplantation. Clin Infect Dis. 1993;16(5):677–88.
17. Gupta KL. Fungal infections and the kidney. Indian Nephrol. 2001;11:147–54.
18. Benbow EW, Stoddart RW. Systemic zygomycosis. Postgrad Med J. 1986;62:985–96.
19. Gupta KL, Radotra BD, Sakhuja V, et al. Mucormycosis in patients with renal failure. Ren Fail. 1990;11:195–9.
20. Nampoory M, Khan Z, Johny K, et al. Invasive fungal infections in renal transplant recipients. J Infection. 1996;33:95–101.
21. Hamdi T, Karthikeyan V, Alangaden GJ. Mucormycosis in a renal transplant recipient: case report and comprehensive review of literature. Int J Nephrol. 2014;2014:950643.
22. Desbois AC, Poiree S, Snanoudj R, et al. Prognosis of invasive aspergillosis in kidney transplant recipients: a case-control study. Transplant Direct. 2016;2:e90.
23. Fitzsimmons EJ, Aris R, Patterson R. Recurrence of allergic bronchopulmonary aspergillosis in the posttransplant lungs of a cystic fibrosis patient. Chest. 1997;112:281–2.
24. Denning DW. Diagnosis and management of invasive aspergillosis. Curr Clin Top Infect Dis. 1996;16:277–99.
25. Kramer MR, Denning DW, Marshall SE, et al. Ulcerative tracheobronchitis after lung transplantation. A new form of invasive aspergillosis. Am Rev Respir Dis. 1991;144:552–6.
26. Silveira FP, Kusne S. The AST Infectious Diseases Community of Practice. *Candida* infections in solid-organ transplantation. Am J Transplant. 2013;1:220–7.

27. Jha V. Infections in dialysis and transplant patients in tropical countries. Kidney Int. 2000;57:S85–93.

28. Fishman JA. Prevention of infection due to *Pneumocystis carinii.* Antimicrob Agents Chemother. 1998;42:995–1004.

29. Radisic M, Lattes R, Chapman JF, et al. Risk factors for *Pneumocystis carinii* pneumonia in kidney transplant recipients: a case-control study. Transpl Infect Dis. 2003;5:84–93. [online] Available from https://www.uptodate.com/contents/epidemiology-clinical-manifestations-and-diagnosis-of-pneumocystis-pneumonia-in-hiv-uninfected-patients/abstract/34.

30. Martin S, Fishman J. AST Infectious Diseases Community of Practice. Pneumocystis pneumonia in solid-organ transplant recipients. Am J Transplant. 2009;9:S227–33.

31. Vilchez RA, Fung J, Kusne S. Cryptococcosis in organ transplant recipients: an overview. Am J Transplant. 2002;2:575.

32. Lee SC, Dickson DW, Casadevall A. Pathology of cryptococcal meningoencephalitis: analysis of 27 patients with pathogenetic implications. Hum Pathol. 1996;27:839.

33. Dismukes WE, Cloud G, Gallis HA, et al. Treatment of cryptococcal meningitis with combination amphotericin B and flucytosine for four as compared with six weeks. N Engl J Med. 1987;317:334.

35

Fungal Diseases of the Lungs

Ashish Jain

INTRODUCTION

Fungal pneumonia has a minor share of lung infection in immunocompetent individuals; but in immunocompromised, the fungal infections have a significant importance. This is not only due to difficulty in diagnosis but also for the fact tha t fungal diseases are a major cause of morbidity and mortality. The incidence is on the rise in critically ill but otherwise immunocompetent individuals due to prolonged stay in intensive care unit (ICU) and indiscriminate use of antibiotics. In addition, the environmental exposure and preexisting lung conditions also predispose to different ailments of fungal etiology.

The major risk factors for fungal pneumonia include myeloproliferative malignancies, solid organ malignancy, bone marrow transplant, heavy immunosuppression, prolonged corticosteroid therapy, and neutropenia from various causes amongst others.

CLINICAL PRESENTATION

Broadly, the fungal infections can be classified into opportunistic and endemic infections. While the opportunistic infections, such as *Aspergillus* and *Candida*, are pathogenic in neutropenic and nonneutropenic immunosuppressed patients, the endemic fungal infections are seen in population inhabiting a specific geographical area.[1] Fungi, such as histoplasmosis, coccidioidomycosis, and blastomycosis, are more commonly seen in North America than any other part of the world. Individuals who inhale aerosolized spores of these fungi acquire illness. Immunosuppressed patients may develop life-threatening infection while the healthy individuals generally experience few nonspecific symptoms and recover quickly. Among endemic mycoses frequent in India, histoplasmosis and penicilliosis are common in immunocompromised patients.[2] *Penicillium marneffei* is restricted to Manipur, Nagaland, and Mizoram. *Histoplasma* has been isolated from the banks of Hooghly River near Kolkata.[3]

Due to their ubiquitous presence in soil, air as well as on indoor surfaces and even on human skin, fungi can easily colonize skin and respiratory tract. Presence of *Candida* in a sputum sample does not always mean infection. Depending on the immune status of the individual, the fungus can present itself in a variety of clinical presentations making it difficult for the treating physician to diagnose. A high clinical suspicion always helps in early diagnosis.

CANDIDA

Candida species are eukaryotic opportunistic pathogens that reside on the mucosa of the gastrointestinal tract as well as the mouth, esophagus, and vagina even without producing disease.[4] Thus isolation of *Candida* from respiratory sample alone in a nonneutropenic patient should be considered nonpathogenic.[5] However, they are known to cause superficial and life-threatening infection in post-transplant and immunocompromised patients. Critically ill patients with intravenous catheters, total parenteral nutrition, invasive procedures, and on broad-spectrum antibiotics or cytotoxic chemotherapies are predisposed to *Candida* infections.[4] *Candida albicans* is the most common species causing invasive fungal infection; however, the incidence of non-*albicans* species is also increasing. The common non-*albicans* *Candida* are—*Candida glabrata, Candida parapsilosis, Candida tropicalis,* and *Candida krusei.*

To diagnose infection, biopsy with demonstration of tissue invasion is more reliable than mere isolation of organism.[6]

The colonization of the respiratory tract by *Candida* species is common in patients receiving mechanical ventilation for periods of longer than 2 days. This occurs due to hematogenous spread or pulmonary aspiration of the contents of colonies of oropharyngeal or gastric origin.[4] Blood stream *Candida* infection is more common than pneumonia.[6] Majority of *Candida* pneumonia cases are secondary to hematological dissemination of *Candida* organisms from a distant site, usually the gastrointestinal tract or skin.[7] The presence of *Candida* in respiratory samples can be a part of multifocal colonization. In a patient with risk factors, it has a high incidence of bloodstream candidiasis. High-risk factors for candidemia in an intensive care setting are: (1) peritonitis, (2) complicated or repeat abdominal surgery, (3) use of broad-spectrum antibiotics, (4) total parenteral nutrition, (5) invasive catheters, (6) prior *Candida* species colonization, (7) renal replacement therapy, (8) mechanical ventilation, (9) chemotherapy-induced neutropenia, (10) radiation-induced tissue injury, (10) hematopoietic stem-cell transplantation (HSCT), etc.[8]

The pathogenicity of *Candida* species is attributed to certain virulence factors, such as the ability to evade host defenses, adherence, biofilm formation (on host tissue and on medical devices), and the production of tissue-damaging hydrolytic enzymes, such as proteases, phospholipases, and hemolysin. The ability of *Candida* species to form drug-resistant biofilms is an important factor in their contribution to human disease.[4]

Absence of any specific clinical and radiological presentation makes the diagnosis of *Candida* pneumonia difficult. There is no clear definition or clinical predictive model to differentiate *Candida* pneumonia with other forms of candidiasis or colonization.[7] Usually, fungal pneumonia manifests as a fever in patients who do not respond to antibiotic therapy, especially in the cases of prolonged catheter use or other major risk factors as noted above or in patients with septic shock and multiple organ dysfunction.[9]

ASPERGILLUS

Aspergillus is a ubiquitous and hardy organism. It grows best in moist environments, although spore aerosolization and dispersion occur most effectively in dry climates. Spores survive harsh external conditions and adapt to a range of internal environments.

Aspergillus causes a variety of clinical syndromes which depends on the immunity of the patient and interaction of fungus with the host, preexisting lung condition, and quantum of fungal exposure. Classical risk factors for invasive pulmonary disease are prolonged antibiotic therapy, steroid therapy, ICU stay, mechanical ventilation, and renal transplantation. Patients with acquired immune deficiency syndrome (AIDS) have been reported to acquire the disease. However, the incidence of this fatal fungal infection in immunocompetent individual is also rising.[2]

Unlike the Western world and temperate countries where *Aspergillus fumigatus* (AF) is the foremost pathogen, *Aspergillus flavus* is the most common etiological agent for fungemia in India.[2] *Aspergillus terreus* is a common cause of invasive aspergillosis (IA) in some institutions and is amphotericin B resistant. *Aspergillus niger* is an occasional cause of IA or *Aspergillus* bronchitis but is also a proportionately more common colonizer of the respiratory tract.[10]

Aspergillus lung infections are acquired by inhalation of spores. In a normal host, it fails to produce any disease. While in preexisting cavitary lung lesion in an immunocompetent host, it leads to the formation of fungal ball, aspergilloma. In a patient with chronic lung disease or with mild immunocompromised status, the fungus may cause chronic necrotizing aspergillosis. In patients suffering from atopy, asthma, or cystic fibrosis (CF), exposure to fungus may lead to hypersensitivity manifestation as allergic bronchopulmonary aspergillosis (ABPA). Invasive pulmonary aspergillosis (IPA) develops not only in severely immunocompromised host but also in critically ill patients and with chronic obstructive pulmonary disease (COPD).

Invasive Aspergillosis

Invasive aspergillosis implies invasion of the lung tissue by hyphae. It was first described in 1953. The classic risk factor for IA is neutropenia, and the likelihood of IA correlates with its duration and depth. Platelets may also be important in defense against IA, and thrombocytopenia tends to parallel neutropenia.[10] The mortality rate of IA exceeds 50% in neutropenic patients and reaches 90% in HSCT recipients (Box 35.1).

Several other factors predispose patients with transplantation to acquire IPA: multiple immune defects including prolonged neutropenia in the preengraftment phase of HSCT; the use

---

Box 35.1: Classical risk factors for invasive pulmonary aspergillosis.

- Prolonged neutropenia
- Lung transplantation, HSCT and other transplantation
- High-dose corticosteroid therapy for more than 3 weeks
- Hematological malignancy
- Chemotherapy
- AIDS
- Chronic granulomatous disease

Adapted from M Kousha, R Tadi, AO Soubani. Pulmonary aspergillosis: a clinical review European Respiratory Review. 2011:20:156-74.

of multiple antirejection or anti-graft-versus-host disease therapy (such as corticosteroids and cyclosporine); parenteral nutrition; use of multiple antibiotics; and prolonged hospitalization.[11]

Invasive aspergillosis occurs in a wide range of nonneutropenic hosts. The most common risk factors are long-term steroid therapy, hepatic cirrhosis, dialysis, near-drowning, or diabetes; sepsis due to bacterial, viral, or parasitic agents; chronic granulomatous disease and severe post-sepsis immunoparalysis.[12] IPA is relatively uncommon in patients with human immunodeficiency virus (HIV) infection, especially with the routine use of highly active antiretroviral therapy. A low CD 4 count (<100 cells/mm^3) is present in almost all cases of AIDS-associated aspergillosis, and half of HIV-infected patients with IPA have coexistent neutropenia or are on corticosteroid therapy.[11]

Patients with COPD have increased susceptibility to IPA for several reasons, including structural changes in lung architecture, prolonged use of corticosteroid therapy, frequent hospitalization, broad-spectrum antibiotic treatment, invasive procedures, mucosal lesions and impaired mucociliary clearance, and comorbid illnesses, such as diabetes mellitus (DM), alcoholism, and malnutrition. It is also possible that abnormalities or deficiencies in surfactant proteins, and alveolar macrophages play a role in the pathogenesis of IPA in some patients with COPD. COPD also predisposes airway colonization with *Aspergillus*.

The occurrence of *Aspergillus* infection has been clearly related to building hygiene and construction work. Building activities have been shown to increase the concentration of *Aspergillus* conidia in the air with subsequent development of IA. Although this conjunction is still under discussion, the use of high-efficiency particulate air filtration units with laminar air flow could markedly reduce the amount of contamination with *Aspergillus* conidia and the subsequent development of IA.[12]

Aspergillus is usually introduced in the lungs via inhalational route to cause IPA. Less commonly, IPA may start in other locations, such as gastrointestinal tract, skin, or sinuses. Clinical signs are nonspecific, but characteristic. The occurrence of fever despite appropriate antibiotic therapy for >96 h in neutropenic patients is suspicious for IA. Chest pain during breathing and cough are present in ~20% of IPA cases. Patients may also present with pleuritic chest pain due to vascular invasion leading to thromboses that cause small pulmonary infarcts.[11]

Hemoptysis is not an initial symptom of IPA. It occurs when granulocytopenia resolves. The leukocyte reconstitution leads to an overwhelming inflammatory response in the infected lung with local necrosis of the pulmonary parenchyma. Life-threatening pulmonary bleeding may occur; and therefore, hemoptysis is regarded as a poor prognostic sign in IPA.

Diagnostic Criteria for Invasive Pulmonary Aspergillosis

Several classifications have been proposed to define the diagnostic level of certainty reached for IPA (proven, probable, and possible). The European Organization for Research and Treatment of Cancer/Mycoses Study Group has proposed new criteria for the classification of invasive fungal infections (Table 35.1).

These diagnostic criteria proved to be useful in research and practice in severely immunocompromised patients but are not without serious drawbacks. The open lung biopsy is

Table 35.1: Diagnostic criteria for invasive pulmonary aspergillosis
According to the EORTC/MSG and the clinical algorithm
EORTC/MSG criteria
Proven IPA:
Microscopic analysis on sterile material: Histopathologic, cytopathologic, or direct microscopic examination of a specimen obtained by needle aspiration or sterile biopsy in which hyphae are seen accompanied by evidence of associated tissue damage.   *Culture on sterile material:* Recovery of *Aspergillus* by culture of a specimen obtained by lung biopsy
Probable IPA (all three criteria must be met):
Host factors (one of the following):
1. Recent history of neutropenia (<500 neutrophils/mm3) for 110 days
2. Receipt of an allogeneic stem cell transplant
3. Prolonged use of corticosteroids at a mean minimum dose of 0.3 mg/kg/day of prednisone equivalent for 13 weeks
4. Treatment with other recognized T-cell immunosuppressants
5. Inherited severe immunodeficiency
Clinical features (one of the following three signs on CT):
1. Dense, well-circumscribed lesion (s) with or without a halo sign
2. *Air crescent sign (Fig. 35.1):*   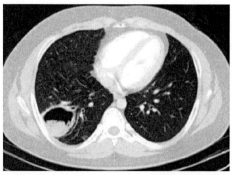   **Fig. 35.1:** Computed tomography (CT) scan image of thick-walled cavity with aspergilloma showing air crescent sign.
3. Cavity
Mycological criteria (one of the following):
1. Direct test (cytology, direct microscopy, or culture) on sputum, BAL fluid, bronchial brush indicating the presence of fungal elements or culture recovery *Aspergillus* spp.
2. *Indirect tests (detection of antigen or cell-wall constituents):* Galactomannan antigen detected in plasma, serum, or BAL fluid

Contd...

Contd...

According to the EORTC/MSG and the clinical algorithm
Possible IPA:
Presence of host factors and clinical features (cf. probable IA) but in the absence of or negative mycological findings
Alternative clinical algorithm
Proven IPA:
Idem EORTC/MSG criteria
Putative IPA (all four criteria must be met)
1. *Aspergillus*—positive lower respiratory tract specimen culture (=entry criterion)
2. *Compatible signs and symptoms (one of the following)*:
• Fever refractory to at least 3 days of appropriate antibiotic therapy
• Recrudescent fever after a period of defervescence of at least 48 h while still on antibiotics and without other apparent cause
• Pleuritic chest pain
• Pleuritic rub
• Dyspnea
• Hemoptysis
• Worsening respiratory insufficiency in spite of appropriate antibiotic therapy and ventilatory support
3. Abnormal medical imaging by portable chest X-ray or CT scan of the lungs
4. Either 4a or 4b
4a. *Host risk factors (one of the following conditions)*:
• Neutropenia (absolute neutrophil count <500/mm^3) preceding or at the time of ICU admission
• Underlying hematological or oncological malignancy treated with cytotoxic agents
• Glucocorticoid treatment (prednisone equivalent >20 mg/day)
• Congenital or acquired immunodeficiency
4b. Semiquantitative *Aspergillus*-positive culture of BAL fluid (+ or ++), without bacterial growth together with a positive cytological smear showing branching hyphae
Aspergillus respiratory tract colonization
When ≥1 criterion necessary for a diagnosis of putative IPA is not met, the case is classified as *Aspergillus* colonization.
BAL, bronchoalveolar lavage; CT, computed tomography; EORTC/MSG, European Organization for the Research and Treatment of Cancer/Mycosis Study Group; ICU, intensive care unit; IA, invasive aspergillosis; IPA, invasive pulmonary aspergillosis. *Adapted from*: Bolt et al., ARJCCM Vol 186, No 1, Jul 01, 2012.[13]

not possible in all sick patients to prove the diagnosis. Moreover, the definition of possible and probable is validated only in immunocompromised individuals leaving behind the critically ill patients in ICU who may develop IA without the classically described host factors. Similarly the radiological findings in mechanically ventilated patients are nonspecific and difficult to interpret. Finally, the galactomannan test is of little value in nonneutropenic patients. The lack of specific criteria for diagnosing IPA in critically ill patients hampers timely initiation of appropriate antifungal therapy and may, as such, compromise the odds of survival.[13] The algorithm was evaluated in a multicenter trial by Bolt et al. With histopathology as the gold standard, the algorithm demonstrated 61% specificity and 92% sensitivity. Because the prevalence of IPA in ICU patients remains uncertain and may vary according to the risk profile of the index population, predictive values were calculated for different possible prevalences. For an assumed IPA prevalence of 40%, the positive predictive value (PPV) and negative predictive value were 61% and 92%, respectively. The need for a modified diagnostic approach for IPA in ICU patients has been repeatedly underlined (Flowchart 35.1).[12]

Flowchart 35.1: Diagnosis of IPA in ICU.

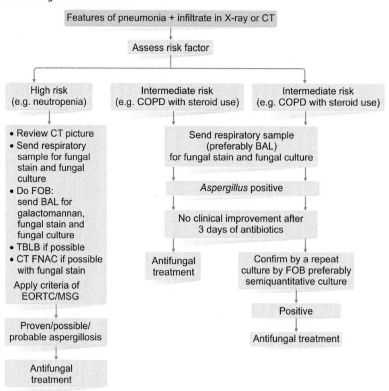

ICU, intensive care unit; IPA, invasive pulmonary aspergillosis; CT, computed tomography; FOB, fiberoptic bronchoscopy; BAL, bronchoalveolar lavage; TBLB, transbronchial lung biopsy; FNAC, fine needle aspiration cytology; EORTC/MSG, European Organization for Research and Treatment of Cancer/Mycoses Study Group; COPD, chronic obstructive pulmonary disease.
Courtesy: Shamim et al.[8]

Aspergilloma

Pulmonary aspergilloma is a saprophytic form of aspergillosis, and the diagnosis is usually based on radiological findings, such as thickened cavitary wall and fungus ball, and on positive serum antibody. Aspergilloma may manifest as an asymptomatic radiographic abnormality in a patient with preexisting cavitary lung disease due to sarcoidosis, tuberculosis, or other necrotizing pulmonary processes or cystic areas resulting from prior *Pneumocystis jirovecii* pneumonia (PCP) in patients with HIV infection.

The most common symptom in this disorder is productive cough and hemoptysis, which may be massive and life-threatening. Dyspnea could be related to their preexisting disease. Few patients experience systemic symptoms, such as fever, malaise, and weight loss. Over half of the patients will have clubbing.

Of the 23 patients retrospectively analyzed by Rafferty et al. in Northern General Hospital, Edinburgh from 1953 to 1982, hemoptysis occurred in 12 patients, which was fatal in two. IA occurred in five patients and two of them died.[14]

Chronic Necrotizing Pulmonary Aspergillosis

In the early 1980s, chronic necrotizing pulmonary aspergillosis (CNPA), also called semi-invasive or subacute IPA, was first described as a distinct type of pulmonary aspergillosis. In between the spectrum of saprophytic colonization of aspergilloma and IA, there appears to be definite existence of intermediate form such as semi-invasive or chronic IA in immunocompetent or marginally immunocompromised patients.[15]

Chronic necrotizing pulmonary aspergillosis was described as an indolent, cavitary, infectious process of the lung parenchyma secondary to local invasion by *Aspergillus* species, usually AF. CNPA tends to affect persons with abnormal pulmonary defense mechanisms as a result of underlying lung disease or immunocompromise.[16] It is an uncommon manifestation of aspergillosis that usually affects in middle-aged and elderly individuals with altered local defenses, associated with underlying chronic lung diseases, such as COPD, previous pulmonary tuberculosis, thoracic surgery, radiation therapy, pneumoconiosis, CF, lung infarction, or sarcoidosis. It may also occur in patients who are mildly immunocompromised due to DM, alcoholism, chronic liver disease, prolonged low-dose corticosteroid therapy, malnutrition, or connective tissue diseases, such as rheumatoid arthritis and ankylosing spondylitis.[17]

Chronic necrotizing pulmonary aspergillosis is slowly progressive over weeks to months and can eventually involve an entire lung, spread to contralateral hemithorax or invade pleura, mediastinum or chest wall. Patients appear chronically ill with respiratory symptoms and weight loss. Fever may be present (Table 35.2).

As against IPA, CNPA does not have any vascular invasion or dissemination to other organs. However, in contrast to aspergilloma, there is local invasion of lung tissue, and a preexisting cavity is not needed for CNPA to develop.

Aspergillomas may show progression over time causing destruction of wall of cavity and local parenchymal tissue invasion, especially in patients suffering from AIDS, mimicking CNPA. Aspergillomas are present in 50% cases of CNPA. Due to this overlap, Pasquallato et al. have grouped CNPA and aspergilloma as chronic cavitary pulmonary aspergillosis—which

Table 35.2: Diagnostic criteria for chronic necrotizing pulmonary aspergillosis.

Diagnostic criteria	Characteristics
Clinical	■ Chronic pulmonary or systemic symptoms such as weight loss, productive cough, or hemoptysis ■ No overt immunocompromising conditions ■ No dissemination
Radiological	■ Cavitary pulmonary lesion with surrounding infiltrates ■ Formation of new cavity, or ■ Expansion of cavity size over time
Laboratory	■ Elevated levels of inflammatory markers such as C-reactive protein or erythrocyte sedimentation rate ■ Either a positive serum Aspergillus precipitin test or isolation of Aspergillus spp. from the pulmonary or pleural cavity ■ Other pulmonary pathogens with similar disease presentation like mycobacteria and endemic fungi, should be excluded.

Adapted from: Hae-Seong Nam, et al. International Journal of Infectious Diseases, 2010.

is semi-invasive/noninvasive *Aspergillus* disease in immunocompromised host with chronic lung disease.

Allergic Bronchopulmonary Aspergillosis

Allergic bronchopulmonary mycosis is an immunological hypersensitivity lung disease caused by a hyperimmune response to the endobronchial growth of certain fungi and is considered to occur most commonly in atopic patients with asthma. If the disease is not adequately treated, irreversible damage occurs to the airways and lungs.

Hypersensitivity lung diseases include allergic asthma, hypersensitivity pneumonitis, and ABPA; all result from the exposure to allergens of AF. *Aspergillus* spores on inhalation trigger an immunoglobulin E (IgE)-mediated allergic inflammatory response in the bronchial airways, leading to bronchial obstruction and asthma.

Hypersensitivity pneumonitis is characterized by dyspnea due to pulmonary restriction and "influenza-like" syndrome due to fever and fatigue.

Serum IgE titers are usually very low in hypersensitivity pneumonitis, and eosinophilia is often insignificant.

Allergic bronchopulmonary aspergillosis develops from sensitization to allergens from AF present in the environment. Development of allergy to AF depends on the mode and frequency of exposure. Sensitization to AF allergens usually occurs in combination with other aeroallergens. In atopic persons, exposure to fungal spores and hyphal fragments leads to the production of specific IgE.[18] Repeated inhalation of *Aspergillus* spores, principally AF, leads to airway colonization in susceptible hosts that elicit an allergic response. Although type I (IgE-mediated) hypersensitivity is common, type III [immunoglobulin G (IgG)-mediated immune complex] and type IV (cell-mediated) reactions have also been observed; however, tissue invasion does not occur.[19]

Criteria For Diagnosis of Allergic Bronchopulmonary Aspergillosis

In 1977, Rosenberg and Patterson proposed criteria for the diagnosis of ABPA. Based on clinical, laboratory, and radiological features, it had a set of eight major and three minor criteria. Although there is no single test that can confidently establish the diagnosis, except presence of central bronchiectasis with tapering normal bronchi. This feature is considered pathognomonic of ABPA.

In 2002, Greenberger proposed a set of minimally essential criteria, which includes: (1) asthma, (2) immediate cutaneous reactivity to AF, (3) total serum IgE 1,000 ng/mL (417 kU/L), (4) elevated specific IgE-/IgG-AF, and (5) central bronchiectasis in the absence of distal bronchiectasis. When central bronchiectasis is not present, the disease entity is termed as serological ABPA, which could possibly be an earlier or a milder form of presentation. Greenberger in 2013 further suggested that minimal essential criteria 1–3 and 5 could possibly be considered "truly minimal" diagnostic criteria.

The International Society for Human and Animal Mycology Working Group has recently proposed another criterion. Here the items are classified as "obligatory" and "other" criteria. The obligatory features are: (1) positive cutaneous hypersensitivity reaction to *Aspergillus* antigen or high IgE specific to AF, (2) total IgE levels more than 1,000 IU/mL. These two features are essential for the diagnosis of ABPA. Other criteria include: (1) presence of IgG antibodies against AF in serum, (2) radiographic pulmonary opacities consistent with ABPA, and (3) raised total eosinophil counts (>500).

The frequency of *Aspergillus* sensitization in asthmatic subjects varies from 16% to 38% in different geographical regions. According to internationally available data, ABPA may be found in up to 6% of all asthmatic patients. In CF, the prevalence of ABPA ranges from 2% to 15%.

Allergic bronchopulmonary aspergillosis is usually seen in 20–40-year-old patients, but it has been rarely reported in children, and even in infants. The presentation can range from mild asthma, with very few symptoms, to extensive lung disease that may manifest as respiratory failure. Most of the patients will have repeated episodes of exacerbation of asthma, followed by periods of remission of various duration, usually after treatment with steroids. Cough, breathlessness, and wheezing are most prominent symptoms. Usually the patients may complain of expectorating yellowish brown mucus plugs that are pathognomonic of ABPA. More than one-third of the patients may present with hemoptysis.

◼ *PNEUMOCYSTIS JIROVECII* PNEUMONIA

Despite decreasing incidence, *Pneumocystis jirovecii* pneumonia (PCP) is the most common opportunistic infection in HIV-infected patients. Defective T-cell immunity is the primary risk factor for PCP.

On a background of predisposing factors, patients usually present with nonproductive cough, progressive exertional breathlessness, fever, and chest discomfort. The classic triad of fever, dyspnea, and nonproductive cough is present in half of the patients. Symptoms may progress slowly over weeks. The physical findings are nonspecific and at times unremarkable. Bilateral mild crackles or rhonchi may be present on auscultation. Sometimes these patients present with rapidly worsening hypoxemia. Small minority of the patients may also present with spontaneous pneumothorax.

DIAGNOSIS OF FUNGAL INFECTIONS

Diagnosis of fungal infection is difficult, painstakingly time and resource consuming and frustratingly low-yielding. High index of suspicion is usually rewarding. The paucity of specific signs of infections and the low sensitivity of conventional culture-based methods for its diagnosis contributes to delayed initiation of antifungal therapy.

The routine hematological and biochemistry of blood will point toward the underlying pathology. Patients with neutropenia and hematological malignancy are more commonly affected by fungal infection and so are the diabetics and renal failure patients. Therefore, respective changes will be shown in the routine hematology and biochemistry.

Raised eosinophils, IgE, and IgG specific to AF may help in differentiating allergic conditions due to *Aspergillus*. Eosinophilia and high IgE levels are seen in atopic conditions with ABPA. IgE specific to AF are present in ABPA but absent in aspergilloma. In contrast, raised IgG is seen in both ABPA and aspergilloma but not in *Aspergillus* asthma.

Routine blood cultures identify only 50–60% of disseminated candidiasis cases and typically require a 2-day to 5-day period of incubation and are rarely successful in identifying hematogenous aspergillosis. Therefore, negative blood cultures cannot readily exclude invasive fungal disease. Moreover, when blood cultures are positive, they are more commonly contaminants than real infection.

1. *Microbiological diagnosis*: Systemic fungal infections, according to standard criteria, are established when histopathologic examination with special stains confirms fungal tissue involvement or when the etiologic agent is isolated from clinical sterile specimens by culture. Conventional mycological methods include direct microscopic examination and the culture of samples in the mycology laboratory.
2. *Direct microscopy*: Direct microscopy of the clinical specimen is an initial, quick, and low-cost reliable tool which does not require expensive instruments. This method can promptly recognize many invasive fungal infections.

Although a negative direct examination cannot rule out fungal disease, visualization of fungal elements in specimens can often secure initial information helpful in the selection of empiric antifungal therapy.

The specimens from respiratory system for fungal examinations are oral swab, sputum, tracheal aspirate, bronchoalveolar lavage (BAL), and, at times, even computed tomography (CT)-/ultrasonography-guided aspirate from consolidation/abscess situated close to pleura. Pleural fluid/intercostal drain can also be sent for fungal examination and culture in appropriate clinical setting.

Analysis of expectorated sputa lacks both sensitivity and specificity for the diagnosis. Sputum study may show fungal hyphae or yeasts. However, the results must correlate with the clinical situation, because saprophytic colonization occurs in the oropharyngeal or respiratory tract of some patients and may not necessarily indicate invasive infection. BAL is superior to sputum study. In one study by Kahn et al., *Aspergillus* hyphae were identified in 9 of 17 BAL samples from patients with IPA and from 3 of the remaining 65 study patients without this diagnosis. Thus, the presence of *Aspergillus* hyphae in BAL samples had a 53% sensitivity, 97% specificity, and 75% PPV for the diagnosis of IPA. BAL fungal cultures were positive in only 4 of 17 cases (23% sensitivity).

The proper and timely selection, collection, and transport of specimens are imperative, and clinicians are responsible for appropriate specimen selection to ensure optimal chances of recovery of pathogens.

Specimens should be placed into transport media if the sample size is small or if only a small number of organisms are thought to be present. The immediate processing and culturing of clinical specimens for the isolation of fungi are highly desirable and, whenever possible, should always be the rule. However, some pathogenic fungi can be recovered from sputum specimens that are not processed and cultured immediately. Delayed specimen should not be rejected because of a time factor if transported under normal environmental conditions and planted on proper media.

The specimen is prepared by using 10-20% potassium hydroxide (KOH) that degrades the proteinaceous material leaving the fungal cell wall intact. The visibility of fungi within clinical specimens can be further enhanced by the addition of calcofluor white, a fluorophore, which binds to the chitin in fungal cell walls or lactophenol cotton blue, which stains the outer cell wall. Other stains are frequently used in direct microscopy, such as the India ink wet mount which is useful for visualization of encapsulated fungi, particularly *Cryptococcus neoformans*.

Pneumocystis jirovecii pneumonia can be diagnosed in direct microscopy by using various stains, such as KOH, Grocott-Gomori methenamine silver, newer immunofluorescent antibody stains, and highly sensitive direct fluorescent antibody.

Morphology of Different Fungi

Culture

Culture of fungus is an important tool for isolation and identification of pathogenic fungi in the evaluation of a suspected case of fungal disease even if the organism could not be identified by direct microscopy.

Fungi are difficult to cultivate despite proper handling of the specimen and appropriate culture methods. In one study, up to 70% of tissue samples with invasive septate hyphae visualized on histopathology did not grow a mold in culture. In another, approximately one-third of zygomycetous molds visualized on histopathology failed to grow.

In general, for respiratory samples, the most purulent and/or bloody portions of the specimen are inoculated directly onto specialized fungal culture media containing antibiotics to inhibit overgrowth with bacteria. Centrifugation of respiratory samples is not recommended.

The solid media are employed for fungal culture as broths are not usually recommended except for blood culture. The medium commonly used is Emmons modification of Sabouraud dextrose agar. The media may be supplemented by antibiotics to minimize bacterial contamination. Fungi grow relatively slow, and cultures are usually incubated for at least 4 weeks before being discarded as sterile. Usually positive cultures are obtained between 7 days and 10 days. In *Candida* and *Aspergillus* species, growth appears within 24-72 h. Unlike the isolation of fungi from sterile specimen, such as blood, cerebrospinal fluid (CSF), and pleural fluid, the results of fungal culture from respiratory secretions must be interpreted with due care. Importance must be given to quantity of fungus isolated, and further investigations must be undertaken. On the other hand, in severely immunocompromised individuals, no isolate should be lightly discarded, presuming it to be contaminant.

Failure to recover the organism does not negate diagnosis as this may be due to insufficient specimen collection, delayed transport, incorrect isolation procedures or inadequate temperature, and incubation periods.

- Susceptibility testing—Recovery and identification of the infecting fungal pathogen in culture also provides the opportunity for antimicrobial susceptibility testing and standardized procedures for testing both yeasts and molds have been established. Susceptibility testing is increasingly used to guide the selection of therapy, particularly for pathogens with unpredictable antifungal activity profiles and to rule out resistance in the setting of prior antifungal exposure and/or clinical failure.

Histopathological Diagnosis

Visualization of fungal elements within tissue samples provides definitive evidence of invasive infection. When fungal infection is suspected, care must be made to specifically request fungal cultures of the fresh tissue specimen. A diagnostic mycology laboratory should have sufficient feedback from its histopathology division. This is essential because most of the time, it is difficult to decide if fungal isolate in culture is significant or merely a contaminant.

Histopathologic examination of tissues can detect fungal invasion of tissues and blood vessels and also the host reaction to fungal infection.

The advantages of obtaining these specimens have created a series of diagnostic challenges because of the limited amount of tissue obtained and the architectural distortion produced by these new procedures.

Nonculture Methods

Fungal cultures have low sensitivity and long turn-around time. Noncultural methods are fundamental for a rapid diagnosis of invasive fungal diseases. These provide more rapid and sensitive results. These include:

- Antibodies detection
- Antigen detection (galactomannan, *Aspergillus* lateral-flow device, [1,3]-β-D-glucan, mannan)
- Molecular tests
- Fungal metabolites.

Detection of specific host antibody response provides information for the diagnosis of invasive fungal infection. However, such tests are not usually used for detection of *Candida*, *Aspergillus*, or *Cryptococcus* due to their poor sensitivity and specificity. Antibodies to these fungi are usually present in colonized but noninfected patients; and moreover, the host antibody response in severely immunosuppressed patient is poor and inadequate. However, the detection of antibody response is often used to detect the presence of endemic mycoses, such as blastomycosis, histoplasmosis, coccidioidomycosis amongst others. There are also problems associated with false positives generated through prior exposure either through skin testing or to the organism itself and cross-reactivity, and with false negatives resulting from the development of infection in immunocompromised patients. Serologic testing for *Coccidioides* is reasonably effective, and utilizing multiple serological testing modalities (complement fixation, immunodiffusion, and enzyme-linked immunosorbent assay) may be necessary for immunocompromised patients.

Tests to detect antigen are available for cryptococcosis in serum and CSF; and, for dimorphic fungi, such as histoplasmosis, coccidioidomycosis, and blastomycosis, in serum and urine. Some of these tests are available in reference laboratories and suffer from cross-reactivity.

1,3-β-D-glucan, a fungal cell wall constituent, can be detected in serum or plasma during invasive fungal infection. Unfortunately, the specificity is limited as this antigen is also produced by *Pseudomonas* and *Streptococcus*. 1,3-β-D-glucan elevation is a good predictor of *P. jirovecii* infection in immunocompromised patients, especially in the specific setting of AIDS patients with respiratory symptoms.

Galactomannan is an antigen detected in body fluids of experimental animals and patients with IA. It has been shown to correlate with clinical diagnosis and response to antifungal therapy. Unfortunately, it can be detected only in advanced disease.

Radiological Diagnosis of Fungal Infections

Chest X-ray is usually the first test ordered in a suspected case of lung infection and presents with symptoms of lung infection. On a background of immunosuppression, a high index of suspicion is required to diagnose a fungal infection. The X-ray not only helps in early detection but also can be used to follow up the progress. The chest CT scan is usually ordered if the X-ray is abnormal or even if when the X-ray is normal but the patient is breathless and/or hypoxemic in a given setting. The radiological investigations add value by suggesting infections caused by certain organism based on distinguishing features, thereby initiating early therapy as microbiological diagnosis takes few days to weeks to yield results.

Different fungi throw up different phenotypic characteristics on chest radiology, which under a given setting, may be suggestive of particular fungi; however, there is a considerable amount of overlap.

Parenchymal consolidation may be seen in blastomycosis, histoplasmosis, and cryptococcosis. In blastomycosis, the consolidation is usually central abutting the mediastinum.[21] Pulmonary blastomycosis may present as focal or patchy consolidations, and nodules that do not calcify. Patchy airspace consolidation is seen more frequently in IA (84%) at times along with tree in buds appearance than in candidiasis (50%) as noted by Althoff Souza et al. while evaluating high-resolution CT (HRCT) findings of IA and candidiasis in *Journal of Thorax Imaging*, 2006.

Halo Sign and Reverse Halo Sign

The halo sign is a CT finding of ground-glass opacity (GGO) surrounding the circumference of a pulmonary nodule or mass.[22] The halo sign is most commonly associated with IPA along with other infections and noninfectious conditions, such as neoplastic and inflammatory processes. The nodule or the mass in halo sign represents angioinvasion by *Aspergillus* leading to thrombosis and subsequent ischemic necrosis of the lung parenchyma while the GGO is due to hemorrhage due to infarction. Halo sign is the earliest manifestation in IA but it is transient and disappears after 3 days. Therefore, an early CT in suspected individuals is essential so that appropriate therapy can be started to improve the outcome. The presence of halo sign even precedes the detection of biomarkers, such as galactomannan.[22] Apart from halo sign, in a severely immunocompromised patient, IPA may present itself as a pulmonary nodule (>1 cm in diameter), cavitation of nodule or mass and appearance of crescent sign depending on the stage of the disease and timing of the thin section CT scan. The air crescent sign is a late sign due to retraction of necrotic tissue from the lung parenchyma after the neutrophilic infiltration and resolution of parenchyma. Thus the air crescent sign is diagnostically a useful sign for IPA but has a very little impact on the management. Segmental or peribronchial consolidation, tree-in-bud opacities, cavitary lesions, pleural effusions, nonspecific GGOs, and atelectasis are other nonspecific findings on radiology in a patient suffering from IPA. The lesions are distributed bilaterally but asymmetric. These nonspecific findings and even the halo sign are also seen in host of other fungal infections, such as *Candida*, and less commonly seen mucormycosis, but they are usually unifocal and in upper lobes. Mucormycosis may also exhibit the reverse halo sign, which is a focal rounded area of GGO surrounded by a crescent or complete ring of consolidation.[20] Histologically, there is an infarcted lung tissue with greater amount of hemorrhage at the periphery than at the center. The consolidation has a propensity to cavitate.

Aspergilloma, in immunocompetent individuals, is seen in preexisting lung cavity or ectatic bronchi. Radiologically, it can be seen as an oval or round soft tissue mass within the cavity separated by a layer of thin crescent of air from the walls of the cavity. This is called air crescent sign or monads sign. The position of fungal ball moves with the position of the patient and can be demonstrated on X-ray or CT scan by changing the posture of the patient. The walls of the cavity are thick, and adjacent pleural thickening may also be present.

Allergic bronchopulmonary aspergillosis typically presents itself radiologically as recurrent or transient patchy consolidation, central bronchiectasis, and mucoid impaction, manifesting itself as tubular "finger in glove" opacities, postobstructive atelectasis, and air trapping.

Candida presents itself as randomly distributed miliary or multiple large nodules when there is hematogenous spread or as bronchopneumonia with patchy bilateral consolidation. Peripherally distributed nodules or masses with cavitation and focal consolidation may be seen in cryptococcosis. In PCP, the initial X-ray may be normal; however, the patient will be symptomatic. As the disease progresses, the chest radiographs may show bilateral perihilar interstitial pattern. In HRCT chest, the most characteristic finding is bilateral GGO with patchy or confluent diffuse distribution. Often it has mosaic or geographic distribution with normal secondary pulmonary nodules adjacent to diseased one. In 10–30% of AIDS patients with PCP, multiple cystic lesions of various shapes, sizes, and wall thicknesses can be seen. Eventually these cysts are the cause of spontaneous pneumothorax in these patients. Other atypical findings in PCP are nodules or masses, interstitial fibrosis, lobar consolidation, or lymphadenopathy. Pleural effusion is extremely rare.

Active histoplasmosis presents itself as consolidation and lymphadenopathy. Calcified pulmonary granuloma may be seen as a sequel of the disease, seen in endemic areas. The disseminated disease may appear as tiny nodules in miliary or random distribution. Lymphadenopathy may also be seen in acute coccidioidomycosis along with multilobar consolidation. Occasionally, an area of consolidation may resolve and then appear elsewhere, this is called phantom consolidation.

▉ TREATMENT

For the infections caused by fungi, use of antifungals remains the cornerstone of the treatment. Adjunctive treatments include reversal of immunosuppression, whenever possible, and surgery in selected indications. For allergic reactions caused by *Aspergillus*, use of steroids is recommended.[23]

Less severe histoplasmosis can be treated with itraconazole, while severe or disseminated form in immunosuppressed patients may need amphotericin B. Usually liposomal preparations are preferred as they are significantly less nephrotoxic. Chronic pulmonary nodules of histoplasmosis may mimic malignancy but do not require any treatment if *Histoplasma* cannot be cultured. Fibrosing mediastinitis by *Histoplasma* may need a 12-week course of itraconazole. Here, the role of steroids or antifibrotic agents is unclear. Similarly, a 6–12-month course of itraconazole is sufficient for immunocompetent patients with pulmonary and nonmeningeal blastomycosis. More severe life-threatening forms of blastomycosis may need use of amphotericin B, preferably liposomal.

For IA, reversal of immunosuppression, e.g. withdrawal of steroids is recommended whenever possible. Immunotherapy, such as use of granulocyte/macrophage colony-stimulating factor, offers some protection. Surgery may be considered if aggressive antifungal therapy fails. Therapy is prolonged and needs to be individualized as per patients' clinical condition which may even last up to more than a year. Initial treatment is intravenous voriconazole or amphotericin B until patient improves clinically, followed by oral voriconazole or itraconazole until resolution or stabilization of all clinical and radiological manifestation. Intravenous caspofungin or micafungin or posaconazole may be used as a salvage therapy. The response can be monitored by serum galactomannan levels. There is insufficient data to support combination therapy though many clinicians use this as a last option.

Azoles are recommended for cases of mild-to-moderate chronic semi-IA until clinical or radiological resolution/stabilization. Intravenous amphotericin B is reserved for severe cases. Surgery can be considered based on severity of disease, anatomical consideration, and response to antifungal therapy.

Allergic bronchopulmonary aspergillosis is a noninvasive hypersensitivity disease. The treatment is therefore aimed at prevention of acute exacerbations and end-stage fibrotic disease. Cornerstone of the therapy is systematic steroids. Starting dose is usually 0.5 mg/kg/day which can be tapered as and when there is clinical improvement. Inhaled steroids, bronchodilators, and leukotriene antagonists are used for symptom control. Chronic steroids therapy is required to manage repeated exacerbations. It is important to monitor serum IgE levels at regular intervals, such as once in 2 months. Itraconazole therapy is sometimes used as steroid sparing and lead to early symptomatic improvement. But antifungal therapy has limited role in aspergillomas, which are fungal balls in the preexisting cavities of the lung. Hemoptysis is a dangerous complication, which may be life-threatening. Bronchial artery

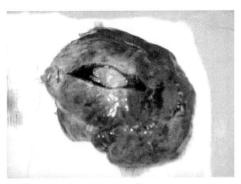

Fig. 35.2: Resected specimen of lung cavity with aspergilloma.

embolization may be required and is lifesaving. Rebleeding is common after embolization. Definitive treatment is surgical resection but is associated with high morbidity and mortality (Fig. 35.2).

Candida pneumonia is reported rarely. Pneumonia is secondary to aspiration of *Candida*-laden oropharyngeal secretion or as a result of hematogenous spread in an immunocompromised host. Isolation of *Candida* from respiratory secretions alone is insignificant and does not merit any treatment. But candidemia needs to be treated aggressively. Change of central venous catheter or hemodialysis catheter needs to be removed or changed to a new site. Candidemia can be treated with azoles, amphotericin B, or echinocandins, or a combination of fluconazole and amphotericin B. The choice of these agents is dependent on multiple factors including clinical status of patient and presence of liver or renal dysfunction. Species of *Candida*, drug susceptibility, and local epidemiologic data should be considered while choosing antifungal treatment. Fluconazole should be avoided if the incidence of non-*albicans Candida* is more than 10%.

Pneumocystis jirovecii pneumonia is an important cause of morbidity and mortality in immunosuppressed individuals. All patients with documented infection require urgent treatment. Trimethoprim (TMP)-sulfamethoxazole (SMX) is the most effective regimen for treatment. The clinical improvement after institution of proper treatment may take up to 7–10 days, which should be continued for at least 3 weeks. Second-line agents such as primaquine plus clindamycin or atovaquone or intravenous pentamidine, if available, should be considered if the patient fails to improve or in the case of clinical deterioration or intolerance/side effects due to SMX/TMP. In HIV patients with PCP and hypoxemia, adjunctive corticosteroids are instituted and tapered off over 3 weeks. Steroids are known to improve the outcome and reduce mortality. Prophylaxis by TMP/SMX in immunosuppressed patients has reduced the burden of the disease. Alternative to TMP/SMX combination for prophylaxis are dapsone, pyrimethamine, leucovorin, atovaquone, and pentamidine.

◼ REFERENCES

1. https://www.thoracic.org/patients/patient-resources/breathing-in-america/resources/chapter-9-fungal-lung-disease.pdf.

2. Chakrabarti A, Chatterjee S, Rudramurthy S. Overview of opportunistic fungal infections in India. Nihon Ishinkin Gakkai Zasshi. 2008;49:165-72.

3. Randhawa HS, Khan ZU. Histoplasmosis in India; current status. Indian J Chest Allied Sci. 1994; 36:193-213.

4. Sardi JC, Scorzoni L, Bernardi T, et al. *Candida* species: current epidemiology, pathogenicity, biofilm formation, natural antifungal products and new therapeutic options. J Med Microbiol. 2013;62 (Pt 1):10-24.

5. Brunke S, Hube B. Two unlike cousins: *Candida albicans* and *C. glabrata* infection strategies. Cell Microbiol. 2013;15(5):701-8.

6. Meersseman W, Lagrou K, Spriet I, et al. Significance of the isolation of *Candida* species from airway samples in critically ill patients: a prospective, autopsy study. Intensive Care Med. 2009;35:1526-31.

7. Shweihat Y, Perry J, Shah D. Isolated *Candida* infection of the lung. Respir Med Case Rep. 2015;16:18-9.

8. Shamim S, Agarwal A, Ghosh BK, et al. Fungal pneumonia in intensive care unit: when to suspect and decision to treatment: a critical review. J Assoc Chest Physicians. 2015;3(2):41-7.

9. Silva RF. Chapter 8: fungal infections in immunocompromised patients. J Bras Pneumol. 2010; 36(1):142-7.

10. Kosmidis C, Denning DW. The clinical spectrum of pulmonary aspergillosis. Thorax. 2015;70:270-7.

11. Kousha M, Tadi R, Soubani AO. Pulmonary aspergillosis: a clinical review. Eur Respir Rev. 2011; 20(121):156-74.

12. Azoulay E, Afessa B. Diagnostic criteria for invasive pulmonary aspergillosis in critically ill patients. Am J Respir Crit Care Med. 2012;186(1):8-10.

13. Blot SI, Taccone FS, Van den Abeele AM, et al. A clinical algorithm to diagnose invasive pulmonary aspergillosis in critically ill patients. Am J Respir Crit Care Med. 2012;186:56-64.

14. Rafferty P, Biggs BA, Crompton GK, et al. What happens to patients with pulmonary aspergilloma? Analysis of 23 cases. Thorax. 1983;38:579-83.

15. Panda BN. Fungal infections of the lung—the emerging scenario. Indian J Tuberc. 2004;51:63-9.

16. Nam HS, Jeon K, Um SW, et al. Clinical characteristics and treatment outcomes of chronic necrotizing pulmonary aspergillosis: a review of 43 cases. Int J Infect Dis. 2010;14:e479-82.

17. Kaymaz D, Ergün P, Candemir İ, et al. Chronic necrotizing pulmonary aspergillosis presenting as transient migratory thoracic mass: a diagnostic dilemma. Respir Med Case Rep. 2016;19:140-2.

18. Ishiguro T, Takayanagi N, Uozumi R, et al. Diagnostic criteria that can most accurately differentiate allergic bronchopulmonary mycosis from other eosinophilic lung diseases: a retrospective, single-center study. Respir Investig. 2016;54(4):264-71.

19. Ishiguro, Takashi & Takayanagi, Noboru & Uozumi, Ryuji & Baba, Yuri & Kawate, Eriko & Kobayashi, Yoichi & Takaku, Yotaro & Kagiyama, Naho & Shimizu, Yoshihiko & Morita, Satoshi & Sugita, Yutaka. (2016). Diagnostic criteria that can most accurately differentiate allergic bronchopulmonary mycosis from other eosinophilic lung diseases: A retrospective, single-center study. Respiratory Investigation. 54. 10.1016/j.resinv.2016.01.004.

20. Georgiadou SP, Sipsas NV, Marom EM, et al. The diagnostic value of halo and reversed halo signs for invasive mold infections in compromised hosts. Clin Infect Dis. 2011;52(9):1144-55.

21. Reichenberger F, Habicht JM, Gratwohl A, et al. Diagnosis and treatment of invasive pulmonary aspergillosis in neutropenic patients. Eur Respir J. 2002;19(4):743-55.

22. Orlowsk HLP, McWilliams S, Mellnick VM, et al. Imaging spectrum of invasive fungal and fungal-like infections. Radiographics. 2017;37:1119-34.

23. Limper AH, Knox KS, SarosAm GA, et al. An official American Thoracic Society statement: treatment of fungal infections in adult pulmonary and critical care patients. J Respir Crit Care Med. 2011;183:96-128.

36

Fungal Infections of Central Nervous System

Tanmay Trivedi, Puneet Agarwal

INTRODUCTION

Fungi are a diverse group of eukaryotic single-celled or multinucleate organisms that live by decomposing and absorbing the organic material in which they grow. Only a small group of fungi are pathogenic in humans. Invasive fungal infections of the central nervous system (CNS) are associated with high mortality and morbidity, particularly in immunocompromised hosts. Clinical presentation may range from acute and fulminant among the immunocompromised to indolent and insidious among the relatively immunocompetent. Incidence of CNS fungal infections is on a rise due to aging population, pandemic of human immunodeficiency virus (HIV), increasing malignancy, usage of chemotherapeutic drugs, and diabetes mellitus, immunosuppression with steroids and biologicals, organ transplant, and hepatorenal insufficiency.

They may result in meningitis, cerebritis, cerebral abscess, granuloma, and meningeal vasculitis. Computed tomography (CT) and magnetic resonance imaging (MRI) of the head and brain may show certain unique radiological characteristics aiding the diagnosis, but the findings are nonspecific in a large number of cases. Early diagnosis facilitates prompt initiation of treatment that is vital in disease control.

EPIDEMIOLOGY AND CLASSIFICATION

Precise information of the prevalence of fungal CNS infection is not available. A miniscule amount of species are pathogenic in humans, and even fewer caused invasive CNS infection. Although fungi are generally considered to be ubiquitous, there are species endemic to certain geographical areas. Examples are Blastomycetes, *Coccidioides*, *Paracoccidioides*, *Histoplasma*, *Sporothrix*, etc. Whereas fungi, such as *Aspergillus fumigatus*, *Candida albicans*, *Cryptococcus neoformans*, *Rhizopus arrhizus*, are ubiquitous in distribution. Infection with ubiquitous fungi does not provide any long-term immunity to the patients; and hence, relapses are noted.

Fungi are found as (1) molds (colonies of branching hyphae–mycelium), (2) yeasts (colonies of single cells), and (3) intermediate forms.

Some fungi are thermodimorphic and transform from mold to yeast based on environmental conditions. Clinically important examples are Blastomycetes, *Coccidioides*, *Histoplasma*, *Sporotrichum*, and *Paracoccidioides*. *Cryptococcus* remains as an encapsulated yeast in all environmental conditions.

PATHOGENESIS

Fungi selectively grow on organic matter in the presence of moisture. They produce enzymes that digest the macronutrients of organic matter and utilize the products for sustenance and proliferation.

The CNS is protected from pathogenic organisms by a relatively impermeable blood–brain barrier (BBB). The BBB acts as a physical barrier and deters fungal infestation. Under normal circumstances the microglia and CNS macrophages maintain immune surveillance with the help of activated T lymphocytes. However, in immunocompromised states, these anatomical and functional barriers are easily overcome by opportunistic pathogens, such as fungi, leading to clinical manifestations as described above. The fungi infiltrate the vessel wall deriving nutrition from the plasma. Inflammation of the vessel wall and fungal proliferation lead to ischemia of brain tissue. Liquefaction necrosis thus produced acts as a source of nutrition for the fungi leading to a vicious cycle.

CANDIDA SPECIES

Candida albicans is the most common pathogen in humans, followed by *C. parapsilosis*, *C. glabrata*, and *C. tropicalis* in that order. Candidemia is the fourth most common infection found in blood culture in patients with sepsis and has a crude mortality rate of 40%.[1] CNS infection is uncommon; however, postmortem studies in patients with candidemia show incidence of about 50%.[2] Risk factors in addition to neutropenia include advanced age, indwelling catheters, total parenteral nutrition, malignancy, immunosuppressive drugs, prolonged use of broad-spectrum antibiotics, and mucosal disruption.[1] Source of infections can be endogenous in immunocompromised patients and exogenous in the case of postsurgical and instrumentation-related infections.

It is the most common cause of scattered brain microabscesses after *Staphylococcus aureus* in adult population[3] with little involvement of the meninges and is chronic, whereas, in neonates, it presents as an acute meningitis.[4] Rarely, CNS *Candida* can present as a brain abscess with vascular involvement and basilar artery thrombosis or subarachnoid hemorrhage from rupture of mycotic aneurysms or vascular invasion (Fig. 36.1).[5]

Cerebrospinal fluid (CSF) examination shows pleocytosis characterized by a neutrophilic or monocytic predominance, reduction in glucose, and elevations in protein. Immunocompromised patients show less pleocytosis, which is a poor prognostic marker. CSF culture is frequently negative with increased yield in high volume, centrifuged samples.[6] Detection of 1,3-β-D-glucan, a component of fungal cell wall, has been used in the diagnosis of iatrogenic meningitis. Its presence is not specific for *Candida*.[7,8]

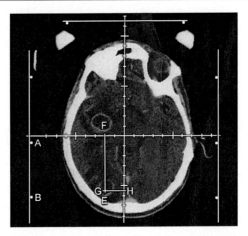

Fig. 36.1: A computed tomographic axial scan following contrast administration in a case of disseminated candidiasis showing a right temporal abscess and an occipital abscess, or both, treated with computed tomography (CT)-guided stereotactic surgery.

Magnetic resonance imaging has been useful in visualizing microabscesses that can identify biopsy targets and help monitor the therapy.

Treatment

Candidemia is treated with intravenous (IV) echinocandins (Caspofungin 70 mg loading, followed by 50 mg once daily).

For CNS infection initial treatment, liposomal amphotericin B (AmB), 5 mg/kg daily, with or without oral flucytosine, 25 mg/kg four times daily, is recommended. For step-down therapy after the patient has responded to initial treatment, fluconazole, 400–800 mg (6–12 mg/kg) daily, is recommended. Therapy should continue until all signs and symptoms and CSF and radiological abnormalities have resolved. Infected CNS devices, including ventriculostomy drains, shunts, stimulators, prosthetic reconstructive devices, and biopolymer wafers, which deliver chemotherapy, should be removed if possible. For patients in whom a ventricular device cannot be removed, Amphotericin B deoxycholate (AmBd) could be administered through the device into the ventricle at a dosage ranging from 0.01 mg to 0.5 mg in 2 mL 5% dextrose.[9]

■ *CRYPTOCOCCUS* SPECIES

The genus *Cryptococcus* consists of encapsulated yeast that lacks myecelium.[10] Primary infection involves lung parenchyma with subsequent dissemination to brain parenchyma and meninges in 40–86% cases.[11] *C. neoformans* and *Cryptococcus gattii* are the two main pathogenic fungi in HIV and non-HIV host and have a predisposition to involve dopaminergic tracts. The fungus inhabits the soil and uses the virulence factor laccase to protect itself from phytotoxins in its role as a plant pathogen of seedlings. During human infections, it uses this same laccase as a neurotropic virulence factor, oxidizing neurocatecholamines within dopaminergic tracts, particularly the basal ganglia, to produce immunosuppressive compounds, such as melanin.[12] Patient with acquired immune deficiency syndrome (AIDS) has much higher risk of infection (2.9–13%) as compared with non-HIV-infected patient (0.2–0.9%). Major risk factors in non-HIV population consist of hematological malignancies, diabetes mellitus, use of steroid, and biologicals for immunosuppression.[13] Approximately 13–18% of patients with cryptococcal disease may have no known underlying immunocompromising conditions but contribute up to 35–50% of the attributable mortality owing to delays in diagnosis from slow presentations in an unsuspected host.[14,15] *Cryptococcus* may have an indolent clinical course in immunocompetent host, leading to delay in diagnosis and sequelae, such as cranial neuropathies and cognitive impairment.

Clinical presentation in the form of subacute to chronic meningitis with fever, mental status changes (often confused with dementia), seizures, or basilar meningeal signs may occur; in the absence of fever, these presentations make the diagnosis of cryptococcal disease difficult. Cranial neuropathies that affect cranial nerves II through VIII are not uncommon and may be related to elevated intracranial pressure (ICP) manifested by papilledema, direct fungal invasion, or inflammation. Hearing loss, vision loss, gait ataxia with or without urinary incontinence may accompany obstructive or nonobstructive hydrocephalus.

Cerebrospinal fluid examination is the most important test for diagnosis and to determine efficacy of treatment. It classically demonstrates low glucose, elevated protein, and high IgG indices, although cell counts can be quite low, especially in HIV-related cases. Low cell count is a poor prognostic sign, as are persistent fungal growth and elevated ICP.[16] Serum and CSF may be tested for the presence of cryptococcal antigen using enzyme assay or latex agglutination test. This test is significant in culture negative cases. In 2009, a low-cost and single-point lateral flow assay test was introduced for the detection of cryptococcal antigen, which has shown high level of agreement with traditional tests.[16] An India ink preparation is commonly used with CSF to identify the organism and to support a presumptive diagnosis.[17] If performed correctly, 25–50% of patients with cryptococcal meningitis show cryptococci. Diagnosis depends on detecting the organism with culture; therefore, it always confirms positive smears with cultures. Culture-centrifuged CSF specimens on three or more occasions are to increase the yield.[18]

Magnetic resonance imaging may reveal focal mass, such as cryptococcomas or granulomas, leptomeningeal enhancement, hydrocephalus with or without transependymal flow, and dilated Virchow–Robin perivascular spaces with gelatinous pseudocysts[19,20] (Fig. 36.2).

Medical Management[9]

Human Immunodeficiency Virus-infected Patients

Induction: AmB 0.7–1 mg/kg/day (can substitute liposomal amphotericin 4–6 mg/kg/day) + flucytosine 100 mg/kg in four divided doses × 4–6 weeks (minimum).
Successful treatment to be considered only after CSF culture negative at 4 weeks.
Consolidation: Oral fluconazole 400 mg/day × 8 weeks (minimum).
Maintenance: Oral fluconazole 200 mg/day × 1 year (minimum).

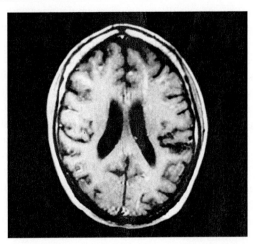

Fig. 36.2: A T1-weighted axial magnetic resonance (MR) image following contrast infusion, in a well-diagnosed case of cryptococcal meningitis, showing small multiple enhancing areas in the white matter in both the cerebral hemispheres representing foci of cryptococcal infection.

Organ Transplant Patient

Induction: Lipid formulation—Amphotericin + flucytosine × 2 weeks (minimum).
Consolidation: Oral fluconazole 400–800 mg/day × 8 weeks.
Maintenance: Oral fluconazole 200–400 mg × 6–12 months.

Immunocompetent Host

Induction: AmB + flucytosine × 4 weeks. The 4-week induction therapy is reserved for persons with meningoencephalitis without neurological complications and CSF yeast culture results that are negative after 2 weeks of treatment. In complicated cases, induction phase to continue for 6 weeks.
Consolidation: Oral fluconazole 400–800 mg/day × 8 weeks.
Maintenance: Oral fluconazole 200–400 mg × 6–12 months.

Raised Intracranial Pressure (Any Group)

If ICP ≥ 25 cm H_2O and symptomatic, then remove CSF via lumbar puncture (LP) to closing pressure of ≤20 mm H_2O or ≤50% of opening pressure (OP), if OP very high, recheck OP daily until stable × 2 days.

Surgical Management

Temporary ventriculostomy or lumbar drain if requiring daily LP for ICP management and for the management of hydrocephalus.

ASPERGILLUS SPECIES

They are ubiquitous septated molds which have a higher propensity to invade the tissue and vasculature in immunosuppressed host. *Aspergillus* species cause both allergic and invasive syndromes.[21] *A. fumigatus* is the most common pathogenic species responsible for 90% of clinical syndrome. *Aspergillus flavus, Aspergillus nidulans,* and *Aspergillus terreus* are other non-*fumigatus Aspergillus* species, the incidence of which is on the rise.[22] Risk factors include quantitative and qualitative neutropenia, hematologic malignancies, chronic granulomatous disease, end-stage AIDS, transplantation, and autoimmune diseases requiring corticosteroids.[23] The lungs and paranasal sinuses are the primary routes of infection with intracranial dissemination in 10–20% of cases.

Fever, headache, changes in mental status, hemiparesis, and seizures may occur. Cavernous venous thrombosis and skull base involvement may lead to multiple cranial nerve palsies. Nasal stuffiness, ear discharge, and periorbital pain may occur in the trans-sinus route with subsequent proptosis, ophthalmoplegia, chemosis, and visual loss. Angioinvasion usually involves anterior and middle cerebral arteries resulting in stroke syndromes that present acutely. In addition, brain parenchymal aspergillosis may cause mycotic aneurysms or hemorrhage, ring lesions with abscess formation via hematogenous dissemination, and direct tissue plane invasion from the paranasal sinuses. Relatively immunocompetent hosts demonstrate a contained fibrous capsule.[24] Case-fatality proportion is 50–100% in case series with complications, such as cavernous sinus thrombosis requiring prompt surgical intervention.

Diagnosis is made via tissue biopsy culture and histopathology, but biomarkers such as serum galactomannan and 1,3-β-D-glucan or polymerase chain reaction are becoming increasingly used with high negative predictive values. These biomarkers have not yet been sufficiently validated for the CSF, although reports supporting their successful use exist.[25] CSF sampling may be difficult when a mass effect is present. If invasive pulmonary aspergillosis is suspected in a patient, performing CT scanning of the chest, regardless of chest radiography findings, is recommended. Bronchoscopy with bronchoalveolar lavage is also recommended in these patients to obtain samples for histopathology and culture. The brain MRI findings include infarction, abscess like ring-enhancing lesions following infarction, dural, or vascular infiltration from paranasal sinus or orbit and extradural occupying infiltrates. Ischemic lesions may be visualized using MRI diffusion-weighted imaging. Irregular space-occupying lesions that are hypointense or isointense on T1 but bright on postgadolinium T1 and dim on T2, correlate with brain tissue coagulative necrosis[26] (Fig. 36.3).

Medical Management

If invasive aspergillosis (IA) is suspected, antifungal therapy should be initiated while diagnostic evaluation is ongoing. Voriconazole is recommended for primary treatment of IA, although combination therapy with voriconazole and echinocandin may be warranted for some high-risk patients. Antifungal therapy for IA should continue for at least 6–12 weeks.

Alternative therapies include liposomal AmB, isavuconazole, or other lipid formulations of AmB. Combination antifungal therapy with voriconazole and an echinocandin may be considered in select patients with documented IA. Primary therapy with an echinocandin is

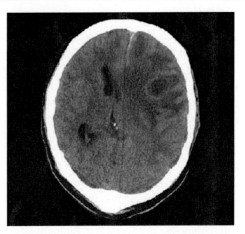

Fig. 36.3: An axial plain computed tomography (CT) brain scan showed a left frontal abscess with extensive edema and mass effects with subfalcine herniation in a case of aspergillosis.

not recommended. Echinocandins (micafungin or caspofungin) can be used in settings in which azole and polyene antifungals are contraindicated.[27]

■ *MUCORMYCOSIS* SPECIES

Mucormycosis is a disease caused by a group of clinically aggressive aseptate molds that infect the same patient populations as *Aspergillus*. Mucormycosis must be distinguished from aspergillosis because of its aggressive course, requirement for surgical debridement, and poor response to voriconazole therapy. Delayed diagnosis results in significantly higher mortality.[28] Mucormycosis should rise in the differential in patients with prolonged neutropenia, especially in the setting of leukemia, high-risk hematopoietic stem cell transplantation. Diabetic ketoacidosis and corticosteroid-associated hyperglycemia, IV drug use, and iron overload states (e.g. massive transfusions following major trauma) as well as deferoxamine chelation are also unique risk factors for mucormycosis.[29] Rhinocerebral disease is the major CNS manifestation, especially in uncontrolled diabetes mellitus or stem cell transplant recipients. The mold traverses tissue planes inferiorly to the palate and sphenoid sinus, laterally to the cavernous sinus and orbits, and cranially via the orbital apex or cribriform plate to the brain. Sinusitis, periorbital cellulitis, and facial numbness or pain with or without associated ocular cranial neuropathies in a susceptible host should trigger a high index of suspicion and early intervention.[30] Findings on imaging include rhino-orbital disease, with or without cerebral invasion, accompanied by bony destruction.[31] A strong tropism for invasion of blood vessels also results in a propensity for infarction and necrosis in both neurologic and pulmonary lesions.[32] All such immunosuppressed patients should have rapid evaluation by otolaryngology and biopsy of suspicious lesions. Typically, sinus lesions are necrotic, but this sign is unreliable, especially early in the disease; thus, absence of tissue necrosis in the appropriate host should not preclude tissue biopsy.

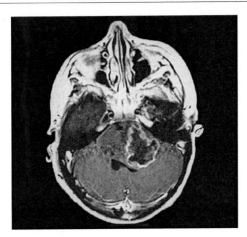

Fig. 36.4: An axial T1-weighted magnetic resonance (MR) scan in a known fatal case of extensive sino-cranio-orbital mucormycosis showed a large left pontine abscess with variegated irregular abscess capsule.

Sinus CT may show fluid-filled sinuses, bony destruction is a late finding. MRI is more sensitive and can identify cavernous sinus thrombosis and perineural intradural spread[30] (Fig. 36.4). On biopsy, lack of septa in the hyphae, with irregular diameters, is an important histologic feature that distinguishes *Mucorales* from *Aspergillus*, evident on Gomori methenamine–silver stain as well as by calcofluor-white fluorescent stain. CSF offers poorer yield.

Therapy normally includes aggressive debridement with clean surgical edges and high-dose liposomal AmB-based regimens accompanied by reductions in immunosuppression with or without adjunctive therapy, such as cytokine support, granulocyte transfusions, or hyperbaric oxygen.[31] Posaconazole has activity against certain species and may be used effectively as salvage or in combination with liposomal AmB but has poor CNS penetration; serum levels must be monitored. Mortality remains high at 25–40%.[30]

EXSEROHILUM ROSTRATUM

It was identified as the major pathogen (20% or more) in the largest recorded fungal outbreak to date. This was the consequence of contamination of compounding pharmacy with lots of preservative-free methylprednisolone acetate for epidural, spinal, or paraspinal injections to treat chronic musculoskeletal pain. A total of 751 iatrogenic cases were identified by the Centers for Disease Control and Prevention with 64 deaths (case fatality ratio = 8.5%).[33] Symptoms began approximately 40 days following exposure. One-third of those affected developed meningitis; while 5% had posterior circulation strokes (ischemic more often than hemorrhagic). Although the majority of cerebrovascular events affected the vertebrobasilar system, many affected the basal ganglia, and 85% of deaths were associated with stroke. Forty-three percent had spinal or paraspinal infections presenting as epidural abscess, vertebral osteomyelitis/discitis, arachnoiditis, and cauda equina syndrome. Accordingly, fever, headache, and back pain were the most common symptoms.[34]

Dimorphic Endemic Fungi

These fungi are geographically restricted and exist as tissue-invasive yeast forms at human body temperature but as molds in the environment. The main etiologies in North America include *Blastomyces dermatitidis* in the United States Midwestern states and Canadian provinces that border the Great Lakes and St Lawrence River, as well as Southeastern and South Central states; *Histoplasma capsulatum* around the Ohio and Mississippi river basins; and *Coccidioides immitis* and *Coccidioides posadasii* in the arid Southwestern United States. The use of tumor necrosis factor-α antagonists increases the risk for disseminated disease in all these following inhalation of the fungus.[35]

Progressive disseminated histoplasmosis may occur after exposure to soil contaminated by avian droppings or bat guano from endemic areas, or among patients with AIDS or other cellular immune deficits, the latter of which may be subclinical. Among those with disseminated histoplasmosis, CNS disease may occur in 5–10% as manifested by focal parenchymal lesions of the brain or spinal cord and chronic meningoencephalitis with or without ischemic strokes due to emboli or small-vessel vasculitis, as can be seen in cryptococcosis and the other endemic mycoses. CSF reveals high protein and hypoglycorrhachia with a myeloid pleocytosis. Urine, serum, and CSF *Histoplasma* galactomannan antigen (quantitative enzyme immunoassay) may be positive, but cross-reaction with *Blastomyces* is frequent. CSF culture requires multiple high-volume sampling to increase the yield.[36] Biopsy of mass lesions may be positive by culture and histopathology.[37] Corticosteroids may be inadvertently given rather than antifungal therapy for presumed noninfectious vasculitis, which can lead to clinical deterioration.[38] Liposomal AmB (5 mg/kg/day for a total of 175 mg/kg given over 4-6 weeks) followed by itraconazole (200 mg two or three times a day) for at least 1 year is the suggested treatment for CNS histoplasmosis, with monitoring of itraconazole trough serum levels and CSF *Histoplasma* antigen. Voriconazole or posaconazole may be effective step-down alternatives.[31] Lifelong suppressive therapy with such triazoles may be necessary in those for whom effective immune reconstitution is not possible, as relapse may occur.

Disseminated coccidioidomycosis occurs after exposure to dust from endemic areas, especially among high-risk groups, such as African Americans, Filipinos, Hispanics, those in late pregnancy, and those who are immunocompromised because of AIDS or transplant conditioning or genetic mutations. CNS involvement may occur in up to half, presenting as a chronic basilar meningitis with headache, low-grade fever, weight loss, and mental status changes, but one-third of patients may lack meningismus. Hydrocephalus and ischemic vasculitis may complicate up to 40% of cases months later.[3] MRI may reveal predominantly leptomeningeal enhancement of the basilar cisterns and middle cerebral artery cisterns. Hydrocephalus with transependymal flow may require shunting. Spinal nerve root enhancement and clumping that may be asymptomatic occurs in one-third of cases.[39] CSF may occasionally reveal an eosinophilic pleocytosis with elevated protein and low glucose, but culture is positive in only about 15%, requiring complement fixation titers that may have a diagnostic yield of greater than 70%.[3] The clinical microbiology laboratory should be notified if this diagnosis is suspected so that appropriate specimen handling may be performed. Fluconazole is the drug of choice, affording nearly 80% clinical response, but intrathecal AmB has also been advocated.[36] Lifelong suppressive therapy may be needed, as relapse can occur. Nonetheless, 40% mortality has remained in the postazole era.[3]

CONCLUSION

Central nervous system fungal infections are associated with high mortality and morbidity. Clinical manifestations are varying depending on host immune status. High degree of suspicion and astute investigation can facilitate timely diagnosis. Early and efficacious treatment with appropriate antifungals and surgery, if required, can improve clinical outcome and reduce the mortality.

REFERENCES

1. Pfaller MA, Diekema DJ. Epidemiology of invasive candidiasis: a persistent public health problem. Clin Microbiol Rev. 2007;20(1):133-63.
2. Lipton SA, Hickey WF, Morris JH, et al. Candidal infection in the central nervous system. Am J Med. 1984;76(1):101-8.
3. Pendlebury WW, Perl DP, Munoz DG. Multiple microabscesses in the central nervous system: a clinicopathologic study. J Neuropathol Exp Neurol. 1989;48(3):290-300.
4. Faix RG. Systemic *Candida* infections in infants in intensive care nurseries: high incidence of central nervous system involvement. J Pediatr. 1984;105(4):616-22.
5. Burgert SJ, Classen DC, Burke JP, et al. Candidal brain abscess associated with vascular invasion: a devastating complication of vascular catheter-related candidemia. Clin Infect Dis. 1995;21(1):202-5.
6. Voice RA, Bradley SF, Sangeorzan JA, et al. Chronic candidal meningitis: an uncommon manifestation of candidiasis. Clin Infect Dis. 1994;19(1):60-6.
7. Lyons JL, Erkkinen MG, Vodopivec I. Cerebrospinal fluid (1,3)-β-D-glucan in isolated candida meningitis. Clin Infect Dis. 2015;60(1):161-2.
8. Litvintseva AP, Lindsley MD, Gade L, et al. Utility of (1-3)-β-D-glucan testing for diagnostics and monitoring response to treatment during the multistate outbreak of fungal meningitis and other infections. Clin Infect Dis. 2014;58(5):622-30.
9. Perfect JR, Dismukes WE, Dromer F, et al. Clinical practice guidelines for the management of cryptococcal disease: 2010 update by the Infectious Diseases Society of America. Clin Infect Dis. 2010;50(3):291-322.
10. Halliday CL, Bui T, Krockenberger M, et al. Presence of alpha and a mating types in environmental and clinical collections of *Cryptococcus neoformans var. gattii* strains from Australia. J Clin Microbiol. 1999;37(9):2920-6.
11. Perfect JR, Casadevall A. Cryptococcosis. Infect Dis Clin North Am. 2002;16:837-74, v-vi.
12. Williamson PR. Laccase and melanin in the pathogenesis of *Cryptococcus neoformans*. Front Biosci. 1997;2:e99-107.
13. Husain S, Wagener MM, Singh N. *Cryptococcus neoformans* infection in organ transplant recipients: variables influencing clinical characteristics and outcome. Emerg Infect Dis. 2001;7:375-81.
14. Bratton EW, El Husseini N, Chastain CA, et al. Comparison and temporal trends of three groups with cryptococcosis: HIV-infected, solid organ transplant, and HIV-negative/non-transplant. PLoS One. 2012;7(8):e43582.
15. Brizendine KD, Baddley JW, Pappas PG. Predictors of mortality and differences in clinical features among patients with cryptococcosis according to immune status. PLoS One. 2013;8(3):e60431.
16. Lindsley MD, Mekha N, Baggett HC, et al. Evaluation of a newly developed lateral flow immunoassay for the diagnosis of cryptococcosis. Clin Infect Dis. 2011;53(4):321-5.
17. Rivet-Dañon D, Guitard J, Grenouillet F, et al. Rapid diagnosis of cryptococcosis using an antigen detection immunochromatographic test. J Infect. 2015;70(5):499-503.
18. Ogundeji AO, Albertyn J, Pohl CH, et al. Method for identification of *Cryptococcus neoformans* and *Cryptococcus gattii* useful in resource-limited settings. J Clin Pathol. 2016;69(4):352-7.

19. Starkey J, Moritani T, Kirby P. MRI of CNS fungal infections: review of aspergillosis to histoplasmosis and everything in between. Clin Neuroradiol. 2014;24(3):217-30.

20. Hansen J, Slechta ES, Gates-Hollingsworth MA, et al. Large-scale evaluation of the immuno-mycologics lateral flow and enzyme-linked immunoassays for detection of cryptococcal antigen in serum and cerebrospinal fluid. Clin Vaccine Immunol. 2013;20(1):52-5.

21. Marr KA, Patterson T, Denning D. Aspergillosis. Pathogenesis, clinical manifestations, and therapy. Infect Dis Clin North Am. 2002;16:875-94, vi.

22. Lass-Florl C, Griff K, Mayr A, et al. Epidemiology and outcome of infections due to *Aspergillus terreus*: 10-year single centre experience. Br J Haematol. 2005;131:201-7.

23. Panackal AA, Bennett JE, Williamson PR. Treatment options in invasive aspergillosis. Curr Treat Options Infect Dis. 2014;6(3):309-25.

24. Song E, Jaishankar GB, Saleh H, et al. Chronic granulomatous disease: a review of the infectious and inflammatory complications. Clin Mol Allergy. 2011;9(1):10.

25. Barton RC. Laboratory diagnosis of invasive aspergillosis: from diagnosis to prediction of outcome. Scientifica (Cairo). 2013;2013:459405.

26. Shamim MS, Enam SA, Ali R, Anwar S. Craniocerebral aspergillosis: a review of advances in diagnosis and management. J Pak Med Assoc. 2010;60(7):573-9.

27. Patterson TF, Thompson GR 3rd, Denning DW, et al. Practice guidelines for the diagnosis and management of aspergillosis: 2016 Update by the Infectious Diseases Society of America. Clin Infect Dis. 2016;63(4):e1-60.

28. Lass-Florl C, Resch G, Nachbaur D, et al. The value of computed tomography-guided percutaneous lung biopsy for diagnosis of invasive fungal infection in immunocompromised patients. Clin Infect Dis. 2007;45(7):e101-4.

29. Garcia-Vidal C, Upton A, Kirby KA, Marr KA. Epidemiology of invasive mold infections in allo-geneic stem cell transplant recipients: biological risk factors for infection according to time after transplantation. Clin Infect Dis. 2008;47(8):1041-50.

30. Petrikkos G, Skiada A, Lortholary O, et al. Epidemiology and clinical manifestations of mucormycosis. Clin Infect Dis. 2012;54(Suppl. 1):S23-34.

31. Vehreschild JJ, Birtel A, Vehreschild MJ, et al. Mucormycosis treated with posaconazole: review of 96 case reports. Crit Rev Microbiol. 2013;39(3):310-24.

32. Ben-Ami R, Luna M, Lewis RE, et al. A clinicopathological study of pulmonary mucormycosis in cancer patients: extensive angioinvasion but limited inflammatory response. J Infect. 2009;59(2):134-8.

33. Centers for Disease Control and Prevention. Multistate outbreak of fungal meningitis and other infections. [online] Available from www.cdc.gov/hai/outbreaks/meningitis.html. Updated October 23, 2013 [Accessed October 2, 2015].

34. Chiller TM, Roy M, Nguyen D, et al. Clinical findings for fungal infections caused by methyl-prednisolone injections. N Engl J Med. 2013;369(17):1610-9.

35. Smith JA, Kauffman CA. Endemic fungal infections in patients receiving tumour necrosis factor-alpha inhibitor therapy. Drugs. 2009;69(11):1403-15.

36. Galgiani JN, Ampel NM, Blair JE, et al. Coccidioidomycosis. Clin Infect Dis. 2005;41(9):1217-23.

37. Wheat LJ, Musial CE, Jenny-Avital E. Diagnosis and management of central nervous system histoplasmosis. Clin Infect Dis. 2005;40(6):844-52.

38. Saccente M. Central nervous system histoplasmosis. Curr Treat Options Neurol. 2008;10(3):161-7.

39. Galgiani JN, Catanzaro A, Cloud GA, et al. Fluconazole therapy for coccidioidal meningitis. The NIAID-Mycoses Study Group. Ann Intern Med. 1993;119(1):28-35.

NEW FRONTIERS IN MYCOLOGY

37

Vaccines, Immunotherapies, Nanobiotechnology and Newer Antifungals

Monica Mahajan

▨ INTRODUCTION

The field of mycology is expanding at a fast pace with frequent identification of new human fungal pathogens. Unfortunately, the treatment of these infections is still limited to the four conventional groups of antifungals—azoles, polyenes, echinocandins and flucytosine. These drugs have inherent issues in their usage, including efficacy against a limited number of fungi, drug interactions, toxicity, resistance, duration and expense of treatment, including need for hospitalization. The antifungal drug development has not matched pace with the dramatic rise in the cases of invasive fungal infection (IFI). Longevity is increasing, but it also implies a burgeoning number of immunocompromised patients undergoing chemotherapy and organ transplant. Human immunodeficiency virus (HIV) and acquired immune deficiency syndrome epidemic increased the incidence of pathogens, such as *Cryptococcus neoformans*, whereas the development of highly active antiretroviral therapy (HAART) has subsequently decreased the incidence. In the underdeveloped nations, cryptococcal meningitis continues to be a major cause of morbidity and mortality since a large number of people do not have access to HAART. In contrast, most cases of IFI in the developed countries are nosocomially acquired. Widespread use of broad-spectrum antibiotics is adding to the woes. Cadaveric and live donor transplants are increasing. The exact incidence of IFI is not known due to nonspecific symptoms, gaps in knowledge, underdiagnosis, and underreporting. However, it is estimated that there are at least 1.5 million cases of IFI annually worldwide. These include infections from molds, yeasts, and dimorphic fungi. There are rare and emerging fungal diseases that are adding to the numbers. The antifungal drugs focus on targeting the pathogen and aim at curing the disease. We need preventive strategies if we wish to reduce the burden of IFIs. Multifactorial drug resistance is a concern. Vaccines have been developed against bacteria and viruses and are a part of universal immunization program. Trials on fungal vaccines began in the 1980s with clinical trials being conducted on vaccine against coccidioidomycosis. However, no fungal vaccine has been approved till date against any fungal pathogen. There is a relative lack of funding for research and development for human fungal vaccines. Most fungal vaccines developed till now do not meet with the stringent efficacy and safety measures set for approval of vaccines.

■ FUNGAL VACCINES—THE UNMET NEED

A vaccine should have a high benefits to risks ratio, few side effects and provide long-term protection. The efforts to develop effective fungal vaccines have faced many hurdles. Majority of the patients susceptible to IFI are immunocompromised. It is debatable whether their immune system will be able to develop an adequate response on active immunization. Moreover, the vaccine may do more harm than good by putting them at an increased risk of opportunistic fungal infection. The route and timing of vaccination may have to be individualized in specific situations, such as neutropenia, thrombocytopenia or organ transplant. This is in contrast to vaccines against bacteria, which have a specific dose, route of administration, timing and length of protection.

There are technical challenges in developing fungal vaccines. Various cellular components have been targeted for vaccine development. These include the whole cell, cell wall, cytoplasmic extracts, dendritic cells (DCs) and recombinant proteins. These vaccines have shown promising results against various fungi, including *Candida* and *Aspergillus* species in immunocompromised animal models. The issue remains whether the results can be replicated in immunocompromised human hosts. Vaccines for *Candida albicans, Cryptococcus neoformans, Aspergillus fumigatus,* and *Paracoccidioides brasiliensis* have been tested in animal models but have not been endorsed for human use due to technical issues. Novel vaccines against *C. albicans* and *C. neoformans* offered immunity in neutropenic Balb/C mice and in CD4$^+$ and/or CD8$^+$-depleted Balb/C mice, respectively. Two recombinant protein vaccines against *Candida* species are in clinical trials. Other vaccines are in the stages of preclinical development.

Fungi, such as *C. albicans* are asymptomatic commensals. There can be a symbiotic relationship between the fungus and the host. Altering this relationship can be disadvantageous.

Vaccinating against fungi, such as *Cryptococcus* and *Coccidioides*, entails the risk of reactivating these infections since these have a clinical latency phase in the host. The risks may outweigh the benefits while vaccinating for allergic conditions, such as allergic bronchopulmonary aspergillosis.

Animals and fungi have evolutionary similarities and fungi resemble animals much more than resembling plants. The fungi have numerous molecular similarities with humans. This limits the number of unique fungal antigens which may be targeted for vaccine development. Biomolecules targeting fungi can be toxic to humans.

Fungi have the capability to change their morphological types, antigenic profile, virulence factors, and genetic makeup enabling them to develop resistant/mutant strains. This enables them to evade an attack by the immune system and may result in failure of the candidate vaccines. The molecular mechanisms regulating the vaccine immune response have not been fully understood in the case of fungal pathogens.

The killed and attenuated vaccines work on the principles that exposure to these killed or attenuated pathogens generates immunological memory. These can be very effective in combating opportunistic and endemic fungi once the safety concerns have been addressed.

Killed Vaccines

Killed vaccines contain previously virulent pathogens that have been destroyed with chemicals, heat or radiation. Heat-killed *Saccharomyces cerevisiae* yeasts (HKY) are used as subcutaneous injections. These direct immune cells to recognize common polysaccharide epitopes in the cell wall, including glucans and mannans. These vaccines are found to be protective against *C. albicans* and *A. fumigatus*. Formalin-killed *Coccidioides immitis* spherules (FKS)-based vaccine was found to be effective in animal models but failed placebo-controlled phase III clinical trials.

Attenuated Vaccines

Attenuated vaccines contain live, attenuated fungi that have been cultivated under conditions that disable their virulent properties. These may also use closely related but less dangerous fungal strains to produce an immune response. Attenuated vaccines carry the risk of producing an infection in an immunocompromised patient. These vaccines are more useful for the prevention of endemic fungal infections since these fungi cause infections in immuno-competent individuals. An attenuated vaccine for *Blastomyces dermatitidis* has been tested for immunization in mice models with low CD4+ T-cell counts. A mutant produced by deletion of *Blastomyces* adhesion-1 is used as subcutaneous injections to offer protection from a lethal inoculum. Another live vaccine has been developed by engineering a *C. neoformans* strain to produce murine interferon-γ (H99γ). These live attenuated vaccines are genetically engi-neered to produce cytokines and generate a robust immune response.

Recombinant Protein Vaccines

Recombinant protein vaccines are subunit vaccines that are specifically formulated to elicit a protective immunological response. Acellular vaccines are formulated with an adjuvant to increase their immunogenicity potential. Alum has been approved as an adjuvant for human vaccines since it induces a strong antibody response to admixed antigens. These recombinant protein vaccines are safer than attenuated vaccines when administered in immu-nocompromised states. The antigen must be present on all strains of the fungus while designing the vaccine. The challenge faced with this strategy is that the T-cell responses to the antigens may differ as a function of the human leukocyte antigen (HLA) haplotype. NDV-3 is an anti-*Candida* vaccine found to be effective not only for oropharyngeal, vaginal, and invasive candidiasis but also for *Staphylococcus aureus* infection due to structural homology. Thus one vaccine can possibly target two of the most notorious nosocomial infections. The shell of a virus can also be used as an adjuvant for fungal vaccines. The virosome acts as a carrier for the fungal antigen to be delivered at the desired target site. It also activates antigen-presenting cells (APCs). A virosome-based vaccine is being developed against *Candida* species.

Conjugate Vaccines

Conjugate vaccines are based on the principles that conjugating proteins to polysaccharides enables the immune system to recognize the cell wall components of the fungal pathogen. If saccharide epitopes like β-glucans are targeted, it may be possible to develop a universal vaccine against a wide range of fungal pathogens. A conjugate vaccine against invasive can-didiasis and aspergillosis is being tested.

■ IMMUNOTHERAPY

Various exogenous agents can be used to enhance the immune attack against a fungal infection.

Monoclonal Antibodies

Due to the presence of a rigid cell wall, fungi can resist lysis on activation of the complement cascade. However, deposition of complement on the surface of the fungal cell leads to "opsonization." The phagocytic cells are aided in ingestion of pathogens opsonized by antibodies or complement. This leads to killing of the fungi and offers protection to the host.

Monoclonal antibodies (mAbs) may target specific fungal antigens. The antibodies may recognize different epitopes, which determine the efficacy of these antibodies in fighting an infection. Some mAbs have antifungal properties that are not dependent on immune cells activation. 2G8 (IgG2b) prevents attachment of *C. albicans* to host epithelial cells and is fungistatic when tested in mouse models for invasive and vaginal candidiasis. 2G8 also prevents formation of capsule when incubated with *C. neoformans*. It also demonstrates in vivo activity against pulmonary cryptococcosis. Another approach that has been tested is to label an intracapsular mAb, IgG1 mAb targeting *C. neoformans* with radioisotopes. When these [213]bismuth and [188]rhenium isotopes are used, these emit α and β particles, respectively. These have demonstrated improved survival in mice with disseminated cryptococcosis.

The potential advantage of the fungistatic 2G8 antibodies and the radiolabeled antibodies is that they offer protection irrespective of the host's immune status. Thus these are an excellent adjuvant therapy and may form the backbone of protective vaccines in the future.

Antibody-based therapy has certain limitations. *Cryptococcus* species are unique since they shed their capsule only during infection. This poses a problem since the anticapsular antibody may form immune complexes with the circulating capsule. So the antifungal activity of the antibody is lost.

Passive antibody therapy provides variable levels of protection. The fungi may mask their target-binding sites causing resistance against the mAbs. Antibodies that are dependent on neutrophil activity for protection can be ineffective in neutropenic patients.

Dendritic Cell Immunotherapy

Dendritic cells are found in tissues, which come in contact with the external environment. These include the Langerhans cells in the skin, linings of nose, lungs and intestines. These cells have branched projections or dendrites. These are a type of antigen-presenting cells (APCs). On activation, the DCs move to the lymph tissue. The cells interact with the B cells and T cells to develop an adaptive immune response. The DCs have the capacity to capture the antigens from invading pathogens, process them and then present them on their cell surface. This induces a primary immune response in the inactive T lymphocytes. DCs have a role in release of cytokines, B-cell activation and B-cell immune memory by formation of antigen–antibody complexes.

Dendritic cell immunotherapy involves incubating or pulsing DCs with selected fungal antigens in vivo and then infusing them back into the host circulation to offer protection. DC immunotherapy involves use of this strategy after the onset of infection, whereas dendritic vaccines are meant to be administered to prevent an infection from happening. DCs act as APCs on major histocompatibility complex molecules and also upregulate cytokines. Based on the specific cytokines produced, CD4+ T cells differentiate into specific T-helper cells. Various peptides have been tested as antigens for DC immunotherapy. Experiments have been conducted with DCs pulsed with *A. fumigatus* conidia. P10 is a synthetic oligomer that has been used for pulsing DCs against *P. brasiliensis*. DC immunotherapy can be useful as an adjuvant strategy in times to come. DC vaccines combine these cells with fungal antigens. These vaccines may not be cost-effective for widespread prophylaxis but may be used in specific target populations, such as bone marrow transplant recipients.

NANOBIOTECHNOLOGY

Drug delivery systems containing nanoparticles have the potential advantage of enhancing antifungal potency, improving drug bioavailability and reducing toxicity. Smart delivery systems target specific organs. These nanoparticles facilitate entry into the cell and direct attack on the intracellular pathogens. These particles may be coated with substances, such as polyethylene glycol (PEG). This offers advantages, including prolonging their circulation time and masking these from phagocytic attack. This prevents the opsonins from attaching on these nanoparticles containing drugs.

The potential advantages of nanobiotechnology for drug delivery include:
- Better/organ-specific drug targeting
- Intracellular activity
- Prolonged circulation time
- Improved pharmacokinetics
- Prevention of early degradation
- Reduced toxicity
- Reduced cost of therapy due to effective drug delivery
- It can be useful as adjuvant in vaccines.

Nanostructures being explored for drug delivery include polymeric nanoparticles, solid lipid nanoparticles, liposomes and magnetic nanoparticles (Table 37.1).

Nanotechnology increases the bioavailability of both topical and systemic antifungals and is an attractive strategy for effective and more targeted drug delivery.

Use of nanotechnology for improving efficacy as well as reducing infusion-related side effects of amphotericin B has been studied since the 1980s. Three different lipid formulations of amphotericin B have been introduced. Other formulations which have been developed include nanosomal amphotericin B using phosphatidylcholine and sodium cholesterol sulfate, anionic and PEG lipid nanoparticle for intravenous amphotericin B, nano-disk or ND-AMB which is a super-aggregate of protein-phospholipid bioparticle. Voriconazole has been encapsulated with polylactic-*co*-glycolic acid (PLGA). It has demonstrated higher drug levels in the lungs with early release and a well sustained level in murine models. PLGA-encapsulated itraconazole has been conjugated with dimercaptosuccinic acid to target the lungs. Miconazole penetration is improved when ultraflexible liposomes carry the drug. Solid lipid nanoparticles (SLNs) have a role in delivery of topical antifungals. SLN-bearing hydrogel formulation of miconazole causes less irritation to the skin compared with

Table 37.1: Properties of nanoparticles being developed as drug delivery systems

Nanoparticle	Properties
PNPs	■ Polymeric colloidal systems in which the drug can be dispersed, encapsulated or coated ■ Nanoparticles are coated with natural polymers (chitosan and alginate) or synthetic polymers (PLA, PGA, PLGA) ■ Protect drug against gastrointestinal pH, degradation enzymes and efflux pumps ■ Degradation of nanoparticle polymer for incorporated drug release at target site
SLNs	■ Spherical nanoparticles coated with physiological biodegradable lipids, such as stearic acid ■ Allow delivery of insoluble drugs with higher efficiency, physical stability, and lower toxicity ■ Studied for topical drug delivery
Liposomes	■ Particles made by natural or synthetic phospholipids ■ On contact with aqueous medium, liposomes form a spherical structure with a lipid layer surrounding an aqueous nucleus ■ Can deliver both hydrophobic and hydrophilic substances ■ Better protection against external degradation by enzymes ■ Sensitive to pH variations, so drug can be released at a specific pH ■ LAmB uses liposomes
Magnetic nanoparticles	■ Particles are amenable to manipulation by a magnetic field to target specific tissues ■ Ferrous compounds used to make these particles include cobalt, manganese and zinc ferrites, magnetite and maghemite ■ Can be combined with liposomes or PNPs

LAmB, liposomal amphotericin B; PGA, polyglycolic acid; pH, hydrogen ion concentration; PLA, polylactic acid; PLGA, polylactic-co-glycolic acid; PNPs, polymeric nanoparticles; SLNs, solid lipid nanoparticles.

conventional hydrogel and suspension. Topical ocular use of itraconazole aided by SLNs showed higher antimicrobial efficacy in animal models. SLN fluconazole has shown efficacy in fluconazole-resistant *Candida* species.

■ NEWER ANTIFUNGALS

Some of the existing drugs, such as protease inhibitors for HIV treatment and antihelminthic mebendazole, have been found to have significant antifungal activity. The emphasis is on discovery of newer classes of antifungal drugs. Randomized controlled trials are needed to study the real-world data on efficacy and safety of these drugs.

Albaconazole

Albaconazole is a broad-spectrum triazole antifungal that has shown strong efficacy against *Candida, Aspergillus* and *Cryptococcus.* It has been found to be effective in vaginal candidiasis. It has been used in treatment of onychomycosis and tinea pedis. It is expected to be available as a topical and oral formulation. Once weekly 100–400 mg albaconazole has been found to be effective in the treatment of onychomycosis in phase II clinical trials.

Biafungin (CD101)

Biafungin (CD101) is a new echinocandin molecule, which has an unusually long half-life. It has been tested in multiple animal species. The half-lives of biafungin and anidulafungin were found to be 81 h and 30 h, respectively, in studies conducted on chimpanzees. It had a very slow clearance in chimpanzees, dogs, monkeys and rats and displayed significant drug levels after 1 week of intravenous administration of a dose. It may hold promise as a novel antifungal with potential for weekly administration rather than daily dosing.

Biafungin (CD101) topical is the first topical agent in the echinocandin class and exhibits fungicidal activity against *Candida* species. In May 2016, the Food and Drug Administration (FDA) granted qualified infectious disease product (QIDP) and fast-track designation to CD101 topical for the treatment of vulvovaginal candidiasis (VVC) and the prevention of recurrent VVC.

Orotomides

Orotomides are a new class of antifungals researched and developed by the University of Liverpool and F2G Limited. It was found to be effective against *Aspergillus, Scedosporium prolificans, Fusarium, Penicillium* species and *Talaromyces*. The most promising drug candidate in this class is designated F901318. The unique mechanism of action involves stopping pyrimidine biosynthesis in fungal cells thereby blocking the growth of fungal hyphae. This results in reversible inhibition of dihydroorotate dehydrogenase, an enzyme that catalyzes dihydroorotate to orotate. They are named orotomides, combining the names of dihydroorotate they act upon with the chemical group α-ketoamide, which they belong to. The European Medicines Agency Committee for Orphan Medicinal Products granted orphan designation to F2G for F901318 for the treatment of scedosporiosis and invasive aspergillosis in 2016. In 2017, it was shown to be useful for acute sinopulmonary aspergillosis caused by *Aspergillus flavus* in phase 1 clinical trials.

SCY-078

SCY-078 (formerly MK-3118) is a semisynthetic derivative of a natural product enfumafungin. Triterpenoids is a new class of structurally distinct glucan synthase inhibitors with activity against multidrug-resistant *Candida auris, Pneumocystis* and other species of *Candida* and *Aspergillus*. SCY-078 is the first representative of this class and is being developed as both oral and intravenous formulation. It may have the potential to show efficacy in refractory IFI cases. An ongoing open-label study is being conducted to study its efficacy and safety in *C. auris* infection. The FDA has granted both QIDP and fast-track designations for invasive candidiasis, invasive aspergillosis and VVC. It has been given orphan drug designation for invasive candidiasis and invasive aspergillosis.

Phendione

Metal-based drugs, including 1,10-phenanthroline-5,6-dione (phendione) and its Ag^+ and Cu^{2+} complexes have been studied for their role in management of chromoblastomycosis. It causes ultrastructural changes, such as surface invaginations, cell shrinkage and disruption.

It inhibits metallopeptidase activity and reduces ergosterol content disrupting transformation of conidia of *Phialophora verrucosa* into mycelia.

C7a

Biphosphinic cyclopalladate C7a was previously developed as a chemotherapeutic agent but has now been found to be active against *P. brasiliensis, Paracoccidioides lutzii, C. neoformans, C. albicans* and parasite *Trypanosoma cruzi.* It is fungicidal at low minimum inhibitory concentrations and has shown in vitro activity against fluconazole-resistant *Candida.* It causes structural alterations in cellular organelles, mitochondrial swelling, marginalization of chromatin into the nuclei and disruption of cell wall. It has shown survival benefits in disseminated candidiasis in mice. It reduces biofilm formation and decreases the viability of yeast in mature biofilms.

■ CONCLUSION

There is an urgent need for the development of vaccines, immunotherapeutics, and newer antifungal agents. There are a few molecules in different phases of clinical trials, but the pace needs to match the requirement for effective therapy for IFI, particularly in the immuno-compromised host. There is a need to explore new avenues and newer therapeutic strategies in fungal therapy. Vaccines, immunotherapy, nanobiotechnology and new antifungal drugs may offer an option.

■ SUGGESTED READING

1. Butts A, Krysan DJ. Antifungal drug discovery: something old and something new. PLoS Pathog. 2012;8:e1002870.
2. Carvalho A, Cunha C, Iannitti RG, et al. Host defense pathways against fungi: the basis for vaccines and immunotherapy. Front Microbiol. 2012;3:176.
3. Cassone A. Fungal vaccines: real progress from real challenges. Lancet Infect Dis. 2008;8:114-24.
4. Das PJ, Paul P, Mukherjee B, et al. Pulmonary delivery of voriconazole loaded nanoparticles providing a prolonged drug level in lungs: a promise for treating fungal infection. Mol Pharm. 2015;12:2651-64.
5. Gajbhiye M, Kesharwani J, Ingle A, et al. Fungus-mediated synthesis of silver nanoparticles and their activity against pathogenic fungi in combination with fluconazole. Nanomedicine. 2009;5:382.
6. Gupta M, Goyal AK, Paliwal SR, et al. Development and characterization of effective topical liposomal system for localized treatment of cutaneous candidiasis. J Liposome Res. 2010;20:341.
7. Horký Pavel, Skalickova S, Baholet D, et al. Nanoparticles as a solution for eliminating the risk of mycotoxins. Nanomaterials. 2018;8(9):727.
8. Kumar A, Jena PK, Behera S, et al. Multifunctional magnetic nanoparticles for targeted delivery. Nanomedicine. 2010;6:64-9.
9. Ng SMS, Yap YYA, Cheong JWD, et al. Antifungal peptides: a potential new class of antifungals for treating vulvovaginal candidiasis caused by fluconazole-resistant *Candida albicans.* J Pept Sci. 2017; 23:215-21.
10. Nosanchuk JD, Taborda CP. Vaccines and immunotherapy against fungi: the new frontier. Front Microbiol. 2013;4:6.

11. Nosanchuk JD, Zancopé-Oliveira RM, Hamilton AJ, et al. Antibody therapy for histoplasmosis. Front Microbiol. 2012;3:21.
12. Roemer T, Krysan DJ. Antifungal drug development: challenges, unmet clinical needs, and new approaches. Cold Spring Harb Perspect Med. 2014;4(5):a019703.
13. Roque L, Molpeceres J, Reis C, et al. Past, recent progresses and future perspectives of nanotechnology applied to antifungal agents. Curr Drug Metab. 2017;18(4):280-90.
14. Souza AC, Amaral AC. Antifungal therapy for systemic mycosis and the nanobiotechnology era: improving efficacy, biodistribution and toxicity. Front Microbiol. 2017;8:336.
15. Vecchiarelli A, Pericolini E, Gabrielli E, et al. New approaches in the development of a vaccine for mucosal candidiasis: progress and challenges. Front Microbiol. 2012;3:294.

Index